Pathways in Surgical Management

Pathways in Surgical Management

Second Edition

Michael Hobsley, TD, PhD, MChir, FRCS

David Patey Professor of Surgery, The Middlesex Hospital Medical School;
Surgeon, The Middlesex Hospital and University College Hospital, London;
Examiner, London University BS; lately Penrose May Tutor, Royal College of Surgeons of England

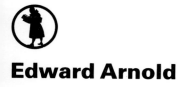

Edward Arnold

© Michael Hobsley 1986

First published in Great Britain 1979 by
Edward Arnold (Publishers) Ltd,
41 Bedford Square,
London WC1B 3DQ

Edward Arnold (Australia) Pty Ltd,
80 Waverley Road,
Caulfield East,
Victoria 3145,
Australia

Edward Arnold,
3 East Read Street,
Baltimore,
Maryland 21202,
USA

Reprinted 1982, 1984
Second Edition 1986

British Library Cataloguing in Publication Data

Hobsley, Michael
    Pathways in surgical management.—2nd ed.
    1. Diagnosis, Surgical
    I. Title
    617′.075   RD35

ISBN 0-7131-4495-5

Text set in 10/11pt Times Roman Linotron 101
by Oxprint Ltd, Oxford
Printed and bound in Great Britain by
Butler & Tanner Ltd, Frome, Somerset.

Preface to the First Edition

The arrangement of this book is unorthodox. Its relationship to a conventional textbook of surgery is comparable with that of a thesaurus to a dictionary.

A dictionary lists words, many of which have more than one meaning, and defines these various meanings. A thesaurus, on the other hand, starts with an idea and then lists all the words and phrases which in general express that idea, although with wide differences in emphasis and specialization.

Similarly, a conventional textbook of surgery lists surgical diseases and describes the symptoms and signs to which they might give rise: most of these symptoms and signs may occur in more than one disease. On the other hand, this volume starts with some common combinations of symptoms and signs such as the surgeon is likely to meet every day, and works backwards to show how one can identify which of several possible diseases produced that clinical picture.

Since the aim of surgical teaching is to make the student competent to deal with patients, and since these present with clinical pictures rather than with diseases, the author hopes that this book may prove helpful both to students of surgery and to their teachers.

1979   M.H.

Preface to the Second Edition

The aims and methods of this book remain as described in the preface to the first editon.

The major changes in this edition are a first chapter on physical signs with reference to lumps, ulcers and tenderness, and increased emphasis on the role of the general practitioner. Many surgical decisions are now easier to make because of the availability of improved investigations such as ultrasound. Factors like these have enabled the text of several chapters, for example that on Jaundice, to be considerably simplified.

1986   M.H.

Acknowledgements

The text has been read and criticized by several surgical and medical colleagues, mainly at The Middlesex Hospital. While I am grateful to them for their help, the responsibility for the views I have expressed is entirely mine.

Most of the photographs were prepared by the Department of Medical Illustration at The Middlesex Hospital. Most of the x-rays came from the Departments of Radiodiagnosis at that Hospital or at Acton Hospital, but I am indebted to Dr R. Dick of the Royal Free Hospital for Fig. 11.2. The original drawings were prepared by the publisher's artist. Copyright material in the illustrations is acknowledged in the appropriate captions.

I am grateful to my secretary, Miss Carol Walters, and to the Librarian of the Boldero Library of the Middlesex Hospital Medical School, Mrs Janet Cropper, and her staff, for much help in the preparation of this second edition.

1986   M.H.

Contents

Flow-charts

Introduction

Problem-solving in medical education

The traditional approach to teaching medicine depends upon the following view of the scientific basis of medicine.

A patient presents to a doctor with certain complaints. The doctor takes the history of the illness, examines the patient for abnormal physical signs, and does appropriate special tests which he has reason to believe may influence his management. This combination of symptoms, physical signs and special tests constitutes the clinical presentation. The doctor then attaches to this presentation a label called a diagnosis, and gives the patient treatment which should do him good, if previous experience or logical argument are to be trusted. If the doctor cannot attach a precise label to the presentation, because the clinical features will fit more than one diagnosis, he makes a differential diagnosis which consists of all the possible diseases that might produce the observed presentation and then does further tests designed to discriminate between them. When he has eliminated all but one possible diagnosis, or has decided on positive grounds that one diagnosis only is correct, he can proceed to rational therapy.

In the light of this approach there are three distinct facets of medical education:

1. The development of the skills involved in gathering information about a particular patient — basically, history taking, clinical examination and special investigations.
2. The acquisition of 'knowledge', the corpus of established facts about disease and their management.
3. Learning to select the correct diagnostic label from one's store of knowledge.

In most medical schools, the emphasis is on items 1 and 2. With regard to item 3, the usual advice given is to construct the differential diagnosis and then narrow down the possibilities. Yet when the medical student qualifies as a doctor he finds that there are problems with the approach via differential diagnosis.

Firstly, a complete list of all possible diagnoses would usually be very long: rarely does even the most deliberate and conscientious of doctors draw up such a list. Secondly, no matter how many possibilities the doctor enumerates, it usually transpires that he has forgotten some, of which one may be the correct diagnosis. Thirdly, the concept of the differential diagnosis is only useful if the doctor, having constructed his list, can then afford to sit back and wait for the results of any investigations that he has ordered for their discriminatory value — in other words, if none of the possible diagnoses require urgent treatment. The immediate and pressing problem posed by the patient is, what must the doctor do, or advise, at that instant?

In place of the *differential diagnosis,* the writer offers the concept of the *working diagnosis.* There is a clear-cut distinction between these concepts. Instead of a list of all the possible diagnostic labels in terms of disease, the working diagnosis presents the key to the management of a clinical situation in terms of the action that the doctor should take. Not often is this diagnosis expressed in the form of exact aetiology or pathology: instead it is the most accurate description of the patient's problem available to the doctor at that moment, and as such it decides the doctor's immediate management. This book describes the management of surgical patients in terms of the concept of the working diagnosis. While it contains much detail, it is primarily a book about ideas and therefore it is aimed at everyone who is interested in surgery — students, practitioners, and surgeons whether in training or fully qualified.

The difference in attitude produced by a working diagnosis compared with a differential diagnosis can be illustrated by considering one of the commonest problems in general surgery — the patient complaining of a lump in the breast. The differential diagnosis of such a lump includes a wide range of conditions, and most of these cannot be diagnosed with certainty on clinical grounds. The doctor seeing the patient in the out-patient surgical clinic has to decide, not so much the exact pathological diagnosis but rather his course of action: should he put a needle into the lump and try to aspirate fluid from it; ask the patient to come into hospital for an urgent operation; put the patient on a non-urgent waiting list for admission; or deliver reassurance that there is nothing seriously wrong and that no treatment is required? A dominant feature of the concept of the working diagnosis is that the principle of 'fail-safe' must be applied: that is, the most serious of the possible diagnoses must be adopted as the working diagnosis. For example, a lump in the breast may have no particular features suggestive of malignancy, but this fact does not exclude the possibility that it is a carcinoma. Unless, therefore, there is unequivocal evidence that the lump is something else such as a cyst or gynaecomastia that needs different handling, it must be assumed to be a carcinoma and urgent steps taken to get a histological diagnosis. The differential diagnosis *includes* carcinoma, but the working diagnosis *is* carcinoma and this decides the immediate management of the patient. Another example concerns the surgeon's attitude to the patient complaining of acute pain in the right lower quadrant of the abdomen. This problem is discussed in detail on page 330, but the surgeon should say, not 'Is there sufficient evidence to justify a diagnosis of acute appendicitis and therefore the performance of an operation?' but 'Am I so sure that this patient has not got acute appendicitis that I am prepared *not* to advise operation?' For practical purposes, a differential diagnosis including acute appendicitis is tantamount to a working diagnosis of 'pain in the right lower quadrant, possibly appendicitis' and results in the advice of an immediate operation.

It is true that in certain clinical situations the doctor follows the same course of action whether he thinks in terms of working diagnosis or differential diagnosis. If the various conditions in the list of differential diagnoses are of approximately the same urgency and do not require any immediate active management, then it is reasonable to ask for investigations designed to discriminate between these possibilities and await the results. However, even here the working diagnosis helps clarity of thought. Consider, for example, another very

common problem — the patient complaining of chronic epigastric pain. Most such patients have no abnormal physical signs, nor can an accurate pathological diagnosis be made from the history. The five commonest conditions responsible for this clinical picture are peptic ulcer, gallstones, hiatus hernia, carcinoma of the stomach and chronic pancreatitis, and a doctor working by differential diagnosis probably makes these five conditions his list. The doctor using working diagnosis thinks of the same five conditions but his working diagnosis is chronic epigastric pain requiring special investigations. In each case, the doctor's action is the same: he requests such investigations as an upper gastrointestinal endoscopy and ultrasound examination of the gall bladder region. If the investigations show that one of the five diagnoses is correct, then the differential diagnosis has performed as well as the working diagnosis. However, all the investigations may be negative. The approach by differential diagnosis seems to suggest only two possible explanations: either serious organic disease has been excluded, or the list of differential diagnoses must be extended. In terms of the working diagnosis, the problem is different: the patient has chronic epigastric pain which has not been diagnosed by the first-line investigations: should he be reassured that nothing serious is amiss; should the investigations be repeated in a few weeks; or should other more elaborate (and probably more uncomfortable and possibly more dangerous) investigations be ordered? The decision is really, how certain is the clinician that the patient has a serious disease? This decision does not depend on the nature of that disease, and is therefore a consideration which the mere differential diagnosis cannot take into account, yet it is the guiding factor in the management of the patient.

The previous example has illustrated another important feature of a working diagnosis: that it is not meant to be a fixed and unchanging label. The working diagnosis is decided at a certain point in time by the relevant clinical data available up to that moment. A line of management is embarked upon, appropriate to the working diagnosis. As a result of, or perhaps despite, this management, the patient's illness develops in a certain way or more clinical data are collected: the working diagnosis has to be modified, and in turn so is the management. In other words, most of the time there may be no such thing as *the* diagnosis of the patient: simply the working diagnosis in the out-patient department, the one in the ward after the results of the special investigations have been received, the modification in the operating theatre, the histological diagnosis, and maybe (and only then, finally) the post-mortem diagnosis. At each stage the new working diagnosis produces a fresh shift in the emphasis or the direction of the scheme of management.

The purpose of this book is to provide schemes of management for some of the commoner clinical presentations in general surgery. Each chapter begins with a discussion of the features which define the particular presentation, whether it be a relatively simple problem such as a lump in a particular anatomical location or a complex disturbance of function such as shock. A scheme is proposed to group the patients into separate treatment categories in the first instance, and then as a result of doing something else — making a further clinical observation, applying a special test, or sometimes just waiting — each category is further subdivided. As each logical YES/NO decision is made, the patient's problem is more clearly and narrowly defined, but the strict pathological diagnosis may not be made until treatment has been completed. At the end of the section or chapter there are one or more pages in which the scheme of management is set out as a flow-diagram or algorithm. These flow-diagrams represent one way (not necessarily the best!) of tackling each presentation, and are an attempt to indicate specifically the methods of diagnosis and treatment followed by experienced surgeons. This is the way surgeons work, this is the way that they should teach.

The author must emphasize a point made in the previous paragraph — that his recommended scheme of management is not necessarily the best solution to every problem discussed. However, this book describes the particular solutions that he has found to work best in his hands. In certain areas where there are important alternative solutions, these are also described. The reader can then make up his mind which solution he prefers,

or perhaps decide to do a controlled trial to decide between them.

The discussion of the management of common surgical situations in the following pages starts from the assumption that a complete and accurate history has been taken and a complete and accurate examination made. Special tests are brought into the picture when their results may have a direct effect on the decision-making in the flow-pathway, and it is assumed that their results are also perfectly reliable. These assumptions are necessary if any useful discussion of management is to follow, but in practice they are not always justified. Ideally, the probability of the accuracy of any special investigation should be known, and its result weighted accordingly in the decision-making. The doctor should never forget that his decisions on management can only be as accurate as the data upon which they are based. However, the data themselves are not enough: the present book demonstrates how to make the best use of the data.

The problem-solving discussed is how to proceed to manage the patient's problem using symptoms, signs and special tests, and a logical method. These processes are usually summarized in the phrase 'clinical acumen', and clinicians usually argue that acumen cannot be taught but that it is a quality which gradually improves as a result of experience and in its highest degree is vouchsafed only to a fortunate, gifted few. The writer does not accept this thesis: he believes that the algorithmic approach of action resulting step by step from a series of logical YES/NO decisions can put the surgical tyro on a par with his teacher.

This book aims to teach so-called 'clinical acumen' to anyone who has, or may be about to have, the surgical care of patients. I apologize in advance for my presumptuousness in attempting such a task.

About this book

The moment a student is qualified as a doctor, he is expected to have some skill in diagnosis and treatment. It is hoped that this book will therefore be useful to medical students, and to all those younger doctors whose clinical experience is not yet so great that they can construct comprehensive schemes of management for themselves, especially

in the stress of having to find the right answer in an urgent clinical situation. Postgraduate students preparing for higher surgical examinations may also find that this approach to common surgical problems helps them to arrange their thoughts in a logical and orderly fashion. Most medical students become general practitioners, and so both the flow-diagrams and the text include guidance as to when the practitioner should refer the patient for a consultant surgical opinion or for immediate admission to hospital.

The book is arranged in two parts. Part I contains a description of nineteen common non-emergency surgical situations. It must be confessed that certain subjects cannot be easily divided into acute and chronic aspects. When this is the case, the subject has been arbitrarily assigned to one or the other part. Thus intestinal obstruction is in Part II, although the appropriate chapter also discusses chronic intestinal obstruction. Despite such difficulties, the main subdivision into acute and chronic situations has been retained in order to emphasize that the surgeon naturally reacts differently to the two different sorts of situation. The leisurely sifting of detailed information obtained by complicated investigations is acceptable in the out-patient clinic, but not in the casualty department. These non-emergency situations are described first because they are usually simpler than emergency situations.

Part II includes the common emergency surgical situations which the general surgeon might meet. The great importance of trauma is acknowledged by devoting the first chapter to a general analysis of the problem presented by the seriously injured patient. The effects of trauma may be so widespread, and involve so many systems, that certain aspects of trauma considered in later chapters entail a considerable overlap. Most of the rest of Part II is concerned with acute abdominal emergencies.

The suggestions for further reading at the end of each chapter are either classical articles introducing stimulating ideas or recent reviews with valuable lists of references. The number of illustrations has been deliberately restricted: those used have been chosen to emphasize features that are either novel, or of crucial importance, or difficult to describe in words. Several books are available which concentrate on illustrations of surgical diseases.*

This book should be used in conjunction with other sources of knowledge, and these will vary according to the category of person reading the book. The medical student will need his textbook of pathology, while the surgeon in training will require a textbook of operative surgery and an acquaintance with some of the articles in the lists for further reading.

Finally, the author suggests with great respect that the experienced surgeon may find the book stimulating as a challenge to justify his own (different) approach to these surgical situations, while the teacher of surgery may wish to consider whether his teaching techniques require modifying!

*For example, Browse, N. (1978). *An Introduction to the Symptoms and Signs of Surgical Disease.* London, Edward Arnold.

Part I

Non-emergencies

Chapter 1

Lumps; Tenderness

The life of a surgeon consists of making a series of decisions about how best to care for his patient, and then implementing each decision. The data on which any decision is made are the history given by the patient of his illness and the findings obtained by the surgeon on his examination of the patient.

By far the commonest situations with which patients present are a *lump*, or else *pain*; of these, pain is a subjective complaint, but it is frequently associated with *tenderness*. This chapter therefore presents some introductory remarks about the assessment of a lump and of tenderness: the principles detailed here are illustrated many times in the rest of the book.

Lumps

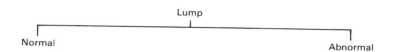

A frequent trap for the unwary is to fail to appreciate that the 'lump' is a normal structure. Normal anatomical features vary in their size, and bilateral pairs are often asymmetrically developed. We should be no more surprised at this than we are to note that some individuals have particularly large hands or feet, or have one ear or breast that is larger than the other. One of the reasons that medical students are encouraged to examine their ward-patients from top to toe is to help them achieve an awareness of the normal ranges.

Apart from natural variations in size, another source of confusion is that the palpability of a lump depends upon its consistency being firmer than that of its surroundings. The mere presence of a structure does not necessarily mean that it is palpable: the parotid covers a large area of the face and neck (Fig. 4.1) yet it is not palpable. Remembering that fact, the student might assume that the submandibular salivary gland is also not palpable, yet that is not true. The normal gland is firmer than the surrounding subcutaneous tissues, and in most individuals is readily palpable. Patients too are often misled, and a normal submandibular salivary gland that happens to be larger than its opposite fellow can lead to much anxiety as a possible cancer.

There are five features of the examination that are generally found to be most helpful in the assessment of abnormal lumps: *site, shape, consistency, layer,* and the neighbouring *lymph nodes.* Many other attributes can sometimes be helpful, but these five require special attention.

Site

The significant feature of location is not its co-ordinates so much as its relation to neighbouring or underlying anatomical structures. To say that a lump lies 7.5 cm medial to the anterior superior iliac spine and 3.5 cm below it may enable someone else to find the lump; but to say that it lies at the mid-inguinal point indicates that it overlies the femoral artery and could be an aneurysm.

Lumps in special anatomical territories, for example, the neck, breast or groin, are considered later in separate chapters. Lumps presenting anywhere else, i.e., where there is no special significance attaching to the site, are considered below.

Shape

Many lumps are irregularly shaped, and their

shape is then no help in diagnosis. However, there are three shapes of special significance.

Spherical lumps are nearly always liquid-containing cysts. As the lump grows, the pressure in the liquid is transmitted equally in all directions, and equal growth in all directions results in the spherical shape. Of course, one cannot be certain that a lump is completely spherical because one can never feel all round the lesion to its deep aspect, but if the palpable half (or maybe two-thirds, because one can usually indent the neighbouring skin sufficiently to feel more than half) is smoothly spherical, it is reasonable to assume that the inaccessible aspect is similar.

Lobulation of the surface, with palpable or visible indentations between the lobules, is typical particularly of the subcutaneous lipoma and the mammary fibroadenoma (p. 63).

Discoid lesions are uncommon, but sometimes sufficiently typical to establish a working diagnosis (see gynaecomastia, p. 62).

Consistency

There are five important aspects of consistency.

1. *Degree of hardness.* It is unwise to strive after too many grades of consistency; the more such grades, the less likely are two different observers to agree because the greater the difficulty in defining each grade. It is probably best to stick to *hard, firm, soft:* hard means not deformable, soft means easily deformable, and firm means not easily deformable within the limits of acceptable pressure, but the observer feels that very little more pressure would succeed in altering the shape of the lump.

2. *Fluctuance.* Pushing the lump in at one aspect results in its border pushing outwards somewhere else (Fig. 1.1). If the lump is mobile, mass movement of the lesion could be confused with fluctuance; it is therefore necessary that the lump be fixed, either by the examiner or by an assistant. Fluctuance is shown by lumps that are constant in volume, and soft enough to be readily deformable. The sign is often claimed to be pathognomonic of a liquid-containing cyst, but some cysts are not fluctuant (wall too rigid, or internal pressure too high, to permit deformation) and some solids, e.g., a subcutaneous lipoma, are soft enough to be fluctuant.

3. *Emptying or reduction.* With the application of external pressure, the lump can be made to disappear. This sign is given by lesions which are in continuity with much larger cavities, so that the contents of the lesion can be squeezed into the cavity and so are removed from the field of examination. Examples include hernias (sometimes reducible into the abdomen) and haemangiomas (reducible into the circulation).

4. *Expansile cough impulse.* The lump becomes larger when the patient coughs (or performs any other act, such as straining, that raises the pressure in the subjacent body cavity). This is a valuable sign of abdominal hernias (Chapter 13), but Figure 1.2 indicates some common errors. It is vital to appreciate the importance of the word *expansile:* if the impulse is expansile, then there must be a lump at rest or there would be nothing to expand; and the element of expansion (rather than simple thrust) cannot be appreciated with a flat hand.

5. *Pulsation.* A lump that throbs in time wih the pulse is an aneurysm if the pulsation is *expansile,*

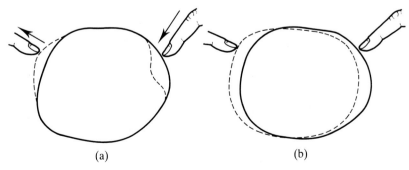

(a)   (b)

Fig. 1.1 *The sign of fluctuance.* (a) When the lump is deformed at one side by pushing the finger into it, it springs outwards at the other side because it is constant in volume. (b) It is important that the lump should be fixed in overall position, otherwise it will move under pressure of the one finger, and this movement may be interpreted by the other finger as bulging.

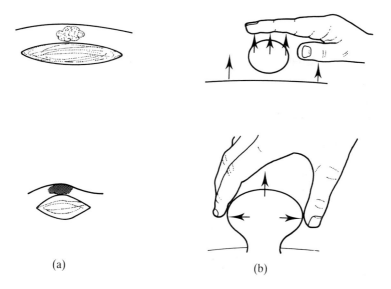

(a) (b)

Fig. 1.2 *The sign of expansile cough impulse.* (a) A soft lump superficial to the muscle may be impalpable until the muscle is contracted. An expansile cough impulse can only be diagnosed if a lump at rest becomes larger on coughing. (b) A common error is to try and diagnose an expansile cough impulse with the fingers flat. With the fingers in this position the examiner can only demonstrate an overall thrust, it needs the cupped fingers and thumb to detect expansion.

or some other lesion overlying an artery if the pulsation is directly outward at all points and therefore *transmitted* (Fig. 1.3). The distinction is often difficult.

Layer

In general there are four layers to consider: *skin, subcutaneous tissue, muscle* and *bone*. In the region of the abdominal wall, one must also determine whether the lesion is *in the abdominal wall* itself, or *within the abdominal cavity*.

1. *Bone.* It is usually obvious that a lesion is in, or attached to, bone. The lump cannot be moved without moving the bone, the bone cannot be moved without the lump moving.

2. *Muscle.* The best evidence that a lesion is attached to a muscle is that the mobility of the lump in a direction at right angles to the line of the muscle when the latter is at rest is reduced when the muscle is contracted (Fig. 1.4a,b). Less valuable is movement of the lump in the line of its movement when the muscle contracts: for example, a muscle producing movement equally in its

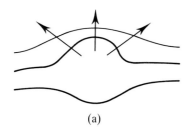

(a)

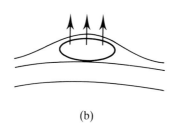

(b)

Fig. 1.3 (a) True expansile pulsation in a lesion in direct communication with an artery. (b) Transmitted pulsation from a lump overlying an artery.

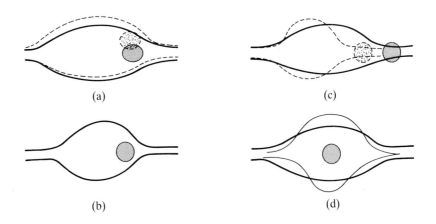

(a)

(c)

(b)

(d)

Fig. 1.4 *Attachment to muscle.* (a) At rest the muscle is flacid and the palpable lump moves from side to side with the muscle when the examiner tests motility at right angles to the muscle fibres. (b) On contraction of the muscle the lump is no longer mobile from side to side. (c) The alternative test when the lump moves proximally with the muscle when it contracts works satisfactorily in this case if the lump is in the region of the tendon. (d) The test illustrated in (c) does not work when the lump is near the centrepoint of the muscle mass.

points of origin and insertion would not move at its midpoint (Fig. 1.4c,d).

A lesion deep within a muscle, or lying actually deep to the muscle becomes less palpable, or even disappears completely when the muscle contracts and hardens, unless its consistency is much greater than that of even the contracted muscle. On the other hand, a lump lying on the superficial aspect of a muscle will become more prominent and feel harder when thrust forward by the expansion outwards of the shortened, but therefore thickened, muscle belly (Fig. 1.2a).

3. *Skin.* It might be thought that the question of whether a lump were in the most superficial layer, the skin, would always be easy to decide. Certainly there is no problem if the skin can be picked up over the lesion and lifted away from it (Fig. 1.5a). The problem becomes more difficult if the skin is naturally tight across the surface of the lump, or if the lesion lies mainly in the subcutaneous layer but is possibly attached to skin at one small region of its superficial aspect. Figure 1.5b,c demonstrates two useful techniques. If there is still doubt, it usually turns out that the lump is indeed attached to skin.

4. *Subcutaneous tissue.* By exclusion, lumps that are not attached to skin but also not attached to muscle or bone lie in the subcutaneous tissue.

5. *Abdomen: wall or cavity?* Since the firmest material of the anterior abdominal wall is muscle, lumps within the abdominal cavity become less prominent, or disappear, when the patient contracts his abdominal wall muscles. Lumps in the muscles become fixed when they contract, and if the lumps are fairly superficial they become harder and more prominent.

Regional lymph nodes

The regional lymph nodes should always be examined as their enlargement or induration may give important evidence of spread from a primarily inflammatory or malignant lesion, and thereby influence management.

Other qualities

Many other qualities of a lump may, in certain instances, help the clinician in his assessment: for example, the colour of a malignant melanoma, the warmth of an abscess, the papillary surface of a wart. However, the five features described above are the most generally helpful.

An approach to the management of the commoner lesions that are not confined to characteristic anatomical sites is now given.

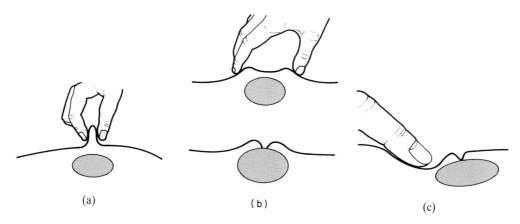

Fig. 1.5 *Attachment to the skin.* (a) A lump not attached to the skin. The skin can be picked up easily over the lump. (b) If the skin is tight in the region of the lump and therefore difficult to pick up, excess skin can be brought in from the periphery as shown (two separate hands can be used if necessary) and it then becomes obvious if the skin is free from or bound down to it. The pit that appears when the skin is bound down to the lump is called 'skin-dimpling'. (c) In the author's experience it is not as reliable as that shown in (b).

Lumps at random sites

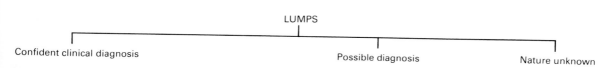

Diagnostic approach

After the history has been taken and the examination made, the clinician finds himself in one of three situations. Either he has made a confident diagnosis of the nature of the lesion, or he makes a working diagnosis which he feels is very likely to be accurate and which modifies his approach to management, or finally, the lump remains an unknown entity. In the first situation, treatment is dictated by one's knowledge of the natural history of the lesion, and indeed there may be no indication for treatment of any kind. In the third situation, the management must be by biopsy or, if the lesion is reasonably small, by excision biopsy. In the intermediate situation, a histological diagnosis is also mandatory but the approach to making this diagnosis may be coloured by the characteristics of the lesion thought most likely to be present.

The immobility of a lump attached to or arising within bone is usually obvious, and most of these lesions are very hard. They will not be further considered here: an orthopaedic opinion should be obtained. Lumps communicating with joints are also usually immobile, although this may not be true if the communication is a narrow pedicle. Their characteristic features are fluctuation, a variation in volume according to the position of the joint, and the possibility in certain positions of the joint of at least partially reducing them into the joint cavity. Most such lesions also fall into the province of the orthopaedic surgeon, though the general surgeon may elect to treat a ganglion (p. 16).

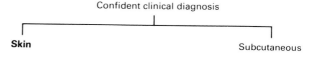

Skin lumps

Everyone displays on his skin a host of pigmented lesions that vary in colour from pink to dark brown. The histological nature of most of these lesions is either angiomatous or naevus cell in origin. Some of these pigmented lesions are not lumps at all, but merely areas of staining of the skin such as the so-called port-wine stain of a cavernous haemangioma or the café-au-lait stain that is often seem in patients with neurofibromatosis. It would not be practicable, even if it were thought desirable, to biopsy all these lesions, and the important principle is to recognize that small pigmented lesions which have remained entirely static in their physical appearance for a long period can safely be left alone. If a particular lesion is so large as to embarrass the patient or to produce symptoms by being, for example, rubbed by his clothing, it should be excised and the opportunity taken for histological confirmation of its benign nature. The question of what constitutes an over-stepping of the clinical dividing line between these lesions and a possible malignant melanoma is considered later.

The *common wart* presents rather different appearances according to whether the lesion is in the sole of the foot (plantar wart) or anywhere else. They are benign papillomas produced by infection with a virus, and they can be diagnosed with confidence from their appearance. Except in the soles, they are domed hemispherical lesions of a mid-brown colour and careful inspection of their surface demonstrates their essential papilliform nature. In the sole, a wart becomes buried under a thick layer of keratin, and presents as a pale yellow or light tan, characteristically translucent nodule that may be exquisitely tender. Warts are usually treated by school medical officers or dermatologists with various chemicals designed to destroy the wart, or with liquid nitrogen or cryosurgery but occasionally a surgeon is requested to deal with persistent or recurrent lesions and diathermy excision is usually effective. For perianal warts, see p. 139.

Sebaceous cyst or epidermal cyst is a spherical lesion which lies mostly in the subcutaneous tissue but can always be demonstrated to have an attachment to the skin while in most cases a punctum can be seen in this region of attachment. The punctum may represent the opening of the sebaceous gland, blockage of which has produced the lesion. These cysts are frequently multiple, and the sites of election are the scalp and the scrotum but they can occur almost anywhere. Excision should be advised because there is always a danger of infection.

Keratoses are roughened brown areas with a papilliform surface that can be partially rubbed off. When they occur in elderly people, usually on the face or the back, they are of no particular significance. However, when they present in younger people, or in the scars of old burns, radiation burns, etc., they should be watched closely because a malignant change to squamous cell carcinoma is possible.

The preceding list, though not exhaustive, covers most of the common conditions which can be confidently diagnosed as requiring no treatment or simple local treatment. To these can be added swellings that are obviously inflammatory in nature, such as boils, styes (infected hair follicles of the eyelids) or carbuncles (multiple confluent boils). We come next to a group of three serious neoplastic lesions which can usually be diagnosed accurately on clinical grounds alone, but which can be confused with other benign conditions. The three malignant conditions are basal cell carcinoma, squamous cell carcinoma and malignant melanoma; the typical diagnostic features of these will be described first and then possible alternative diagnoses mentioned.

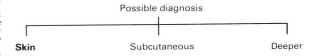

Basal cell carcinoma is often called a *rodent ulcer,* but this synonym should be avoided because ulceration may appear late during the genesis of the lesion. In the earliest stage, the lesion is a slightly raised pinkish nodule without characteristic features so that the correct diagnosis cannot be made with any confidence, although suspicion may be raised by the site of the lesion (they may occur anywhere, but particularly on the skin of the head and neck, especially around the eyes). Later on a very characteristic raised rolled edge becomes manifest, the skin becomes translucent (pearly) and at some time it breaks down to produce an ulcer. This lesion is locally invasive, and if left untreated can produce a horrible mutilation as it erodes cartilage and bone. Metastasis is very rare, and adequate local treatment is usually curative. After biopsy has confirmed the diagnosis, excision and radiotherapy are about equally effective, but radiotherapy should not be used where the lesion is adherent to bone or cartilage because the risk of radionecrosis of these tissues is very high. When surgical excision is used, a margin of 5 mm should be excised all round the visible and palpable limits of the growth. This can be done at the same operation as the biopsy if facilities are available for the examination of frozen sections. It should be remembered that occasionally a lesion diagnosed clinically as a basal cell carcinoma will prove on histological examination to be a squamous cell carcinoma or a melanoma, or occasionally even a non-neoplastic condition.

Squamous cell carcinoma usually develops in skin damaged by x-rays, chemicals, or long-standing sepsis, and hardening and cracking of skin are usually the first indications of malignant change. Soon a mass becomes evident, and ulceration is also an early feature. Dissemination to the regional lymph nodes may also occur quite early in the course of the disease, but it should be remembered that enlarged lymph nodes may be a response to infection entering via the ulcer crater rather than to metastases. Squamous cell carcinoma occurs rather commonly at certain sites where basal cell carcinoma is rare: e.g. the pinna, lip, genitalia and perineum. Once the diagnosis has been confirmed by biopsy, the primary lesion may be treated either by surgery or by radiotherapy, but again the latter is contraindicated by the risk of radionecrosis where cartilage or bone lies close to the lesion. If surgery is used, a margin of at least 1 cm, and maybe more in rapidly growing lesions, must be obtained. If the regional lymph nodes are large, it is wise to wait a few weeks until the primary has been dealt with before proceeding to block dissection, since this permits inflammatory rather than neoplasic involvement of the lymph nodes to subside.

The histological report may fail to confirm the diagnosis of squamous cell carcinoma: there may be evidence only of chronic non-specific inflammation, or of a specific infection, or of some different neoplastic process. A particularly confusing lesion is the keratoacanthoma which, although benign, grows rapidly and may be disfiguring. Around a core of keratinous material, which may later become ulcerated, a spherical lesion develops with a smooth and shiny pink surface. If the histological picture confirms this diagnosis, it is best to await spontaneous resolution which is likely to occur in a few weeks or months, but when the lesion is on an exposed surface the patient usually demands more radical management so the lesion should be excised.

Malignant melanoma is a possibility which must be borne in mind whenever a pigmented lesion changes in its physical characteristics in any way. The change may be a lightening or a darkening in colour, an increase in size, bleeding or ulceration, or the onset of a subjective sensation such as burning or itching. Malignant melanoma has a very bad

prognosis, among the worst of all types of malignant disease, and once this possibility is raised there can be no other management than urgent biopsy. The traditional advice has been that a full excisional biopsy should be performed, on the grounds that cutting into the tumour rather than completely removing it worsens the prognosis by favouring metastatic spread. There is little evidence in favour of this hypothesis, but it is probable that a satisfactory alternative is biopsy and immediate histological examination of a frozen section so that definitive surgery can be carried out during the same anaesthetic. The snag about this alternative is that the histological diagnosis of malignancy in a melanoma is not always easy, and the pathologist may be reluctant to give an opinion on the frozen sections. Should this problem arise, the surgeon has to decide whether to proceed on the assumption it is a malignant melanoma, or to excise the lesion with the sort of margin that would be adequate for a squamous cell carcinoma and await the definitive histological report on paraffin sections.

The margin of excision required in the management of malignant melanoma is larger than that for other malignant lesions of the skin because the growth tends to spread in the intradermal lymphatics, and satellite pigmented nodules frequently arise at the margins of an inadequate excision. It is difficult to lay down exact dimensions for an adequate area of excision. In the case of a melanoma situated on the lower limb, one would on average like to excise a margin of 3 cm all round the lesion. Indeed, there is a correlation between the thickness of a melanoma and the seriousness of the prognosis: 0.75 mm seems to be an important threshold with those below this thickness behaving in relatively benign fashion. Lesions with a thickness greater than 1.5 mm behave in a highly malignant fashion. Various features of the lesion may suggest an increased malignancy and therefore demand a greater than average area of excision. Lesions which are nodular from the start rather than a flat stain tend to be particularly malignant. Melanomas of the genital and anal area or those arising in mucous membranes also tend to be particularly malignant. Melanomas of the exposed regions of the face, and particularly around the eyes, tend to be less malignant; this is just as well because wide skin excision is impractical in these areas without producing severe deformities or destroying important structures. In any case the excision is carried down to the deep fascia, and the repair is usually with a split-skin graft. The better cosmetic effect of more complex grafting procedures can be used if the patient goes a year or two without recurrence, but in the early months it is easier to spot a local recurrence through a thin graft than through a full-thickness one.

The question of management of the regional lymph nodes is becoming more settled now that the results of multicentre trials are becoming available. On the whole, prophylactic block dissection is not recommended unless the primary lesion is very close to the lymph nodes so that both the lesion and the lymph nodes can be readily removed in a monoblock excision. If the regional lymph nodes are clinically involved or lymphangiography suggests that they are the site of metastatic deposits, or if the lesion is rapidly advancing and histological examination shows invasion of the dermal lymphatic channels, block dissection is advised.

Malignant melanomas are not very radiosensitive, but chemotherapy undoubtedly has an important part to play in the management of some cases. Immunotherapy has been explored but does not seem to be an effective weapon. Certainly immune responses in the host can be detected in many patients with melanoma.

A large variety of red, brown or even blue pigmented lesions may be mistaken for a malignant melanoma (and *vice versa*). The best mimic is the *juvenile melanoma* which may for a time grow quite fast and histologically be indistinguishable from a malignant melanoma; nevertheless, before puberty such lesions are nearly always benign in their ultimate behaviour. *Seborrhoeic keratosis* and some haemangiomas are brown and may cause confusion, though the haemangiomas often blanch on pressure with a transparent plate such as a microscope slide. Among the reddish lesions an important one is the *pyogenic granuloma* which results from minor trauma such as the prick of a thorn, and forms a rapidly growing pink nodule which attains its full size within a few weeks and then remains static. Excision and curettage is the correct treatment if histological examination confirms the diagnosis. Haemangiomata may be pink, and benign naevi may be pink or brown (the hairy mole falls into the category of benign naevi). Such naevi may, of course, undergo malignant degeneration at any time. Finally there is an interesting condition called *Bowen's disease* which presents as a pink thickened plaque growing slowly in the skin, with scaling and crusting of its surface. When it occurs on the glans penis or on the foreskin it is called *erythroplasia of Queyrat*. This is a

pre-malignant condition and when diagnosed histologically it should be treated by excision, radiotherapy or cryosurgery. Patients with Queyrat's erythroplasia should be circumcised.

With regard to skin lumps in which no clinical diagnosis can be made with any approach to conviction, there is no point in giving a list of the possible diagnoses. The management is inevitably biopsy or excision biopsy so that a histological diagnosis can be made, after which any treatment appropriate to the condition can be carried out.

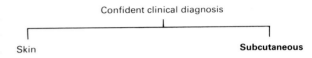

Confident clinical diagnosis

Skin   Subcutaneous

Subcutaneous lumps

There are three lumps of the subcutaneous tissues which can be diagnosed so confidently on the clinical findings that they may be left without a biopsy if the patient does not wish them to be removed. These are the lipoma, the ganglion, and the neurofibromas occurring as part of the multiple neurofibromatosis of von Recklinghausen's disease.

A *lipoma* is a collection of benign fatty tissue. In the subcutaneous region it is possible to be sure of the softness in consistency (these lesions are usually fluctuant), the lack of superficial or deep attachments, and the lobulated outline which characterize the lesion. They are occasionally tender, particularly if multiple, and they can be readily removed through small incisions overlying their centres.

The *ganglion* is a cystic lesion which occurs in relation to the sheaths of extensor tendons and the extensor aspects of small joints in the neighbourhood of the wrist and ankle. A fluctuant swelling in these regions with a demonstrable attachment to the underlying tendon is diagnostic of the condition. Attachment to the joint is usually more difficult to demonstrate, since such an attachment is usually a very narrow pedicle and the contents of the ganglion, although fluid, are so glairy in consistency that they are not readily reduced through this narrow neck into the capsule of the joint. With regard to treatment, many of these lesions can be ruptured by the firm pressure of the examiner's fingers, although they sometimes recur after this manoeuvre. If this technique fails, there is usually no contraindication to leaving them alone. Complications are rare. However, if the patient complains of any symptoms such as weakness of the neighbouring joint, it may be appropriate to excise the lesion. The operation is not one to be undertaken lightly, since it should be appreciated that the communication with a tendon sheath or a joint raises the possible problems of infection of these structures with the serious consequences of such a complication. The operation should preferably be conducted under a general anaesthetic, under tourniquet control to provide a bloodless field, and with full aseptic precautions.

Neurofibroma, when solitary, is a firm and usually rounded nodule in the subcutaneous region which may have no distinguishing characteristics and so may not be diagnosable. On the other hand, the lesion may be tender, and this may lead to a suspicion of the correct diagnosis. In von Reck-

linghausen's disease the lesions are multiple and are often associated with overlying patches of pigmentation of a light brown colour which has resulted in their being called *café-au-lait spots.* The full-blown clinical picture is so classical that no biopsy need be undertaken. But remember that there is some tendency for the neurofibromas of von Recklinghausen's disease to become malignant as time passes and transform into fibrosarcomas. It is important that if the patient complains of any change in size or tenderness of a nodule, it should be submitted to histological examination.

Other tumours are common and cover a wide range of possible diagnoses, but since they are only rarely diagnosable on clinical grounds, and therefore must be submitted to biopsy and histological examination, it is profitless to attempt a list of them.

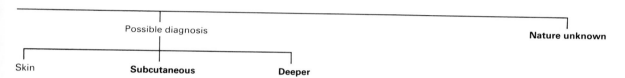

Muscle lumps

For practical purposes all lumps deep to the deep fasica are impossible to diagnose on clinical grounds, and must be subjected to histological ex-

amination. The commonest lesion is probably an intramuscular lipoma, but the typical lobulation of this lesion, although present, is masked by the tough, dense unyielding deep fascia overlying it.

Tenderness

Definition

Tenderness, in surgical parlance, means the complaint of pain in response to local external pressure. This definition corresponds with one of the everyday meanings of the word, but is inadequate in one respect. If the sign is to be of any value to the surgeon in management, it must indicate the presence of an abnormality. Everyone experiences pain if the examiner presses hard enough in the epigastrium: the real question is, with the degree of pressure applied, is an individual's complaint of pain within normal limits for the general population or is it outside those limits?

The problem is not simplified by the wide range of the normal response. One knows that some people have a very low pain threshold while others are remarkably stoic. Other factors include the patient's nervousness, the degree of his confidence in his doctor, how wretchedly ill he feels, and many other psychic factors quite apart from the very small problem of malingering.

It is not surprising that the assessment of this sign, with the necessity to decide how much pain the patient is experiencing on the evidence of what he says and how he reacts (e.g., wincing) requires considerable experience. *Distraction* and *reproducibility* are often valuable aids. In children in particular, success in directing the patient's attention elsewhere may reduce apparent tenderness to the level of the normal range. The child's suspect right lower abdominal quadrant can be re-tested with the clinician's elbow while his fingers press the left upper quadrant! And pain which is not reproducible with the *same degree of pressure* at the *same site* is unlikely to be significant.

Site

The precise zone of tenderness, and the point of maximal tenderness if there is one, are usually crucial to the diagnosis. The tenderness may be in the area of an abnormality — either an anatomical structure that is larger or harder than normal, or a site of pathological change in the tissues such as infection (e.g., an abscess), trauma or neoplasm. In such cases it is unusual for the tenderness itself to be critically important: the lesion must be assessed as a whole. On the other hand, there may be no obvious pathological disturbance at the site of the tenderness, and then the *exact* site must be carefully identified.

In everyday practice, the complaint of tenderness at a precise anatomical site is most often associated with a history of trauma to the musculoskeletal system. Apart from an obvious wound, the common situation is at the point of insertion of a muscle, tendon or ligament into bone. Such points take the main mechanical strain of distracting forces, and with the tenderness there is usually swelling due to traumatic oedema, and sometimes bruising due to bleeding into the tissues from the torn fibres. In the absence of such associated evidence, the surgeon makes the diagnosis from the history of injury, especially the exact nature of the movement involved, and from noting that gentle straining of the muscle, tendon or ligament by reproducing that movement reproduces severe pain. Such lesions, torn muscles or tendons, 'sprained' ligaments, are not always acute: they may become chronic, like the torn fibres of the brachioradialis muscle at the head of the radius and the consequent *tennis-elbow*.

Layer

Much less well appreciated than the importance of site is the importance of *layer*, especially when the point of tenderness is abdominal. It is a common error to assume that if digital pressure on the anterior abdominal wall elicits pain, the tenderness arises in an intra-abdominal structure. Often the tender area lies in the anterior abdominal wall muscles: in such a case, if the patient contracts his abdominal muscles (ask him to raise his head from the bed without the help of his arms) while the clinician is pressing the appropriate spot sufficiently hard to produce mild pain, the contraction greatly increases the pain. Conversely, if the tenderness arises within the abdomen, the firmly contracted muscles prevent the deformation of the abdominal wall that is necessary to reach the diseased structure and so the patient experiences less rather than more pain.

The aetiology of these tender spots in the anterior abdominal wall is unknown, but by analogy with the lesions of the previous section it is reasonable to accept it as traumatic. Certainly, a careful history has usually demonstrated that the pain is related to turning over in bed, bending forwards, carrying heavy shopping, or similar activities.

A common site is at the lateral margin of the right rectus abdominis, at the junction of its lower and middle thirds. The syndrome of chronic pain and tenderness at this site has given rise to the myth of the 'grumbling appendix' and the removal of countless normal appendices. Similarly, in the right *upper* quadrant there may be confusion with chronic cholelithiasis (Ch. 9).

Treatment. Treatment, and also the proof of the diagnosis, is by infiltrating the area of tenderness with a mixture of 1% xylocaine, 1 ml, and hydrocortisone acetate 1 ml containing 25 mg. The point of the needle is moved around until the pain is reproduced, before injecting. Further injections may be needed at 4-week intervals until permanent relief is gained, but the patient should be warned with each injection that when the effect of the local anaesthetic wears off (in 2–3 hours) the hydrocortisone may make the pain worse for a day or two before it makes it better.

Flow-chart 1.1

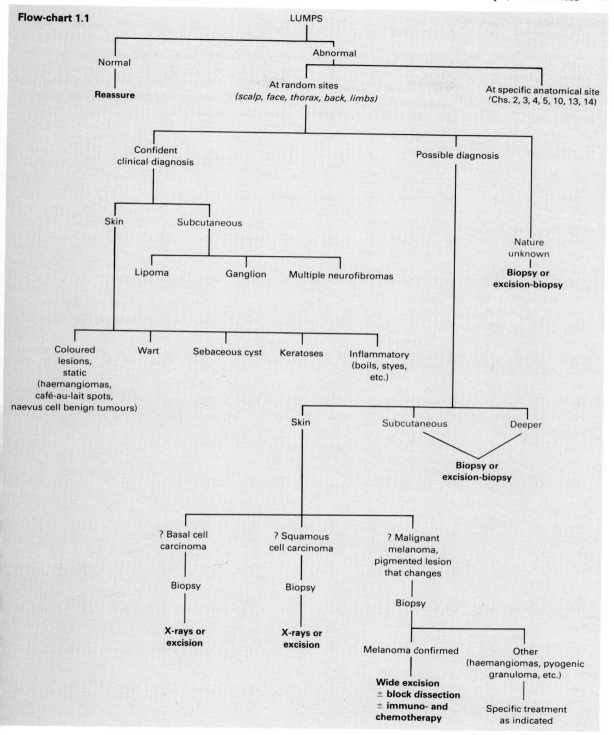

Further reading

Boulter, P. S. (1976). Diagnosis and management of skin tumours. In: *Current Surgical Practice*. Vol I. pp 232–49. Ed. by G. J. Hadfield and M. Hobsley, London, Edward Arnold.

Browse, N. L. (1978). *An Introduction to the Symptoms and Signs of Surgical Disease*. London, Edward Arnold.

Davies N. C. (1985). Melanoma: issues of importance to the clinician. *British Journal of Hospital Medicine* **33,** 166–71.

Chapter 2

Swellings in the Neck

Although the presentations discussed in this first section of the book usually come in chronic form, it is important to consider first the possibility that occasionally they arrive in urgent circumstances. There is no more urgent situation in surgery than a lump in the neck that is a haematoma, resulting from reactionary haemorrhage following thyroidectomy and producing hypoxia by obstruction to the airway (p. 279). Similarly urgent situations arise when spontaneous bleeding occurs into a goitre, especially into a solitary nodule, or when respiratory airways obstruction arises in the post-operative period after elective surgery in a patient with a goitre. The factors producing the obstruction are not always clear-cut in the latter group: they may include that the goitre is asymmetric, and hence tending to buckle the trachea towards the opposite side, that ventilation may be depressed by the lingering effects of anaesthesia upon the respiratory centre, that the cough reflex is similarly depressed, and that there may be oedema of the vocal cords as a result of intubation by the anaesthetist at the recent operation.

The essence of management is that, in the case of recent thyroidectomy, the wound is reopened immediately to allow blood clot to extrude, and that if this procedure does not result in the immediate improvement of the patient's clinical condition, or if there has been no recent thyroidectomy,

an immediate peroral endotracheal intubation or tracheostomy is performed. Once the airway has been re-established, further investigation and treatment of the cause can be carried out as indicated. Thus post-thyroidectomy bleeding requires a check on haemoglobin concentration after the bleed in case transfusion is indicated, and it may be considered worth while to check the normalcy of the haemostatic mechanism; the management of any goitre that seems to have precipitated the obstruction does not differ from the management of other patients with a goitre as discussed in Chapter 3.

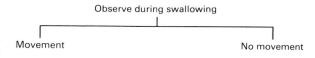

When a cervical swelling presents in chronic fashion, the first step in management is to determine whether or not the swelling moves vertically upwards during the act of swallowing, returning to the resting position as the act is completed. This test should always be applied, even if the lump appears to be far from the anterior mid-line of the neck.

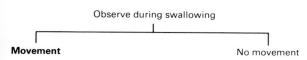

Movement on swallowing

Movement on swallowing indicates that the lump either is in the thyroid gland, or is attached to the thyroid gland by direct continuity of tissue, or is pressed against the gland so tightly by the pretracheal fascia that it cannot help but move with the gland. There is no clinical method of distinguishing between the first and third possibilities: for example, a nodule of abnormal thyroid tissue in the isthmus of the gland is indistinguishable from an enlarged lymph node of the isthmus, although special tests may help to prove the former possibility. The only example of the second possibility that can sometimes be diagnosed on clinical grounds is the thyroglossal cyst.

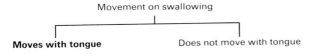

Thyroglossal cyst

If the lump lies in or near the anterior mid-line of the neck, above the level of the thyroid isthmus (i.e. at or above the level of the second ring of the trachea), and distinctly moves vertically upwards when the patient protrudes his tongue, the lump is probably a thyroglossal cyst. Should the lesion clearly manifest the sign of fluctuance, the diagnosis is not in doubt; should there be a possibility that the lump is solid, it is wise to ask for a scan of the thyroid region after a dose of radioactive iodine. Very rarely, a solid lump with the characteristics quoted is an ectopic thyroid gland which has not completed its embryological journey from the tuberculum impar at the root of the tongue to the usual postnatal position, and removal of the swell-

ing by the surgeon unaware of this possibility results in myxoedema and a life-long dependence on exogenous thyroxine.

The thyroglossal cyst is a remnant of the embryological track (Fig. 2.1) and when the cyst presents itself as a cervical swelling it lies anywhere in the mid-line, or near it usually slightly on the left. When removing the cyst, it is important to excise with it all remnants of the track or the cyst may recur. The track consists of a well defined band of fibrous tissue that can be followed for a variable distance upwards and (less often) downwards from the cyst: only very rarely can it be traced between the mylohyoid muscles right up to the tongue. It appears that a very persistent part of the track is usually present in immediate relationship to the back of the centre of the hyoid cartilage, so it is essential to excise this central segment of the cartilage as part of the operation.

Despite the clinical suggestion of movement with the tongue, the author finds that the histological report on a lump removed as a thyroglossal cyst occasionally proves it to be a median (inclusion) dermoid (p. 31).

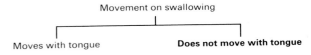

Thyroid and pseudo-thyroid swellings

These are discussed in Chapter 3.

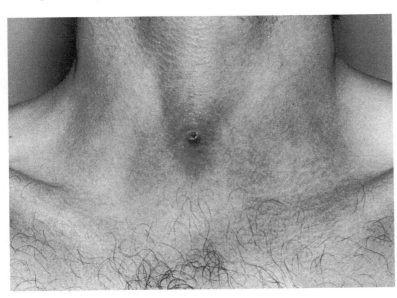

Fig. 2.1 Thyroglossal fistula. When the thyroglossal tract remains patent at its lower end, presenting with an external opening in the skin of the lower part of the neck in the mid-line, there is usually no cystic lesion (thyroglossal cyst). In the case of the young man shown, the tract extended upwards behind the hyoid bone, but there was no extension to the base of the tongue.

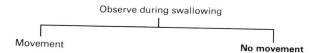

Observe during swallowing

Movement   **No movement**

No movement on swallowing

Having excluded a thyroid origin by observation, the next step is to define lumps occurring in easily definable regions so that they can be further subdivided. The most accurately definable of these regions is the parotid, and swellings in the parotid region are described in Chapter 4. The remaining definable regions are the submandibular salivary gland, the anterior triangles, the posterior triangles, and the submental triangles. Finally, there remain lesions which cannot be classified easily according to their presentation in one of these regions.

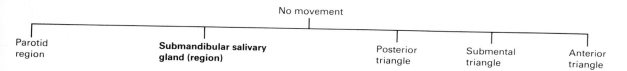

No movement

Parotid region | **Submandibular salivary gland (region)** | Posterior triangle | Submental triangle | Anterior triangle

Submandibular salivary gland region

A word of explanation is necessary about the definition of this region. A strict anatomical definition of the submandibular region is impossible. However, the normal submandibular salivary gland is a palpable structure and the implication of our classification is that the presenting lump is clearly an enlargement of the submandibular salivary gland or a swelling which at least partly encroaches on the region of the normal gland. Even when the presence of the swelling has greatly distorted the region, and nothing of the normal gland can be felt, the presence of a normal salivary gland on the opposite side helps greatly in orientation.

A swelling in the submandibular salivary gland region may present with or without the signs of acute inflammation.

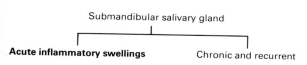

Submandibular salivary gland

Acute inflammatory swellings   Chronic and recurrent

Acute inflammatory swellings

Bilateral

Bilateral presentation of acute pain, tenderness and swelling of the submandibular salivary gland regions is unusual, but practically pathognomonic of mumps since other causes of acute inflammation are most unlikely to be bilateral. Other features of mumps may also be present — parotitis, pancreatitis, orchitis; or there may be circumstantial evidence such as a history of contact or the prevalence of an epidemic.

Unilateral

Unilateral acute inflammatory symptoms and signs may also be due to mumps, but they are much more likely to be due to some other cause and are best treated as a non-specific inflammation. A cause for the condition is sought: a stone in the submandibular duct may be visible and palpable as a hard swelling in the floor of the mouth, lying along the course of the duct, but a stone in the gland itself is unlikely to be palpable during the acute inflammatory state, while inflammation of the submandibular lymph nodes may be secondary to an infective lesion of tongue, floor of mouth, mandible, cheek or neighbouring skin. Any inflammatory lesion found is treated on its merits. The submandibular swelling itself is treated by antibiotics and local anti-inflammatory measures, but the removal of a stone in the duct is probably best not undertaken at this stage.

Usually the inflammation subsides, and further investigation and treatment can be undertaken as considered below for chronic swellings. However, should fluctuation develop, incision to release the pus is necessary. The course of the mandibular branch of the facial nerve renders it liable to damage during this procedure.

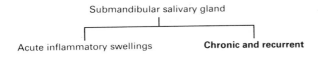

Chronic and recurrent swellings

Bilateral

Bilateral chronic or recurrent enlargement may be part of Sjögren's syndrome or of sarcoidosis. Sjögren's syndrome is described in Chapter 4, but it must be emphasized here that submandibular sialography does not give the typical appearance of punctate sialectasis as seen in the parotids: there is often irregular distortion, enlargement and narrowing of the duct system. The diagnosis of chronic or recurrent bilateral enlargement is probably best made by operative removal of the whole of one submandibular salivary gland. The treatment of Sjögren's syndrome and of sarcoidosis is unsatisfactory: corticosteroid drugs are sometimes effective, but the decision to use them depends very much on how bad the symptoms are.

Occasionally, the histological report indicates some other disease such as tuberculosis, reticulosis, etc., and any specific treatment available for the particular disease is then indicated.

Unilateral

A chronic mass in the submandibular region may be an enlargement and hardening of the whole gland, or a lump in the gland, or a lump superficial to the submandibular salivary gland and obscuring the latter. Remember that this salivary gland is C-shaped, with a superficial portion palpable via the neck, a deep via the mouth, and the concavity of the C is occupied by the posterior edge of the mylohyoid muscle. Thus a swelling of the whole gland is bimanually palpable between a finger in the mouth and the fingers of the other hand on the neck, while any intrinsic swelling of the gland becomes fixed when the patient contracts the mylohyoid muscle. By contrast, a lump superficial to the salivary gland, e.g., a lymph node, is not fixed by contraction of the mylohyoid.

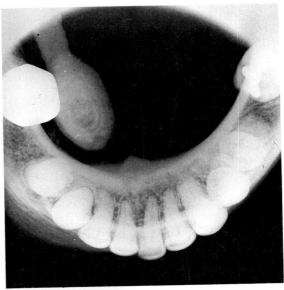

Fig. 2.2   Plain x-ray of the floor of the mouth, showing a large submandibular calculus lying in the submandibular duct near its termination. It would appear likely that the distal oval structure was the primary calculus which, by obstructing the duct, favoured the formation of the tail of secondary calculus which extends proximally.

To get the patient to contract the mylohyoid, ask him to keep his head still and to open his mouth by pushing his lower jaw downwards against your resistance.

If the whole gland is involved, an *associated cause* may be demonstrable. Usually this is a *stone in the submandibular duct*. The typical history is that the patient develops pain and swelling in one submandibular region on eating, and the symptoms subside in a variable length of time after the meal, to recur with the next meal. Occasionally, a history of such recurrent minor symptoms is complicated by an acute attack of sustained pain and swelling for several days, possibly with a constitutional disturbance, and the immediate management of this ascending infection is as described in the section on acute inflammatory swellings. Plain x-rays (Fig. 2.2) and sialography are useful in diagnosis and management.

In a period of chronicity, the stone is removed. If the stone is readily palpable in the anterior 2 cm of the submandibular duct in the floor of the mouth, it can readily be removed through the mouth. However, if the stone is further back in the hilum of the gland, it is usually not palpable in the floor of the mouth and there is always a great risk of operative damage to the lingual nerve if one operates through the mouth: the whole gland and a portion of the proximal duct containing the stone are removed via an incision in the upper cervical skin crease. Even if the stone is readily accessible in the floor of the mouth, a history of much trouble with severe attacks due to ascending infection suggests that the gland is chronically infected and therefore likely to continue to give trouble after the stone has been removed, probably with fresh stone formation. In these circumstances, also, it is wise to remove the whole gland.

Another possible *associated cause* in the floor of the mouth is *ranula*. The possibility of this diagnosis is suggested by the cervical swelling being cystic and transilluminable, and in such cases particular care should be taken in the examination of the floor of the mouth. The oral lesion may be inconspicuous by comparison with the cervical swelling: it consists of a bluish discoloration and dome-shaped swelling of the mucosa in part of the floor of the mouth, and pressure upwards on the cervical swelling makes the oral lesion more prominent and demonstrates their essential continuity. There may be a history of repeated bursting of the ranula into the mouth, with discharge of a little watery fluid, followed by healing. The nature of ranula is still disputed: it has for long been assumed to be a retention cyst of a mucous gland in the floor of the mouth. However, recent evidence suggests that it is an extravasation cyst produced by leakage of saliva from a named or unnamed salivary gland through a tiny hole made by minor trauma of which the patient has not been aware. The leakage of the saliva into the tissues provokes an intense foreign body reaction and explains why the cervical swelling is lined by granulation tissue rather than epithelium.

To cure a ranula, it is essential to remove that part of the floor of the mouth which contains the leaking duct. If the cervical part of the swelling occupies the submandibular salivary gland region, it is very likely that the duct concerned is the submandibular duct, or at least that the submandibular duct will be damaged in the course of the operation. In such cases, therefore, the submandibular salivary gland should be removed from the neck at the same operation. It is interesting to note that it is not necessary to remove the cervical swelling itself: it subsides spontaneously when the causative lesion in the floor of the mouth has been excised.

A wide variety of other associated lesions may be found in the mouth, or indeed in the neighbouring skin and subcutaneous tissues of the cheek, lip and neck, or in the mandible. The nature of these lesions, whether apparently inflammatory or neoplastic, may suggest that the palpable cervical swelling is an enlarged submandibular lymph node rather than an enlarged submandibular salivary gland. In general, the management of this situation is to biopsy (or examine in some other appropriate way) the primary lesion so as to establish the diagnosis: cure of the primary lesion may then be possible without any necessity to treat the lymph node directly. This may be true even if the primary is neoplastic, because enlarged lymph nodes may be involved only by superadded infection and may disappear after the neoplasm has been treated.

Should the lump be near the submandibular salivary gland but not a part of it, a straightforward excision-biopsy is performed. If the lump is *in* the salivary gland and no *associated cause* has been demonstrated, then a histological diagnosis must be sought. Two situations may obtain: that the lump is *clinically benign*, or that there are features of *malignancy*. In this connection it must be pointed out that while malignant tumours of the parotid only constitute about 10 per cent of all parotid tumours, in the submandibular gland the incidence is over 50 per cent of all submandibular salivary tumours. The index of suspicion should be correspondingly high, especially since the operative treatment for a malignant lesion is quite different from that for a benign one.

If the lesion seems benign (long history, slow growth, no pain, no fixity to neighbouring tissues and, particularly, remoteness from the mandible), then a tissue-diagnosis is obtained by excision biopsy, i.e. excision of the tumour with a wide margin of normal tissues. For practical purposes, since the submandibular salivary gland is so small, this means the complete removal of the gland, and even then it may be difficult to achieve a satisfactory margin because a tumour does not have to grow very large before it reaches the surface of the gland. If the histological report confirms that the tumour is 'benign', i.e. non-neoplastic, or neoplastic to as high a level in the scale of malignancy of salivary tumours as the acinic cell tumour (p. 57), no further treatment is needed.

If there are grounds for suspecting malignancy, it is important to achieve a tissue-diagnosis before embarking on surgical treatment. Biopsy carries a strong risk of producing future implantation recurrence, but this risk must be accepted because the incidence of malignancy greater than that of the acinic cell tumour is so high in the submandibular salivary gland. The biopsy may be a preliminary drill biopsy, or may be performed during the definitive procedure when the gland has been exposed. If the biopsy material is reported as benign, operative treatment is undertaken as described above for clinically benign tumours. If the report is malignant, a much wider excision must be carried out, with resection of a segment of mandible in continuity with the specimen. Opinion is divided as to whether a block dissection of the cervical nodes on the same side should be included in the procedure: the author believes it should be done if the histology of the primary is a frank carcinoma, but probably not if it is mucoepidermoid or adenoid cystic carcinoma. Immediate repair of the mandibular defect may be carried out by prosthesis provided that radiotherapy has not been used previously. Postoperative radiotherapy is advised in all malignancies.

Patients with clinically benign tumours treated by wide local excision are a difficult problem if the histology report labels the tumour malignant. Probably radiotherapy and a very careful follow-up is the best compromise, but any suggestion of a local recurrence should lead to radical surgery as described above.

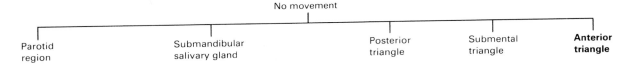

Anterior triangles

Some lesions in the anterior triangles are sufficiently characteristic for the surgeon to be able to make a reasonably confident preoperative diagnosis.

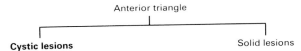

Cystic lesions

If the lump exhibits well marked fluctuance, there are three common possibilities: pharyngeal pouch, branchial cyst, and 'cold' (tuberculous) abscess.

Pharyngeal pouch (Fig. 2.3)

This is the least commmon of the three conditions, but should always be suspected if a patient with a cystic swelling presenting at about the junction of upper and middle thirds of the left (sometimes the right) sternomastoid muscle complains of even very mild dysphagia (see p. 85 for a fuller description).

The condition is cured by operation. The left lobe of the thyroid gland is mobilized by division of the inferior thyroid artery and middle thyroid veins, and the pouch followed behind the gland and behind the trachea to its origin from a defect in the muscle wall of the pharynx just above the pharyngo-oesophageal junction. Immediately below the origin of the pouch is a slip of muscle called

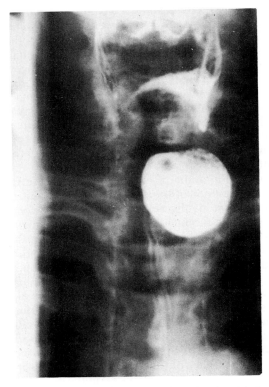

Fig. 2.3 Pharyngeal pouch. A mouthful of barium has been swallowed and outlines the large spherical cavity.

the cricopharyngeus, the lowermost edge of the inferior constrictor muscle, which forms the sphincter at the upper end of the oesophagus. There is evidence that it is uncoordinated spasm of this muscle during the act of swallowing which produces the extrusion of the mucosa immediately proximal to itself. For this reason, after the pouch has been excised, the cricopharyngeus should be divided.

Branchial cyst

A cystic swelling at the same site in the neck as a pharyngeal pouch (but occurring on either right or left sides), but without other characteristic features, is likely to be a branchial cyst. The patient is usually a child or a young adult.

The cyst should be removed, both to confirm the diagnosis and because it is prone to become infected. The origin of these cysts from the vestigial remnants of the branchial clefts results in the frequent presence of a fibrous track of tissue leading upwards from the deep surface of the cyst. Unless this track is completely excised, recurrence is likely. The exact anatomical relations of the track are variable, and depend upon which branchial cleft has given rise to the cyst. Frequently the track may be followed upwards between the external and internal carotid arteries, to finish on the wall of the pharynx in the region of the tonsil.

In association with a branchial cyst, there may be a fistula discharging mucus, often at some distance from the cyst, for example near the root of the neck. The *branchial fistula* may be of congenital origin, or partially an acquired lesion, resulting from infection of a branchial cyst and surgical or spontaneous opening of the resultant abscess, or from incomplete removal of the branchial cyst. The fistulous opening is circumcised, the track dissected up to the cyst, and then any congenital track above the cyst also dissected — all in a single block of tissue.

Cold abscess

A cyst in the same region of the neck, with some mild inflammatory signs but without pain or temperature change in the overlying skin, and with a history that the lump was hard at first and gradually changed in consistency, is likely to be a cold abscess due to breaking down tuberculous lymph nodes. Usually, some solid parts of the lesion are still in existence. A plain radiograph of the neck may show calcification in the soft tissues (in old

infected nodes). The Mantoux test is usually, but not always, positive.

Treatment of this condition is controversial. Some clinicians are satisfied with a clinical diagnosis in the absence of laboratory confirmation of tubercle bacilli, and give antituberculous chemotherapy as a therapeutic trial. Certainly the results can be very satisfactory. However, the author prefers to operate, evacuate the abscess, send scrapings from the granulation tissue of the walls for immediate microscopic examination for acid-fast mycrobacteria and for culture on suitable media for tubercle bacilli, sew up the skin, and then start chemotherapy. The sensitivities of the organisms to chemotherapy are also requested, but while the reports on culture and sensitivity are awaited during the next 2 months, the usual regime of triple therapy is initiated: streptomycin 0·75 g by intramuscular injection daily on 6 days a week plus oral daily doses of isoniazid 300 mg and rifampicin 600 mg in patients weighing at least 50 kg. Streptomycin is usually stopped after 4 weeks, and the rest of the treatment may need to be modified in the light of the sensitivities, but in any case effective chemotherapy should be continued for at least 8 months. In patients over 55 years old, ethambutol orally in a daily dose of 25 mg/kg should be prescribed instead of streptomycin, since the possibility of damage to the eighth cranial nerve from streptomycin is greater in the elderly.

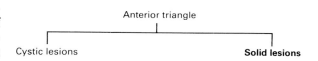

Solid lesions

A solid lump, particularly if more than one lump is present, is likely to be diagnosed as an enlarged lymph node. However, there is at least one characteristic solid lesion of the anterior triangle, and it should be suspected if the lump is situated at the characteristic site of a branchial cyst, but is *pulsatile*. These circumstances are very suggestive that the lump is intimately related to the bifurcation of the common carotid artery, and therefore likely to be a *carotid body tumour*. A tortuous carotid artery may sometimes be confused with such a lesion.

A carotid arteriogram should be requested: splaying apart of the external and internal carotid arteries confirms the diagnosis (Fig. 2.4). The tumour should be removed: at an early stage of the

Flow-chart 2.1

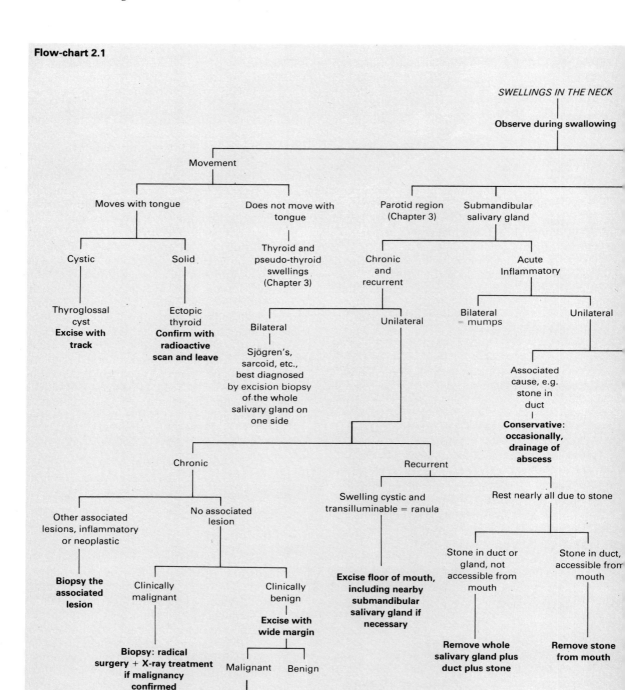

SWELLINGS IN THE NECK

Observe during swallowing

Movement

Moves with tongue — Does not move with tongue — Parotid region (Chapter 3) — Submandibular salivary gland

Moves with tongue:
- Cystic → Thyroglossal cyst **Excise with track**
- Solid → Ectopic thyroid **Confirm with radioactive scan and leave**

Does not move with tongue:
- Thyroid and pseudo-thyroid swellings (Chapter 3)

Parotid region (Chapter 3):
- Chronic and recurrent
  - Bilateral → Sjögren's, sarcoid, etc., best diagnosed by excision biopsy of the whole salivary gland on one side
  - Unilateral

Submandibular salivary gland:
- Acute Inflammatory
  - Bilateral = mumps
  - Unilateral → Associated cause, e.g. stone in duct → **Conservative: occasionally, drainage of abscess**

Chronic:
- Other associated lesions, inflammatory or neoplastic → **Biopsy the associated lesion**
- No associated lesion
  - Clinically malignant → **Biopsy: radical surgery + X-ray treatment if malignancy confirmed**
  - Clinically benign → **Excise with wide margin** → Malignant / Benign

Recurrent:
- Swelling cystic and transilluminable = ranula → **Excise floor of mouth, including nearby submandibular salivary gland if necessary**
- Rest nearly all due to stone
  - Stone in duct or gland, not accessible from mouth → **Remove whole salivary gland plus duct plus stone**
  - Stone in duct, accessible from mouth → **Remove stone from mouth**

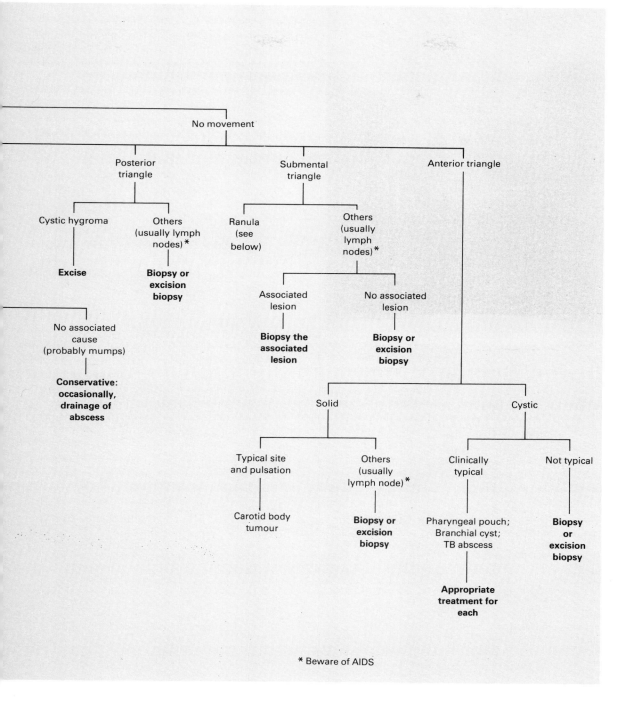

No movement

Posterior triangle | Submental triangle | Anterior triangle

Posterior triangle

Cystic hygroma — **Excise**

Others (usually lymph nodes)* — **Biopsy or excision biopsy**

No associated cause (probably mumps) — **Conservative: occasionally, drainage of abscess**

Submental triangle

Ranula (see below)

Others (usually lymph nodes)*

Associated lesion — **Biopsy the associated lesion**

No associated lesion — **Biopsy or excision biopsy**

Anterior triangle

Solid | Cystic

Solid:

Typical site and pulsation — Carotid body tumour

Others (usually lymph node)* — **Biopsy or excision biopsy**

Cystic:

Clinically typical — Pharyngeal pouch; Branchial cyst; TB abscess — **Appropriate treatment for each**

Not typical — **Biopsy or excision biopsy**

* Beware of AIDS

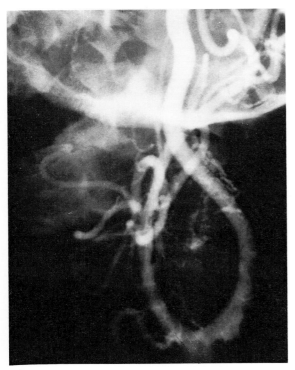

Fig. 2.4 Carotid arteriogram; lateral view, showing the typical splaying apart of the external carotid artery (the vessel with branches) and the internal carotid artery by a carotid body tumour.

operation, tapes are placed around the three main arteries so that control of any severe haemorrhage during the removal is assured.

If the lump is thought to be an enlarged *lymph node,* the possible territories in which a primary source of infection or neoplasia might be present are carefully scrutinized. In particular, the ear and the nasopharynx and oropharynx should be examined by an otorhinolaryngologist, a chest radiograph obtained, and the mouth inspected. Since an enlarged lymph node may be part of a generalized disease of the reticuloendothelial system, it is important to examine the areas of the lymphatic glands elsewhere — axillae and groins — and the spleen, and to ask for a full blood count, including a white blood cell differential count. In the end, it is nearly always necessary to perform excision biopsy. The excised material is divided into two portions: one is sent for histological examination, the other for culture.

There is one condition, suspicion of which is a contraindication to biopsy: *Acquired Immune Deficiency Syndrome* (AIDS) or its associated *Persistent Generalized Lymphadenopathy* (PGL). This condition is due to certain retroviruses known as human T cell lymphotropic virus (HTLV III) and lymphadenopathy associated virus (LAV) — now thought to be the same virus. By its action on T lymphocytes, the virus reduces cell-based immunity and patients suffer opportunistic infections from microorganisms that normally are not pathogenic (e.g., *Pneumocystis carinii* pneumonia) and develop uncommon neoplasms (e.g., Kaposi's sarcoma of skin in patients under the age of 60). There is thought to be an endemic pool of infection with the virus in Central Africa, but the highest incidence at present is in the United States of America. The usual route of infection seems to be via blood or semen, and the main groups at risk are male homosexuals, haemophiliac and other patients who have received clotting factors from pooled serum, and intravenous drug abusers. The disease appears to be uniformly fatal, and the histology of the lymph nodes is not specific. Thus there is no point in surgeons and nurses taking the risk of operating on such patients just to produce biopsy material. The diagnosis is much more safely and efficiently made by serological testing for antibody to HTLV III. Incidentally, not everybody who is antibody-positive develops AIDS or PGL.

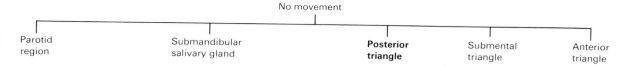

No movement

| Parotid region | Submandibular salivary gland | **Posterior triangle** | Submental triangle | Anterior triangle |

Posterior triangles

There is really only one lesion that is easily di-agnosable on clinical grounds: *cystic hygroma.* If the lump is fluctuant, highly transilluminable and usually lying low in the neck, it is a cystic hygroma (i.e. a benign tumour of lymphatic channels), par-ticularly common in childhood. The mass should be excised.

All other swellings in this region should be ex-cised, and any further treatment depends upon the histology report.

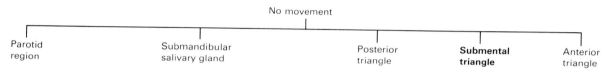

No movement

| Parotid region | Submandibular salivary gland | Posterior triangle | **Submental triangle** | Anterior triangle |

Submental triangles

This region consists of the territory between the hyoid bone below, the mandible above, and the submandibular salivary gland regions on both sides. Although anatomically a part of the anterior triangles, it is convenient to separate it because of the frequent occurrence of two clinically charac-teristic lesions that do not move on swallowing. One is the ranula (p. 25). The other is the median submental (or suprahyoid) dermoid, a cystic sub-cutaneous lesion of the mid-line that does not move on protruding the tongue. This should be removed because it may become infected.

Other lumps will usually be diagnosed as lymph nodes, and the same considerations with regard to management apply as in the case of the similar diagnosis elsewhere in the neck.

Further reading

Albert, G. D. (1963). Branchial anomalies. *Journal of the American Medical Association* **183**, 399–409.

Brown, P. M. and Judd, E. S. (1961). Thyroglossal duct cysts and sinuses: results of radical (Sistrunk) operation. *American Journal of Surgery* **102**, 494–501.

Browse, N. L. (1978). The neck. In: *An Introduction to the Symptoms and Signs of Surgical Disease*. London, Edward Arnold, pp 224–61.

Henzel, J. H., Pories, W. J. and DeWeese, M. S. (1967). Etiology of lateral cervical cysts. *Surgery, Gynecology and Obstetrics* **125**, 1–8.

Kerth, J. D., Sisson, G. A. and Becker, G. D. (1973). Radical neck dissection in carcinoma of the head and neck. *Surgical Clinics of North America* **53**, 179–90.

Thomas, J. M. (1984). Lumps in the neck. *Surgery (Oxford)*, 210–12.

Chapter 3

Goitre

The possibility that a patient with a goitre may present as an acute emergency due to obstruction to the airway is considered on p. 21. In the present Chapter, all other presentations of a goitre are considered.

The operational definition of a goitre — that is, the practical definition which decides how the problem must be handled — is a swelling in the neck that moves on swallowing but not on movements of the tongue. It has been pointed out (p. 22) that certain solitary nodular swellings in the neck not of thyroid origin may be included in this definition, but the true diagnosis becomes clear at the exploratory operation that is mandatory when the goitre is of the solitary nodular type (p. 36).

Preliminary classification

Two major questions must be answered at the outset, before the line of management can be decided: is the goitre diffuse or nodular? and what is the thyroid status of the patient?

Flow-chart 3.1

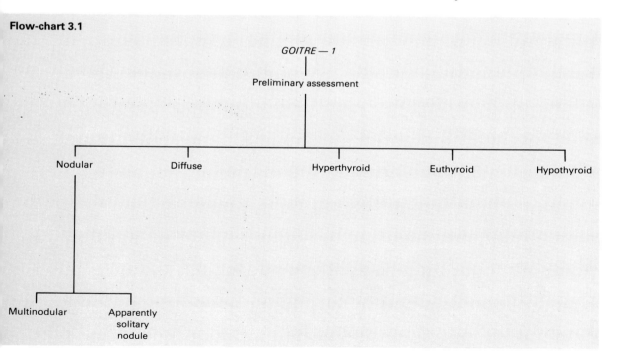

Diffuse or nodular?

Careful palpation is necessary for deciding this question, and it is done most easily and accurately by standing behind the seated patient. The surface of the goitre is palpated gently with the pulps of the fingers to determine smoothness or nodularity.

If the goitre is nodular, the examiner must also decide whether it is a single nodule or multinodular, since this subdivision also greatly influences treatment.

Two points may be made about palpating the thyroid: first, the normal gland is impalpable, even when pushed towards the examining finger from the opposite side; secondly, if a smooth enlargement of one side of the thyroid only is felt, the goitre must be classified as a single nodule. One cannot speak about the diffuse enlargement of one lobe, because one can never be sure that even the largest unilateral goitre is the whole of one lobe: the rest of the lobe may be lying posteriorly, completely overshadowed by the large anterior single nodule.

The sign of fluctuance is most unreliable in goitres, and it is unwise to diagnose a lump in the thyroid as either cystic or solid. The reason is the intervention of the strap muscles, which also render the normal gland impalpable.

Thyroid status

Most patients presenting with a goitre are euthyroid, many are hyperthyroid, while a few are hypothyroid. It is most important to decide a patient's thyroid status because hyper- and hypothyroidism are both dangerous conditions whose presence modifies management.

Hyperthyroidism

The *symptoms* of hyperthyroidism are nervousness, irritability, lability of mood, dislike of heat and tolerance of cold, increased appetite, diarrhoea, palpitations, tiredness of the eyes on reading, and general fatigue.

The *signs* are hyperkinaesia, weight loss despite a normal or increased intake of food, tachycardia (including during sleep), sweating, thinness of the skin, increased muscle tone and limb reflexes, cardiac arrhythmias manifested first as extrasystoles and culminating in atrial fibrillation, a collapsing pulse with a widening of the normal gap of 40 mmHg between systolic and diastolic blood pressure, and specific eye-signs.

The *eye-signs* are exophthalmos, lid retraction, and weakness on convergence.

Many of the symptoms and signs of thyrotoxicosis are present in anxiety state. The author finds that the most useful features to help in the diagnosis of thyrotoxicosis are the combination of weight loss with the fact that food intake has not decreased (and has often increased).

Special tests for the presence of thyrotoxicosis are, for the experienced clinician, often superfluous: most patients are obviously thyrotoxic or obviously euthyroid. However, in the elderly patient with a multinodular toxic goitre hyperthyroidism is often occult; and even in an obviously hyperthyroid patient it is useful to have a baseline estimation of the degree of toxicity in some quantitative form so that the progress of therapy can be assessed. Moreover the surgeon who has to advise operation, a well known cause of the dangerously severe exacerbation of hyperthyroidism known as thyrotoxic crisis, naturally prefers that his clinical judgement that a patient is euthyroid should be reinforced by some laboratory test. Thus all patients with a goitre undergo some form of test for hyperthyroidism.

The tests are multifarious. The rate at which the thyroid gland traps radioactive iodine from a tracer dose given orally has been a useful technique. The isotope ^{131}I, with a half-life of 8 days, is generally used, but in children ^{132}I, with a much shorter half-life of $2\frac{1}{2}$ hours, is safer. The uptake by the gland at 24 hours is measured. The normal range has to be established by each laboratory for the population it serves: higher values indicate hyperthyroidism, lower indicate hypothyroidism. A rapid uptake and high turnover rate of iodine may be encountered in iodine deficiency and after thyroidectomy, so that there can be difficulties in interpretation.

However, it is now possible to measure thyroxine (T4) and tri-iodothyronine (T3) by radioimmunoassay, and so the concentrations of these substances in the plasma, and even their secretion rates, can be measured. There is now a swing in emphasis from uptake tests — which require the patient to attend more than once — to tests based on plasma measurements. The metabolic activity of thyroxine is proportional to the very small proportion of thyroxine carried free in the plasma; the rest of the thyroxine is bound to plasma proteins and is metabolically inactive though in dynamic equilibrium with the free fraction. The free thyroxine index (FTI) is a measurement related to the concentration of free thyroxine. Should the FTI be equivocally raised above the definitely normal but below the definitely thyrotoxic, the decision that thyrotoxicosis is present may be aided by finding a raised T3 concentration.

Hypothyroidism

The *symptoms* of hypothyroidism are apathy, lack of energy and ability to concentrate, tiredness, sensitivity to cold, anorexia, and dryness of the skin.

The *signs* are weight gain, a slow pulse, thickness and dryness of the skin, a non-pitting oedema in many areas including classically the shins, reduced muscle tone and limb reflexes, and loss of hair from the scalp and from the lateral ends particularly of the eyebrows.

Special tests are the same as those for investigating thyrotoxicosis: the FTI is below the normal range. Should the value be in the equivocal boundary zone between normal and hypothyroid, the

finding of a raised thyroid-stimulating hormone (TSH) concentration in the plasma will confirm hypothyroidism.

Further considerations

The answers to these two questions enable patients with goitre to be classified into a number of groups: diffuse toxic, diffuse euthyroid, diffuse hypothyroid; and nodular toxic, nodular hyperthyroid, nodular hypothyroid. The nodular groups can be further subdivided into multinodular and the single nodular type. The management of each of these groups is distinct, although it can be said that hypothyroidism makes less difference to management than does hyperthyroidism. From the surgical viewpoint, the solitary nodule is a definitely surgical challenge. These considerations have been taken into account in the arrangement of subsequent sections of the chapter.

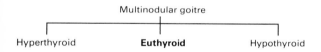

Multinodular goitre

Hyperthyroid · **Euthyroid** · Hypothyroid

Multinodular goitre

Euthyroid

It is generally accepted that a multinodular goitre arises as a sequel to a diffuse goitre. The multiple nodules are degenerative cysts, and they are separated by thyroid tissue showing attempts at regeneration with varying degrees of success. The original diffuse goitre was due to an effective deficiency of iodine, while the attempts at regeneration indicate that at the time seen there has been an improvement in the supply of iodine.

The implication of these factors is that a multinodular goitre is unlikely to improve with treatment with iodine. On the other hand, the size of the goitre may diminish if thyroxine is given because the resulting high blood level of thyroxine damps down the release of TSH from the anterior pituitary. The author's practice is therefore to try thyroxine 0·1 mg daily for 1 month, increased gradually thereafter to 0·3 mg daily or until toxic signs or symptoms appear, and maintained for 6 months.

Indications for surgery

The practical indication is cosmesis: the patient requests relief from an unsightly swelling. The operation performed is bilateral partial thyroidectomy, shaving down both lobes to the level of the front of the trachea. Some surgeons prefer to do a hemithyroidectomy on the more affected side and a partial on the less affected so that if the thyroid enlarges again only one lobe needs to be treated surgically. Following operation, it is probably wise to keep the patient on thyroxine 0·1 mg daily for several years, to reduce any tendency to recurrence.

It is sometimes said that multinodular goitre predisposes to malignant change: this may be true, but it certainly does not constitute an indication for total thyroidectomy as a prophylactic measure in every patient with multinodular goitre. The dangers of total thyroidectomy (damage to recurrent laryngeal nerve, hypoparathyroidism) are so much greater than after partial, or even subtotal, thyroidectomy that one could not contemplate such a radical prophylactic possibility, and any less radical approach (i.e. subtotal thyroidectomy) is clearly illogical since carcinoma may start anywhere in the multinodular gland. A quite different problem is when malignant change is suspected because of a sudden growth in the size of the gland, particularly if it affects only one area of the gland, or because of the development of fixity or of palpable lymph nodes. The management of this situation is discussed later (p. 40).

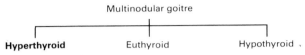

Hyperthyroid

In general, there are three lines of treatment available for thyrotoxicosis. As discussed later (p. 44), there are medical, radiotherapeutic and surgical methods. For toxic nodular goitre, surgery is the method of choice. Toxic nodular goitre tends to occur in elderly subjects, in contradistinction to

thyrotoxicosis with a diffuse goitre, and these elderly subjects are prone to develop cardiac complications so that it is important to control the thyrotoxicosis as soon as possible. The quickest way to achieve this is to give potassium iodide 15 mg (100 μmol) t.d.s. for 10–15 days until signs and symptoms of toxicity have disappeared, and then perform subtotal thyroidectomy. By contrast, radioactive iodine takes about 3 months to make the patient euthyroid, while the antithyroid drugs are uncertain in their effect in the multinodular type of thyrotoxicosis and relapse after some response is also common.

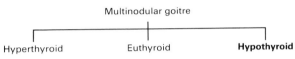

Hypothyroidism

Apart from underlining the need for effective treatment with thyroxine to make the patient euthyroid, hypothyroidism has no marked influence on the management of multinodular goitre.

Apparently solitary nodule

This presentation is surgically the most interesting.

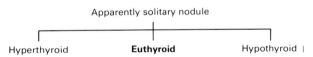

Euthyroid

Assuming that no suggestion of hyperthyroidism or hypothyroidism arises, ultrasonography is the most immediately helpful investigation. This imaging technique is reliable in identifying those patients (approximately half) in whom the apparently solitary nodule is in fact a dominant nodule in a multinodular goitre, or the others in whom the lump is a truly solitary cyst.

If the assessment is that the patient has a *multinodular goitre*, there is no necessity to operate unless mechanical considerations (pressure effects, especially on the trachea, and particularly should there be sudden haemorrhage into the cyst)

seem relevant. If the ultrasound report says that the lesion is a *solitary cyst,* this excludes malignancy. The management then depends on the history — did the cyst appear overnight? If so, it is worth deferring active treatment for a month as long as there is no suggestion during this period that the lump is getting larger. Many simple cysts of the thyroid disappear as rapidly as they appeared.

The treatment of a cyst that developed slowly, or else developed slowly but was of constant or increasing size during a month of observation, is controversial. Some surgeons still advocate an operation to explore the thyroid and enucleate the cyst. Others advise *aspiration,* usually under ultrasound control. After aspiration by percutaneous puncture, a cyst of the thyroid usually does not recur. Should it recur, it is wise to treat the cyst in the same way as a solitary solid lesion, i.e., by excision.

For a *solitary solid* nodule, the author's personal preference is to explore the neck without further ado (p. 39). In many clinics, however, radioactive scanning is performed at this stage.

Flow-chart 3.2

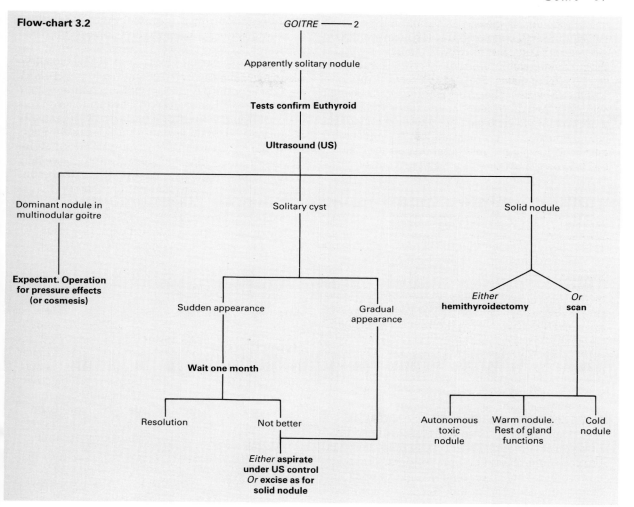

GOITRE ——— 2

Apparently solitary nodule

Tests confirm Euthyroid

Ultrasound (US)

Dominant nodule in multinodular goitre

Solitary cyst

Solid nodule

Expectant. Operation for pressure effects (or cosmesis)

Sudden appearance

Gradual appearance

Either **hemithyroidectomy**

Or **scan**

Wait one month

Resolution

Not better

Autonomous toxic nodule

Warm nodule. Rest of gland functions

Cold nodule

Either **aspirate under US control** *Or* **excise as for solid nodule**

Radioactive scanning

The scans obtained are used to differentiate three types of solitary nodule: the autonomous toxic nodule, the warm nodule, and the cold nodule.

The *autonomous toxic nodule* is represented by a scan in which the clinically palpable nodule concentrates the radioactive iodine but the rest of the gland does not. The interpretation is that the nodule is no longer under the control of the anterior pituitary and is secreting enough thyroid hormone to damp down TSH production by the pituitary and hence thyroxine production by the rest of the gland.

Three features about such a scan require special comment. First, the scan is sometimes said to represent a 'hot nodule'. This nomenclature should be avoided, because other clinicians use this term to indicate the 'warm nodule' described below or,

even worse, to indicate both conditions indiscriminately. Secondly, the production of thyroxine by the autonomous toxic nodule may be large enough to produce clinical thyrotoxicosis (p. 38), but frequently does not: hence the justification for describing this as one type of scan found in the euthyroid group. Finally, the autonomous toxic nodule is never composed of malignant tissue.

The *warm nodule* is represented by a scan in which the nodule can be distinguished by its alteration of the contour of the gland (i.e. it concentrates the radioactive iodine) but the rest of the gland also functions and therefore is also apparent on the scan.

The interpretation of such a scan in terms of histology is less certain. In most cases the lesion is a functioning adenoma, i.e. an adenoma composed of cells which are capable of trapping iodine from the blood in the same way as normal cells; or else it is a nodule in a simple goitre in which some function is still present. However, a small risk, variably estimated between 1 and 5 per cent, exists that the lesion is a carcinoma.

The *cold nodule* is represented by a scan in which the rest of the gland takes up the radioiodine but the lump itself does not. The histology of the nodule may be that it is a nodule in a simple goitre but it no longer retains the ability to concentrate iodine, or a cyst, or (about 15 per cent of cases) that it is a carcinoma.

Possible treatment policies

It is generally agreed that the *cold nodule* must be explored because of the fairly high risk of carcinoma.

The risk of carcinoma in the *warm nodule,* although much smaller, nevertheless indicates exploration, in the author's opinion. In some clinics, an attempt is first made to suppress the nodule by giving T3, 40 μg 8-hourly for a week. Should the scan, repeated after this course, show a reduction in uptake by the nodule, treatment with thyroxine 0·1–0·3 mg daily, is given for several weeks to the limit of producing some toxic symptoms. If the lump does disappear, the patient should be followed up for several months while the dose of thyroxine is gradually reduced. Should the T3 not produce suppression of uptake, or the thyroxine not produce clinical regression and disappearance of the lump, or the nodule recur, exploration is undertaken. The method demands careful follow-up, and in view of the small possibility of cancer, and the greater possibility that the nodule will develop into a toxic adenoma, the author strongly recommends exploration.

For the *autonomous toxic nodule* in an euthyroid patient, opinion is about equally divided between radioactive iodine or surgical resection. The advantages of radioactive iodine are that it should be taken up only in the nodule and not in the rest of the gland, so that when the nodule has regressed under the influence of the radioactive iodine the remaining thyroid tissue should become normally active again. However, most clinicians in Britain are unwilling to use radioactive iodine in a patient under 40 years because of the risk of producing carcinoma in the long term. Surgical resection of the lump with a wide margin (in practice, this usually means a hemithyroidectomy) also cures the patient and is the author's personal choice of

treatment. It obviates the risk of haemorrhage into the nodule more rapidly and more completely than does radioiodine.

The only clear-cut indication for radioactive scanning of the thyroid in an euthyroid patient with a solitary nodule is so that an autonomous toxic nodule can be demonstrated. The incidence of this lesion is only about 1 per cent of all clinically solitary nodules: this means that 99 scans are performed for every 1 that gives useful information. The author's policy that all ultrasonographically solid solitary nodules, including the autonomous toxic nodule, in euthyroid patients should be explored removes the necessity for scanning in the whole group of patients.

The operative procedure for exploring a solitary thyroid nodule is discussed later (p. 39).

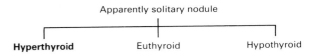

Hyperthyroid

If the clinical evidence suggests the patient is thyrotoxic, and whether or not tests of thyroid activity are confirmatory, the patient should be scanned. The minority of patients are thereby demonstrated to have an *autonomous toxic nodule,* which is treated either by radioactive iodine or by preliminary preparation with antithyroid drugs (p. 44) followed by surgical resection. The majority of patients, however, are shown to have a thyroid gland which concentrates iodine to some extent in all areas. The true situation in such patients is that the apparently solitary nodule is really a particularly prominent nodule in a *toxic multinodular goitre.*

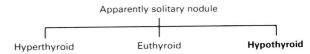

Hypothyroid

The combination of hypothyroidism with a solitary thyroid nodule suggests that the diagnosis is the rare form of Hashimoto's disease (q.v., p. 41) which presents with a solitary nodule instead of diffuse enlargement. If this suspicion is reinforced by the presence of thyroid antibodies in the blood at diagnostic levels, the patient should be first treated by thyroxine in a dosage of 0·1–0·3 mg daily to the limit of toxic symptoms. Under this treatment, if the diagnosis is correct, the lump should disappear in a few weeks; maintenance therapy at a lower dosage will probably be necessary thereafter. Should the lump not respond completely, the treatment is to continue thyroxine sufficiently to keep the patient euthyroid and explore the thyroid as for any solitary nodule.

Exploration for a clinically solitary nodule

The neck is explored through the usual collar incision, and both lobes of the thyroid gland exposed (but not mobilized).

If the lesion is clearly a solitary cyst (this can only be deduced if it is lying at the surface of the gland), it is enucleated and sent for histological examination, and the incision closed. In most patients the cyst will already have been aspirated: recurrent cysts usually contain blood and are difficult to distinguish from solid tumours so the treatment will probably be as for solid tumours.

If the lesion is a particularly prominent nodule in a multinodular goitre, partial thyroidectomy is performed to remove the nodule and shave the lobe down to the level of the trachea. A similar procedure is followed on the other side if the lobe is enlarged to any extent. After operation, the patient is kept on a maintenance dose of thyroxine in an effort to prevent any further development of the goitre. The prominent nodule may be composed of hyperplastic thyroid tissue between areas of degeneration, or may be a large cyst, presumably representing such an area of degeneration.

If the lesion is a truly solitary, solid nodule, the problem is difficult and management controversial. The possible diagnoses are *adenoma* or *carcinoma*, and there are four kinds of carcinoma: *papillary, follicular, anaplastic* and *medullary*. To make things more difficult, some carcinomas show the histological appearance of papillary adenocarcinoma in some areas, follicular in others. The final complicating circumstances are two factors relevant to biopsy: the cells of a thyroid neoplasm, if spilled in a wound, show a very great tendency towards implantation recurrence (they share this propensity with salivary gland, urinary bladder, and large bowel tumours); and the histology of thyroid nodules can be notoriously difficult to evaluate, especially by rapid techniques such as frozen section. The consequence of the first factor is that no form of incision biopsy (including drill or

needle biopsy) is safe; the nodule must be removed with a wide margin of normal tissue. The consequence of the second factor is that following the resection the wound may have to be closed and the result of examination of paraffin sections awaited 24–48 hours later before the diagnosis is established and further treatment can be contemplated.

Notwithstanding the previous paragraph, there is one circumstance in which the pathologist is usually ready to pronounce immediately on the histology of biopsy material examined by frozen section: if one or more lymph glands near the thyroid is enlarged and proves on examination to contain thyroid tissue. In these circumstances there is no doubt that the lesion is malignant since it has metastasized to the lymph node. The type of carcinoma particularly likely to produce lymphatic spread is the papillary.

Behaviour of thyroid carcinomas

Papillary adenocarcinoma particularly affects young people of the second and third decades. Studies of total thyroidectomy specimens have revealed that a solitary palpable nodule is often associated with satellite nodules elsewhere in the same lobe (1 in 3) or even in the opposite lobe (1 in 7). These satellite nodules probably represent lymphatic metastases, and reflect the marked tendency of this tumour to metastasize to neighbouring lymph nodes. Occasionally a patient presents with an enlarged cervical lymph node while the primary in the thyroid is still not palpable: this combination has given rise to the myth of the 'lateral aberrant thyroid'. Despite these features suggesting malignancy, the further progress of the tumour is often slow and patients may live for many years. The tumour is often, surprisingly, under TSH control to the extent that even large masses of tumour often shrink rapidly when thyroxine is given in adequate suppressive dosage. Long-term prognosis is excellent in such cases.

Follicular carcinoma tends to spread by the blood stream rather than by the lymphatics, so distant metastases are more common than with papillary lesions. The lesion is responsive to radiotherapy, although the ultimate prognosis is much less good than with papillary carcinoma. Occasionally follicular carcinoma, both the primary lesion and secondary metastases, weakly concentrate iodine: if the whole primary and the normal thyroid are removed, the secondaries may then concentrate a dose of radioiodine sufficiently to destroy themselves, no matter how widespread they are.

Anaplastic carcinoma usually presents as a diffuse goitre (see below); if encountered as a solitary nodule that has been removed, it is unlikely that further surgery will be of benefit, and postoperative radiotherapy to the neck is usually advised but the prognosis is very poor.

Medullary carcinoma is an interesting condition. It is derived from cells not of the thyroid gland itself but from the parafollicular or C-cells that originate in the neural crest of the embryo and secrete calcitonin, the hormone that depresses serum calcium concentration. The tumour shows no papillary or follicular pattern, no ability to concentrate iodine or manufacture thyroxine, but deposition of amyloid is characteristic. Local lymph node metastases are common, and the lesion usually pursues a benign course for many years but may then become viciously malignant and develop widespread metastases. Associated lesions include phaeochromocytoma, parathyroid adenoma and VIP-oma (vasoactive intestinal polypeptide or VIP is secreted from certain endocrine cells of the gut and produces severe diarrhoea) — one form of the so-called Multiple Endocrine Adenopathy syndrome.

Suggested management of solitary solid nodule

If no enlarged lymph nodes are found locally, the nodule is removed by total lobectomy. This ensures a wide margin, and obviates the need for a difficult operation to move the remnant of the lobe should the subsequent histological report dictate this procedure.

On receiving the report, an adenoma requires no further treatment. If the histology is papillary adenocarcinoma, some authorities advocate the completion of total thyroidectomy. In view of the fact that 6 out of 7 patients do not have lymphatic deposits in the opposite lobe, and that even if they do the prognosis with thyroxine therapy is very good, the author does not advise any further operation. The complications of *total* thyroidectomy (p. 44) are far more common and more serious than those of lobectomy or subtotal thyroidectomy. In either case, long-term thyroxine therapy to the limit of the patient's tolerance is undertaken.

If the histology is reported as follicular carcinoma, total thyroidectomy is completed. After 2 or 3 weeks, during which time hypothyroidism develops and thereby enhances the tendency for any metastases to take up iodine, a tracer dose of radioiodine is given and the whole patient scanned. If there is any evidence of uptake (or even in the absence of any uptake, if metastases have been demonstrated by other means) a curative dose of radioiodine is given. In the absence of any evidence of metastases, the neck is treated by conventional radiotherapy.

If the histology is anaplastic carcinoma, again the neck is irradiated. Medullary carcinoma does not respond to irradiation.

Diffuse goitre

Two main situations may be distinguished: that there is, or is not, a suspicion of malignant change.

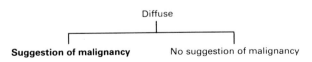

Suggestion of malignancy

Everything in this section applies equally to the similar situation in a multinodular goitre. These suspected malignant cases are never toxic, and usually euthyroid.

Malignancy may be suspected if there is a history of rapid enlargement of the whole gland, or of one part of the gland relative to the rest; if the patient is hoarse, and laryngoscopy confirms a unilateral recurrent nerve weakness; if the gland is painful, or seems to be fixed in one or more areas to surrounding structures so that movement on swallowing becomes less obvious; or if there are hard lymph nodes palpable in the neck or evidence of distant metastases elsewhere. Interference with the airway usually produces the more acute picture described on p. 21 and in any case may occur with non-malignant goitres (the solitary nodule).

If malignancy is suspected because of metastases, the usual reason is that a very vascular, pulsating mass has presented in a bone. Such a metastasis can also arise from the kidneys, and it is important to remember to carry out any investigations of the thyroid and iodine metabolism before asking for an intravenous pyelogram using an iodine compound to opacify the kidney!

If diffuse carcinoma of the thyroid is suspected because of metastasis, an attack on the metastasis may confirm the diagnosis. Whether or not preliminary investigations confirm the suspicion, the neck must be explored and as much of the goitre removed as possible. The management with regard to biopsy, frozen section and subsequent procedures is the same as in dealing with a solid solitary nodule, except that one has to accept a far lesser chance of being able to remove the whole lesion. Ultimately, threatened respiratory obstruction may demand tracheotomy.

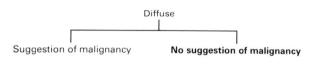

No suggestion of malignancy

The usual subdivision is made according to thyroid status.

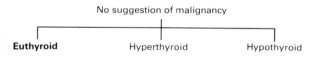

Euthyroid

This is a physician's, rather than a surgeon's, problem, and a few principles only will be mentioned.

The so-called 'physiological' goitre occurs at times of endocrine stress in women: puberty, pregnancy, lactation and the menopause. If there is nothing to suggest Hashimoto's disease (i.e. the gland is soft rather than firm, and thyroid antibodies are not present in the patient's plasma), the wise physician waits for spontaneous regression. If regression does not take place when the period of stress has passed, or if there is no stress in the first place, the condition is either a simple goitre or Hashimoto's disease.

Simple goitre is endemic in certain areas, usually mountainous regions remote from the sea. The cause is iodine deficiency. The richest source of

iodine in food is sea-fish. Iodine in soil exists as inorganic compounds of small molecular weight and great solubility, so the iodides tend to get leached out of the soils of mountainous areas and washed down to the sea. Goitrogenic agents also exist (e.g. in cabbage) which can prevent proper utilization of iodine even when there is enough in the diet. Endemic areas of iodine-deficiency goitre such as Derbyshire in England, or Switzerland, have been more or less wiped out by a policy of iodizing food salts, but still exist in many parts of the world. Sporadic cases of simple goitre still occur occasionally everywhere.

The diagnosis of simple goitre is made by excluding Hashimoto's disease as above: treatment is by iodine or by thyroxine. It would seem logical to try iodine first, but in fact thyroxine is more likely to be successful. When iodine is used, it must be started first in cautious small doses: an iodine-starved gland, hypertrophied under TSH-stimulation, may, if presented a large dose of iodine, form and secrete a large quantity of thyroxine before the feedback mechanism via the pituitary can react to damp down production. The resulting thyrotoxicosis is called the Jod-Basedow phenomenon.

The medical treatment of simple goitre is often disappointing, and for cosmetic reasons the surgeon's aid may be sought.

Hashimoto's disease or *autoimmune thyroiditis* typically produces a firm gland, and ultimately hypothyroidism, but in the early stages the patient is euthyroid or occasionally even thyrotoxic. Antibodies to thyroid tissue are present in high titre in the patient's plasma. The diagnosis should preferably be confirmed by drill or needle biopsy: the histology of the tissue obtained shows the round-celled infiltration typical of immune phenomena. Treatment is with thyroxine, and usually the gland shrinks to normal size.

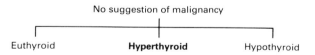

Hyperthyroid

A diffuse goitre with hyperthyroidism is *Graves' disease,* or *primary thyrotoxicosis,* so called because it occurs mainly in young people and to distinguish it from the toxic nodular goitre or secondary thyrotoxicosis of older people.

Flow-chart 3.3

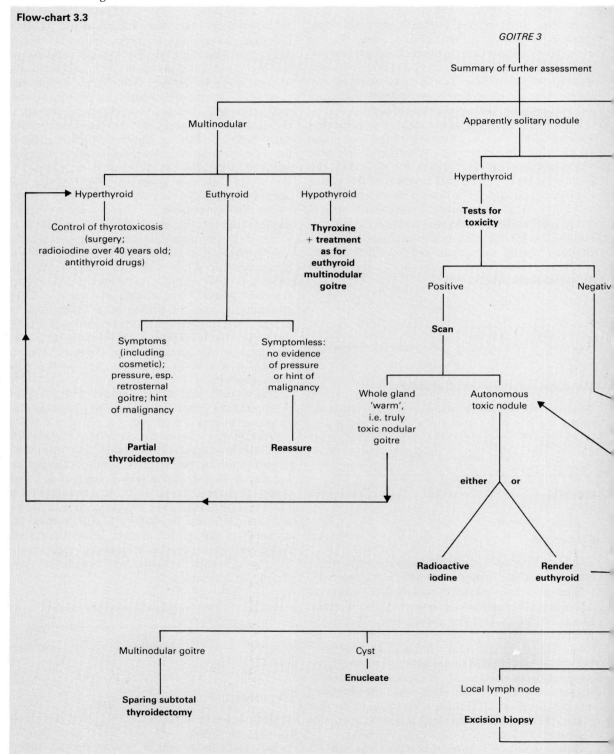

GOITRE 3

Summary of further assessment

Multinodular

Apparently solitary nodule

Hyperthyroid

**Tests for
toxicity**

Hyperthyroid   Euthyroid   Hypothyroid

Control of thyrotoxicosis
(surgery;
radioiodine over 40 years old;
antithyroid drugs)

**Thyroxine
+ treatment
as for
euthyroid
multinodular
goitre**

Positive   Negativ

Scan

Symptoms
(including
cosmetic);
pressure, esp.
retrosternal
goitre; hint
of malignancy

Symptomless:
no evidence
of pressure
or hint of
malignancy

Whole gland
'warm',
i.e. truly
toxic nodular
goitre

Autonomous
toxic nodule

**Partial
thyroidectomy**

Reassure

either   **or**

**Radioactive
iodine**

**Render
euthyroid**

Multinodular goitre   Cyst

Enucleate

Local lymph node

**Sparing subtotal
thyroidectomy**

Excision biopsy

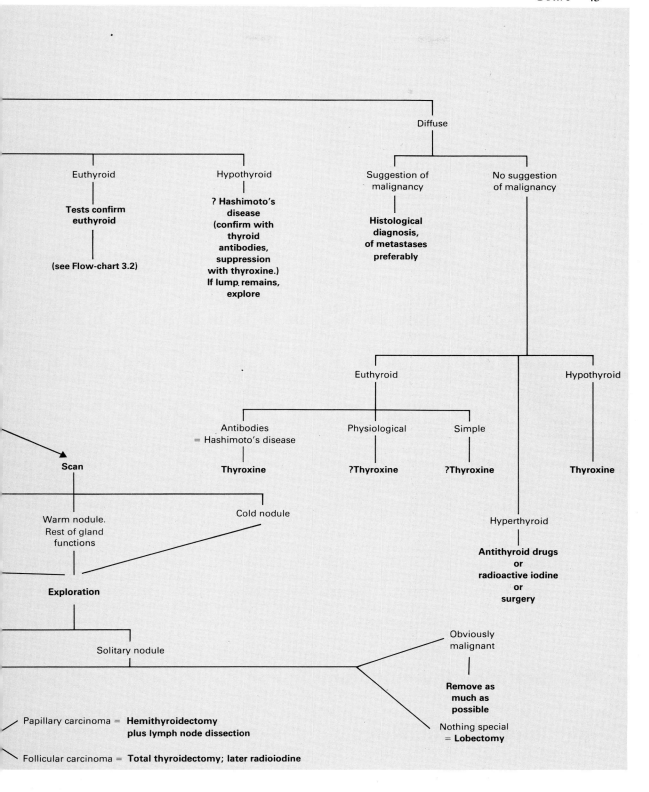

Diffuse

Euthyroid

**Tests confirm
euthyroid**

(see Flow-chart 3.2)

Hypothyroid

**? Hashimoto's
disease
(confirm with
thyroid
antibodies,
suppression
with thyroxine.)
If lump remains,
explore**

Suggestion of
malignancy

**Histological
diagnosis,
of metastases
preferably**

No suggestion
of malignancy

Euthyroid

Antibodies
= Hashimoto's disease

Thyroxine

Physiological

?Thyroxine

Simple

?Thyroxine

Hypothyroid

Thyroxine

Scan

Warm nodule.
Rest of gland
functions

Cold nodule

Exploration

Hyperthyroid

**Antithyroid drugs
or
radioactive iodine
or
surgery**

Solitary nodule

Obviously
malignant

**Remove as
much as
possible**

Nothing special
= **Lobectomy**

Papillary carcinoma = **Hemithyroidectomy
plus lymph node dissection**

Follicular carcinoma = **Total thyroidectomy; later radioiodine**

There are three forms of treatment: by antithyroid drugs, of which the best is carbimazole; by radioactive iodine; and by subtotal thyroidectomy.

In general, the treatment of choice is by antithyroid drugs, but certain exceptions are mentioned below. With carbimazole, 30 mg daily, the patient usually becomes euthyroid in 1–3 months; thereafter a smaller maintenance dose of carbimazole is continued for 12–18 months and then the treatment is stopped. Many patients remain euthyroid, but perhaps one-third relapse and require one of the other two forms of treatment.

Antithyroid drugs are contraindicated if the goitre is markedly retrosternal (because swelling may occur during therapy, and obstruct the trachea or great veins in the mediastinum), or if the patient is judged to be psychologically or socially (perhaps because of distance from medical centres or way of life) unsuited to long-term medical treatment.

Radioiodine is reserved to patients over the age of 40 years because of the long-term risk of inducing malignant change: it also carries a high or inevitable risk of hypothyroidism, and is slow to make the patient euthyroid.

Thyroidectomy carries the risks of any surgical operation plus the special risks of reactionary haemorrhage, recurrent laryngeal nerve damage, and damage to the parathyroid glands with consequent tetany. Thyrotoxic crisis may occur after the operation if the patient has not been made properly euthyroid by antithyroid drugs and/or a final course of potassium iodide for 10–15 days before operation. Propranolol, a β-blocker which prevents the cardiotoxic effects of excess thyroxine, is also useful.

These considerations enable the best line of therapy for each individual patient to be chosen. A particularly difficult problem is posed if the patient is pregnant: radioiodine is clearly ruled out, and surgery must be avoided in the first and final trimesters. If the mother has to be given antithyroid drugs during the puerperium, she cannot be allowed to feed her baby because the drugs are excreted in milk. The baby may be born hypothyroid (cretinous) if antithyroid drugs have to be given in the last trimester.

Fortunately, thyrotoxicosis generally starts early in pregnancy, and usually responds well and rapidly to antithyroid drugs so that these can be reduced or dispensed with in the last few weeks of pregnancy. Occasionally, the response to drugs is poor, and preparation with potassium iodide followed by subtotal thyroidectomy can then be carried out in the middle trimester with little risk to the pregnancy.

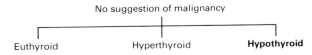

Hypothyroid

Hypothyroidism in *childhood* is called *cretinism,* and the affected child a *cretin.* Most cretins have a goitre, due either to iodine deficiency or to some inborn error of metabolism which makes ingested iodine valueless to the gland. The treatment is thyroxine.

It should be noted that hypothyroidism can occur without a goitre: in children with absence or defective embryological formation of the gland, and in adults as *primary myxoedema* (which is probably allied to Hashimoto's disease as thyroid antibodies are a prominent chemical feature) and as secondary myxoedema after treatment of thyrotoxicosis by any form of treatment. In connection with this last point, many patients with thyrotoxicosis have lymphoid hyperplasia or focal changes of Hashimoto's thyroiditis in the gland, and moderate or weak titres of antibodies: it is these patients who are particularly prone to develop hypothyroidism after treatment, and the surgeon should incline to removing too little rather than too much of the gland at thyroidectomy.

Problems after thyroidectomy

Reactionary haemorrhage

This is described on p. 21.

Injury to recurrent laryngeal nerve(s)

The cords shoud be examined by an expert otolaryngologist *before* thyroidectomy or any similar operation, because the incidence of unsuspected unilateral palsy is not negligible.

The cords are examined again by laryngoscopy a few days after operation. Permanent damage to one cord probably occurs in about 5 per cent of cases, with transient damage in a further 2 per cent. The change in voice is often minimal, just a little tendency to gruffness, because the opposite cord crosses the mid-line.

Bilateral permanent damage results in the cords lying immobile near, and later in, the mid-line: phonation is lost, and tracheostomy is usually necessary, although it may be possible to fix one cord in the abducted position by arytenoidectomy.

Hypoparathyroidism

Early symptoms and signs in cases of damage to or ablation of the parathyroid glands include lethargy, depression, and *tetany*. Tetany may be *latent*, and made manifest by tapping a motor nerve (*Chvostek's sign:* when the facial nerve is tapped the facial muscles twitch), or by reducing the blood supply to an area (*Trousseau's sign:* a sphygmomanometer cuff inflated on an arm to a pressure above the systolic results in carpal spasm); or it may manifest itself as carpopedal spasms. It is important to remember, however, that lethargy and depression after thyroidectomy are much more likely to be due to hypothyroidism than to hypoparathyroidism.

Late signs include cataract, and trophic changes in skin and skin appendages (hair and nails) and in teeth.

The condition is due to a fall in plasma calcium below 2·0 mmol/litre (8 mg/100 ml). Treatment is by vitamin D 400 000 units (10 mg) followed by a daily dose of up to half that amount, or by dihydrotachysterol (AT 10) 3 ml daily at first followed by a much smaller maintenance dose decided by monitoring the plasma calcium level: one aims at a level of 2·2 mmol/litre (9 mg/100 ml). If it is necessary urgently to raise the plasma calcium, this can be done with 20 ml 10 per cent calcium gluconate intravenously.

Thyrotoxic crisis

The mainstays of treatment are intravenous potassium iodide (to prevent any further output of thyroxine from the remnant of the gland), cortisol in massive doses for its antipyrexial effect, propranolol to block the effects of thyroxine on the heart (β-adrenergic blockade), sedation, and physical measures such as tepid sponging to reduce the temperature.

Further reading

Al-Sayer, M. M., Krukowski, Z. H., Williams, V. M. M. and Matheson, N. A. (1985). Fine needle aspiraton cytology in isolated thyroid swellings: a prospective two year evaluation. *British Medical Journal* **290**, 1490–92.

Beaugie, J. M., Brown, C. L., Doniach, I. and Richardson, J. E. (1976). Primary malignant tumours of the thyroid: the relationship between histological classification and clinical behaviour. *British Journal of Surgery* **63**, 173–81.

Britton, K. E., Quinn, V., Brown, B. L. and Ekins, R. P. (1975). A strategy for thyroid function tests. *British Medical Journal* **3**, 350–52.

Cady, B., Sedgwick, C. E., Meissner, W. A., Bookwalter, J. R., Romagosa, V. and Werber, J. (1976). Changing clinical, pathologic, therapeutic and survival patterns in differentiated thyroid carcinoma. *Annals of Surgery* **184**, 541–53.

Evered, D. (1974). Diseases of the thyroid gland. *Clinics in Endocrinology and Metabolism* **3**, London, Philadelphia and Toronto, Saunders, pp. 425–50.

Thijs, L. G. and Weiner, J. D. (1976). Ultrasonic examination of the thyroid gland. Possibilities and limitations. *American Journal of Medicine* **60**, 96–105.

Wade, H. (1974). Solitary thyroid nodule. *Annals of the Royal College of Surgeons of England* **55**, 13–20.

Wheeler, M. H. (1984). Malignant goitre. *Surgery* (Oxford) **1**, 200–206.

Chapter 4

Swellings in the Parotid Region

Apart from the common condition known as mumps, parotid swellings are not frequently encountered by most clinicians. However, when they are encountered, they often prove difficult problems to diagnose and treat. Part of the reason for the difficulty is their relative rarity, so that any one practitioner may see an example of this situation only once or twice a year. Another part, however, is that knowledge of the fairly simple clinical approach which will be outlined in this Chapter is not yet widespread. It is quite true that, even with this approach, a residuum of cases of unknown aetiology will remain to defy empirical treatment. The vast majority can, however, be treated at least logically, though not necessarily successfully.

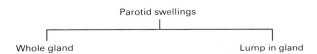

Whole gland versus lump in gland

The most important aid to successful management is a correct decision upon whether the whole parotid salivary gland is enlarged, or whether the presenting swelling is a lump in the parotid salivary region. The decision is crucial, because an enlargement of the whole gland suggests an inflammatory process affecting the whole gland or else a mechanical obstruction of the parotid duct; whereas a lump in the parotid region, unless obviously inflammatory, raises the question of neoplasia. In most instances, the distinction between whole gland and lump in the gland is quite easy: difficulties in management usually arise because the clinician has not attempted to make the distinction.

The parotid region

The key to the correct decision is an appreciation of the position, shape and exact boundaries of the parotid salivary gland. The gland lies in front of the external ear, filling the hollow between the ear and the angle and ascending ramus of the mandible. Above, it rises to the *zygoma*; anteriorly, it spills forwards over the posterior one-quarter to one-half of the *masseter muscle,* and a further extension (the 'accessory lobule') projects forwards in company with the parotid duct, sometimes almost to the anterior border of the masseter muscle. Posteriorly, there is a backward projection covering the *mastoid process,* hidden by the lobule of the pinna. Inferiorly, the lower pole of the gland extends well down into the neck: how far down may best be appreciated by recalling that the inferior tip of the parotid and the posterior tip of the submandibular salivary gland are separated only by a thin band of fascia attached to the angle of the jaw, the *stylomandibular ligament.*

The importance of knowing the exact configuration of the parotid is twofold. First, the normal gland is impalpable but the gland affected by inflammation or by mechanical obstruction becomes hardened and therefore palpable even if it is not greatly enlarged. The woman in Fig. 4.1 suffered from Sjögren's syndrome, and it was easy to work out the boundary of her left parotid by palpation, even though the gland was not visibly enlarged.

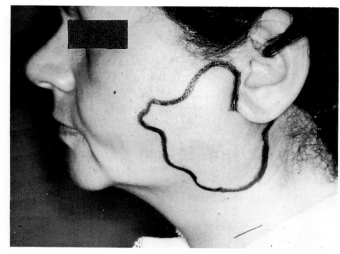

Fig. 4.1 The outline of the parotid salivary gland. This woman's left parotid gland was hardened by the changes of Sjögren's syndrome and therefore easily marked out. Note particularly the extensions forwards along the parotid duct, downwards into the neck behind the submandibular salivary gland, and backwards over the mastoid process (mostly concealed by the pinna). When the whole parotid gland is hardened by inflammation or obstruction, the resultant swelling has this characteristic shape. (Reproduced from *Postgraduate Surgery Lectures* I Ed. John McFarland. London, Butterworth by courtesy of the editor and publishers.)

Even when the parotid enlarges considerably, its characteristic shape, with its zygomatic, masseteric, mastoid and cervical extensions, remains unchanged. By contrast, the boy in Fig. 4.2 had a very large parotid swelling which did not extend backwards over the mastoid process and was thus not an enlargement of the whole parotid gland. The swelling was therefore a lump in the parotid region, and was ultimately proven by histological examination to be a carcinoma.

The second important reason for being able to define the parotid region with accuracy is that it reminds the clinician that a lump near the margins of the parotid region may be of parotid origin. When a nodule presents in the area immediately in front of the ear, the possibility that it is a parotid tumour is obvious; but the same possibility might not occur to the clinician if the lump overlies the mastoid process, or lies low in the neck behind the submandibular gland. The vital importance of appreciating that a lump in the neck or face may arise in the parotid will become manifest as this Chapter proceeds.

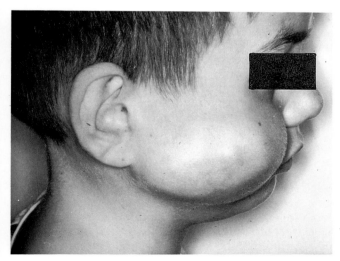

Fig. 4.2 Carcinoma of the parotid. This 11-year-old boy had been treated elsewhere as a case of obstruction of the salivary duct. However, the swelling clearly has no mastoid extension and is therefore a lump in the parotid region rather than an enlargement of the whole gland. The diagnosis of carcinoma was proved by biopsy. (Reproduced by courtesy of the Editor of the *Annals of the Royal College of Surgeons of England*.)

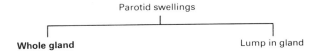

Swellings of the whole gland

Two situations can be considered: the *primary acute* and the *chronic*. In this context, the term 'chronic' should be taken to include *recurrent acute* parotid swelling, because the important causes of recurrent acute episodes may also produce chronic symptoms.

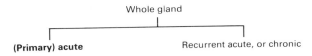

Primary acute

The adjective *primary* must again be emphasized: indeed, the single most important question to ask in taking the history is, has there been any previous attack similar to the present one. A reply in the affirmative means that the clinician is dealing with recurrent parotitis, and a quite different set of possible diagnoses must be entertained.

In primary parotitis, there are really only two possible diagnoses to consider: *mumps* and *ascending parotitis*. A simple but important aid to distinguishing these conditions is afforded by considering whether the affection is *unilateral* or *bilateral*.

Bilateral acute parotitis is almost certainly mumps. On the other hand, *unilateral* acute parotitis is probably mumps as well, but one must consider the possibility of ascending infection. If the inflammation appears to be unilateral, it is important to ask whether there has recently been a similar attack, or even just some mild discomfort, in the opposite parotid region: mumps may affect the two parotids at slightly different times, and with very different grades of severity. By the same token, it is important to watch for involvement of the opposite side as a unilateral parotitis progresses or resolves.

The difficulty about unilateral parotitis is that, while it is usually due to mumps, the exact diagnosis of mumps can usually only be made on the basis of circumstantial evidence. If the patient is a child,

if he has been in contact with another case of mumps 2 or 3 weeks previously, if the disease is epidemic in the district at that time, or if one of the specific complications (pancreatitis or orchitis) should occur, then there is certainly no reason to doubt the diagnosis. The only laboratory test likely to help is the measurement of mumps antibody by a serological technique; even here, only an increase in titre over the course of a week or so is significant, and by that time the disease has probably cured itself anyway.

On the other hand, the possibility that unilateral parotitis is due to infection ascending from the mouth is suggested by the presence of such factors as obvious oral sepsis and by the fact that the patient is weak with malnutrition and/or some other serious illness. The typical patient with ascending infection is elderly, has just undergone a major surgical operation, is too weak to attend to her own oral hygiene, and possibly has inadequate nursing attention in the form of mouthwashes, etc.

The case with bilateral parotitis can confidently be assumed to be mumps, and can equally confidently be presumed to proceed to resolution. Treatment is basically expectant and symptomatic: pain is relieved, constitutional disturbance such as fever treated by antipyretics, oral hygiene given attention to prevent secondary ascending infection, and complications watched for. This expectant treatment is also suitable for cases suspected of being due to ascending infection, provided that the following three further points are taken into account. Systemic antibiotics should be considered; an obstruction at the parotid duct orifice should be sought by inspection and palpation; and evidence of drainage of duct contents through the parotid duct orifice into the mouth should be carefully assessed.

The importance of the first two of these three points is obvious. The importance of the third point is that it is the best guide to whether the parotitis will resolve or proceed to suppuration. As long as a few drops of turbid fluid, or even liquid that looks like pus, can be seen exuding from the orifice of the duct, resolution can be awaited;

however, if the orifice looks dry and if pain and constitutional disturbance increase rather than decrease, a parotid abscess has formed. This must be incised and drained through the cheek, at a point where pain and tenderness are maximal, via an incision parallel to the neighbouring branches of the facial nerve so that the risk of damage to the nerve is reduced.

Patients with bilateral acute parotitis, or with unilateral acute parotitis with clinical features suggesting mumps, may safely be treated at home. By contrast, patients with unilateral parotitis suspected of being due to ascending infection require repeated intraoral examinations to check on the second and third points mentioned, and may well need an operation to remove an obstruction at the duct orifice or to decompress a parotid abscess: they are therefore better referred to hospital.

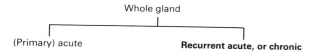

Recurrent acute, or chronic

Following a unilateral, or even perhaps a bilateral, attack of acute parotitis that has been diagnosed as mumps, has been treated expectantly and has resolved, the patient occasionally develops an unexpected recurrence of acute pain and swelling. The practitioner now has a choice of two diagnoses — recurrent mumps, or recurrent acute parotitis of unknown aetiology. There is little doubt that mumps *can* attack the same individual more than once. Nevertheless, this is a rare phenomenon, and must be considered particularly unlikely if the gap in time between the two attacks is only weeks or months rather than years. It is probably safer to assume that the original diagnosis of mumps was in error, and that some other condition is causing recurrent episodes of inflammation.

There are all degrees of severity of recurrent acute parotitis, and sometimes a patient reports recurrent pain and swelling of one or both parotids but there is nothing abnormal to find at the time of the examination. One should be a little cautious about accepting a history of recurrent parotitis in the absence of concrete evidence. Swelling and discomfort in the parotid regions, such as the related salivary symptoms of dryness of the mouth and over-salivation, are notorious as favourite complaints of neurotic subjects. However, if the patient's story seems reliable or there is collateral

evidence such as a convincing description of swelling from a third party, it may be reasonable to make a diagnosis of recurrent acute (or subacute) parotitis.

Finally, one or more parotids may be continuously (although possibly variably) enlarged, and the term 'chronic parotitis' is perhaps best reserved for this situation.

The importance of making a diagnosis of recurrent acute (or subacute) or chronic parotitis is that this requires referral for specialist opinion. The reason for this is that the elucidation of such cases often requires special investigations to which the general practitioner usually has no access. Nevertheless, the features of the history and physical examination used by the specialist in such cases are fundamentally simple, and there is no reason why the practitioner should not elicit them before referral.

The main point at issue is, can the condition be due to mechanical obstruction of the parotid duct? It is intrinsically most unlikely that mechanical factors should occur on both sides, and so great care must be taken to uncover a history of bilateral trouble, even if the presentation is unilateral. Again, parotid duct calculus, the commonest form of mechanical obstruction, is rare in children and young adults. One feature highly suggestive of mechanical obstruction is that the patient describes a sudden spurt of saliva or foul-tasting liquid into the mouth, followed by immediate or rapid relief of pain and swelling in the gland. Others include onset during meals, suddenness of onset and remission, and shortness of duration of the whole attack (a few hours up to 7 days). On the other hand, complaints met with in Sjögren's syndrome (dryness of mouth, dryness of eyes, kraurosis vulvae, rheumatic manifestations), or sarcoidosis (uveitis), may point in the direction of the appropriate diagnosis, while the attacks themselves tend to start and remit gradually, are usually not related to meals and last weeks rather than days.

From the point of view of physical signs, the question of bilaterality is carefully explored by inspection and palpation of both parotid regions. The possible presence of a parotid duct calculus is then investigated by inspection and palpation of the duct from the cheek, as it lies on and hooks round the anterior border of the sternomastoid muscle, and of its oral termination from the mouth. No examination of a parotid problem can be considered complete until the orifice of the duct opposite the second molar tooth has been inspected with a strong light and palpated by a finger in the mouth exerting pressure against the other hand outside the cheek. It is surprising how often this simple manoeuvre leads directly to a diagnosis of parotid duct calculus: sometimes the stone is visible as a projection from the duct orifice, whence it can be lifted with forceps to achieve an immediate and dramatic cure. Or again, sometimes one sees the orifice as a gaping hole with surrounding oedema and inflammation — the stone has passed spontaneously, and the patient can be immediately reassured. Failure to examine the mouth in this sort of case is as bad an error as failure to examine the rectum in a patient with abdominal symptoms.

We now consider the rôle of the surgeon to whose out-patient clinic the patient with recurrent acute or chronic parotitis has been referred. In the light of the history and findings on physical examination as detailed above, the surgeon reaches one of the following decisions: the patient has unilateral or bilateral disease; if unilateral, there is definite or presumptive evidence that a parotid duct calculus is present or that it has recently passed, or there is no such evidence. The next step is to proceed to x-ray studies.

Radiology

If the patient has bilateral disease, the surgeon requests sialography, usually on both sides. The parotid duct is cannulated, and water-soluble contrast medium, e.g. Urografin (sodium diatrizoate with meglumine diatrizoate), injected with gentle pressure until resistance is felt. Usually the amount of injection is only about 0·5 ml into each duct. The typical radiological finding that is being sought is known as 'punctate sialectasis' (Fig. 4.3): the main duct and its branches are normal, but the finer peripheral ducts terminate in blobs of contrast. This appearance can be produced in a normal gland if sufficient pressure is used in injecting the contrast, but if care is taken over the injection the appearance of the blobs, which are lakes of extravasated contrast, indicate special weakness of the walls of the terminal ducts and are almost specific to the histological changes in the gland that are found in Sjögren's syndrome (see below).

If the patient has unilateral disease, the radiological investigations are concentrated upon the affected side. Plain x-rays are carried out in various directions, including a special intraoral view (Fig. 4.4), which shows the oral end of the duct without

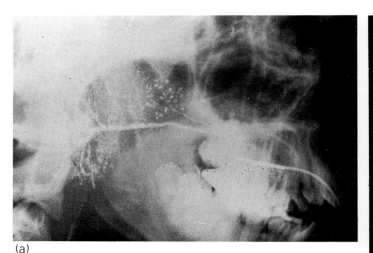

(a)

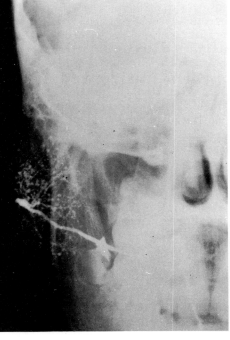

(b)

Fig. 4.3   Punctate sialectasis. (a) Lateral view and (b) anteroposterior view of a sialogram showing the typical picture. The appearance of saccular 'dilatations' has been produced by extravasation of the contrast material through weaknesses at the terminations of the smaller ducts. This condition is almost specific to Sjögren's syndrome.

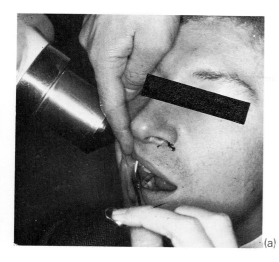
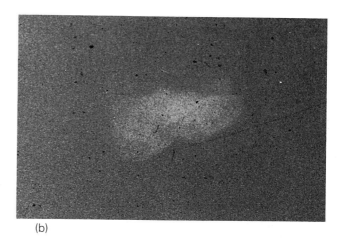

(a)

(b)

Fig. 4.4 Plain x-rays: intraoral view for parotid duct calculus. (a) The patient holds a small dental x-ray plate between his cheek and gums, in the region of the termination of the parotid duct in the mouth, opposite the second upper molar tooth. X-rays are directed through the soft tissues of the cheek without interference from neighbouring bones. (b) An example of the results achieved. The calculus shown measured about 4 mm in length, but it had not been shown in the conventional views because it was overlain by the densities of the facial bones.

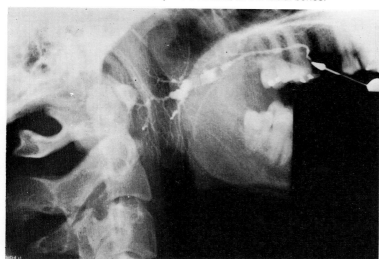

Fig. 4.5 Parotid sialogram showing a stone in the parotid duct. In this example the stone can be seen as a rounded filling defect in the duct near the point where dilatation of the duct commences. Frequently no filling defect is seen, but if a parotid duct is normal in calibre at its distal (oral) end and abruptly enlarges at some point, there must be an obstruction at that point, and in practice the obstruction nearly always proves to be a stone.

Recurrent acute, or chronic

Evidence of obstruction   No obstruction

interference from the neighbouring bones. These plain films may demonstrate a calculus. A sialogram is also done: occasionally this shows the stone as a filling defect, but more often one must diagnose a calculus from the appearance usually described by the radiologist as a 'stricture', with dilatation of the duct system proximal to the obstruction (Fig. 4.5). Again, unilateral disease may turn out to show punctate sialectasis and therefore fall into the group of Sjögren's syndrome.

Further management of unilateral disease

Patients in whom the clinical evidence suggests the stone has passed are seen at intervals for a few months, and if no further trouble occurs, are discharged. Patients in whom the clinical evidence suggests stone but radiology is negative are also observed: usually they settle down, and it may be assumed that a small stone had been passed spontaneously before the patient was seen. Patients with a stone at the parotid orifice are advised to have it removed from the mouth. A stone further back in the duct may occasionally be palpable from the cheek, and it may then be feasible to cut down to the stone through the cheek; branches of the facial nerve run very close to the duct, however, and may even twist around the duct so this is a hazardous procedure. It is probably better to consider that all stones in the parotid duct system that cannot be removed via the mouth should be treated expectantly (i.e. by waiting for them to pass spontaneously or at least reach the accessible oral orifice) unless the patient's symptoms are so severe as to justify superficial parotidectomy (see below).

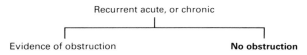

The most important consideration in this non-obstructive group is: does the patient have punctate sialectasis?

Management of patients with punctate sialectasis

Most patients with punctate sialectasis show the histological changes in the parotid characteristic of Sjögren's syndrome, whether or not any of the other possible clinical manifestations of the syndrome (p. 49) are present. These histological changes are proliferation of both the epithelial and the myoepithelial cells of the ducts — so that the latter in the end become converted into solid cords — and a small round-celled infiltration of the whole gland. Very occasionally, the underlying lesion may be a reticulosis such as lymphosarcoma, and if any suspicion of this arises confirmation of the diagnosis of Sjögren's should be sought by biopsy. It should not be necessary to biopsy the parotid gland itself: danger to the facial nerve can be obviated by biopsy of the soft palate or the oral mucosa just below the lower lip. The small unnamed salivary glands in these regions are almost

certain to show the changes of Sjögren's syndrome if that is the condition affecting the parotid.

There is no reliable treatment for Sjögren's syndrome although a minority of patients respond to corticosteroid therapy. Should the severity and frequency of attacks of ascending infection demand symptomatic relief, the safe measure is superficial parotidectomy. Radiotherapy or parotid duct ligation have been tried in this situation, but unless the gland is secreting very little saliva the former may be ineffective and the latter may produce a parotid abscess. The secretory ability of the parotid may be tested by Curry's method. A salivary stimulant is injected intravenously and the secretion from the parotid duct collected continuously for 5 minutes. The normal range of volume produced is 3–13 ml, and with a secretion rate of less than 2 ml/5 minutes it might be safe to tie the duct. It must be emphasized that the surgeon who advises duct ligation should be prepared to perform a very difficult parotidectomy if a parotid abscess ensues.

Management of patients with bilateral disease without punctate sialectasis

The only other method of investigation available is biopsy of the lower pole of the parotid gland itself. Occasionally, this procedure yields a diagnosis of sarcoidosis, which usually responds to steroids. The remainder form an unsolved problem which can only be treated symptomatically and reinvestigated at intervals. It should be stressed, however, that this residual group forms a very small proportion of patients presenting with recurrent acute, or chronic parotitis.

A cautionary note

Occasionally, the parotid is visibly enlarged, but it remains no firmer than its surroundings. In the author's experience this picture is always due to fatty infiltration of the gland and is of no serious significance. Histopathologists refer to this condition as *sialosis*, but *benign lipomatous pseudohypertrophy* is more descriptive.

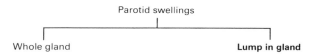

Lump in the parotid region

The most important fact to remember about this situation is that every lump in the parotid region must be considered to represent a potentially dangerous disease, and referred for surgical opinion. This statement applies even if the swelling has been present for years without altering in size, even if it is symptomless, even if the patient says he thinks it is getting smaller, and even if the practitioner elicits physical signs that lead him to believe the lump is in the skin overlying the parotid region rather than in the parotid gland itself. The reasons for this strict injunction will become clear as this section proceeds.

Within the limits of the previous paragraph, however, there is still scope for clinical acumen on the part of the practitioner. The chief points he should consider, because these are the chief points on which the surgeon will concentrate, are: is the lump inflammatory and, if so, is fluctuation present or imminent? is the lump growing very rapidly or has there been a recent increase in the rate of growth? is the lump painful? is it attached to bone? and, finally, is there any weakness of the facial nerve? Depending upon the answers to these questions, he can decide whether the patient should be referred immediately to the casualty department, or to the out-patient clinic as either an urgent or routine referral. If the lump is inflammatory and pointing or threatening to point, the patient should be seen immediately in the casualty department. The presence of any other features mentioned suggests malignancy, and an urgent out-patient appointment should be made. All other cases of lump in the parotid region may reasonably be left to take their place in the queue for a routine out-patient consultation.

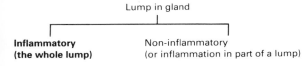

Inflammatory lumps

It is uncommon for a lump in the parotid region to present with the symptoms and signs of inflamma-tion. When this does happen, the most likely diagnosis is that the lesion is basically arising in the skin overlying the parotid (e.g. a sebaceous cyst) and has become inflamed. When the casualty surgical officer sees such a lesion and it appears to require incision and drainage, provided that he is certain of its origin from the skin he should proceed immediately to evacuate the pus. In all other cases, it is probably wiser for him to refer the patient for an immediate surgical opinion.

Inflammatory parotid lumps not arising in the skin can pose difficult surgical problems. For example, the underlying lesion may be a neoplasm undergoing an inflammatory degeneration (this is more likely to happen with benign adenolympho-ma rather than with more malignant lesions), or a stone in the parotid duct. In any case, if a deep abscess needs to be incised, there is always a risk to the facial nerve. Thus if the surgeon decides that the inflammatory area is only part of the lump, he will handle the case as one of a lump requiring urgent *excision* with a wide margin (see next section), rather than one requiring *incision* and drainage. Similarly, to exclude the possibility of an underlying calculus, plain x-rays and sialography should be undertaken as previously detailed. An abscess with a stone lying within it can be evacuated with reasonable safety by incision from the cheek (or orally if it seems to be pointing into the mouth), and the resulting salivary fistula will close spontaneously provided that the surgeon makes sure that there is no distal obstruction.

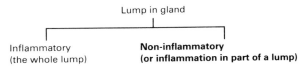

Non-inflammatory lumps

These form the vast preponderance of lumps in the parotid region. Lumps arising in the skin (usually sebaceous cysts) are treated on their merits. For the rest, rarely, they may have *distinctive clinical features* which allow an exact clinical diagnosis to

Flow-chart 4.1

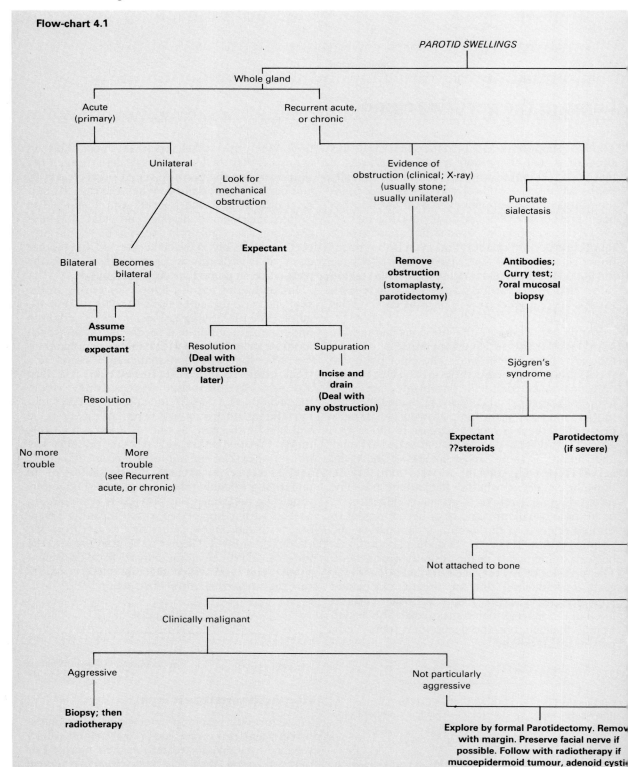

PAROTID SWELLINGS

Whole gland

Acute (primary)

Recurrent acute, or chronic

Unilateral

Look for mechanical obstruction

Evidence of obstruction (clinical; X-ray) (usually stone; usually unilateral)

Punctate sialectasis

Bilateral

Becomes bilateral

Expectant

Remove obstruction (stomaplasty, parotidectomy)

Antibodies; Curry test; ?oral mucosal biopsy

Assume mumps: expectant

Resolution **(Deal with any obstruction later)**

Suppuration

Sjögren's syndrome

Incise and drain (Deal with any obstruction)

Resolution

Expectant ??steroids

Parotidectomy (if severe)

No more trouble

More trouble (see Recurrent acute, or chronic)

Not attached to bone

Clinically malignant

Aggressive

Not particularly aggressive

Biopsy; then radiotherapy

Explore by formal Parotidectomy. Remov with margin. Preserve facial nerve if possible. Follow with radiotherapy if mucoepidermoid tumour, adenoid cysti carcinoma or frank carcinoma

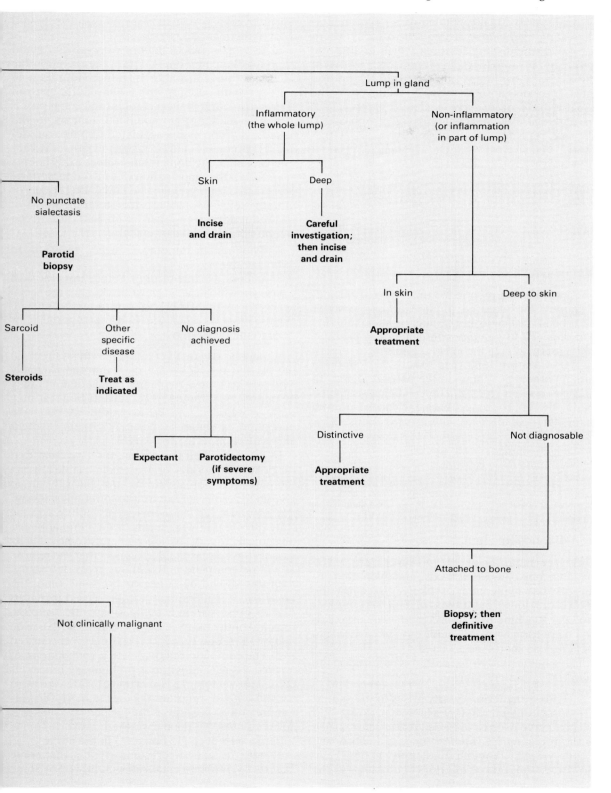

be made; occasionally, the features mentioned as *suggesting malignancy* are present; usually, there are no distinguishing features which enable the nature of the lump to be diagnosed. The fact that in the case of most lumps in the parotid region, the most exact diagnosis that can be achieved by the usual clinical procedures is simply 'lump in the parotid region' cannot be too strongly emphasized. We shall return to this point shortly.

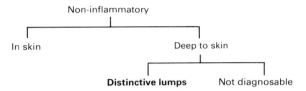

Distinctive lumps

These rarities are mentioned only to be dismissed. Examples encountered in the author's practice have been a calculus in the duct, a haemangioma that changed in volume with changes in posture, and hypertrophy of the masseter muscle, a physiological variation that can easily be confused with a pathological lump in the parotid region. In such cases when an exact clinical diagnosis can be made, the appropriate treatment can be offered immediately or after relevant investigations.

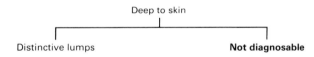

Non-diagnosable lumps

The large majority of parotid lumps cannot be diagnosed by clinical methods, and even the conclusion that malignancy is likely, based on the criteria previously mentioned of pain, recent rapid growth, attachment to bone, and facial nerve palsy, do not form a reliable guide as to what management regime should be adopted.

The scheme used by the author is based upon the following considerations:

1. Unless the lesion clearly arises in the skin, it is impossible to tell whether a lump is in the parotid salivary gland itself or in associated structures such as the investing fat (lipoma) or fascia (fibroma), blood vessels (angioma), lymph nodes, etc. However, about three-quarters of all lumps in the parotid region arise in the salivary gland itself, and most of them are neoplastic.

2. In most series of patient with salivary gland tumours, the commonest type is the pleomorphic adenoma ('mixed tumour'), so that more than 50 per cent of all patients with a lump in the parotid region turn out to have a pleomorphic adenoma.

3. The pleomorphic adenoma appears to the naked eye to be an encapsulated tumour, but detailed histological studies have shown that the capsule is usually incomplete and direct experiments have shown that enucleation of a mixed tumour by blunt dissection may leave behind scattered foci of tumour cells. Moreover, this tumour shows a marked tendency to recur by implantation in the wound if it is biopsied or inadequately excised.

4. The mixed tumour is highly resistant to radiotherapy.

5. Unless a parotid lump bulges into the soft palate (in which case it must be deep to the facial nerve), it is impossible to determine by clinical examination whether the lump is superficial or deep to the facial nerve.

It must be stressed yet again that most lumps in the parotid region cannot be diagnosed clinically with any accuracy. A pleomorphic adenoma may be as soft as a lipoma or as hard as bone; it may grow as rapidly, and be as painful as the most malignant carcinoma, or it may remain indolent and symptomless for 50 years.

In the light of all these facts, it seems clear that the policy one adopts for an undiagnosable lump in the parotid region should be one that is likely to give good results at least for the commonest lesion, the pleomorphic adenoma. The policy can be stated in the following terms: if the lump appears, on clinical grounds, to be completely removable by surgery with a reasonable prospect that the removal will be complete and without gross deformity, then this should be done. At the same time, the facial nerve is identified, and preserved provided that its preservation is compatible with complete removal of the lump — i.e. its removal with a wide margin of tissue that looks normal to the naked eye. The complete removal with a wide margin of normal tissue, and without preliminary biopsy, is consistent with item 3 above and obviates the need for subsequent radiotherapy (see item 4); the preliminary identification of the facial nerve makes it easier to preserve the nerve whether the tumour is superficial or deep (15 per cent) to the nerve.

It must be added for completeness that some experts recommend enucleation followed by some form of radiotherapy, but such a policy is not recommended by the author because it appears to be inconsistent with points 3, 4 and 5 above, and also with the consideration that about 10 per cent of lumps without clinical features suggestive of malignancy turn out to be malignant.

When an operation is undertaken to remove a lump in the parotid region, the facial nerve trunk is exposed and the superficial part of the parotid dissected forwards off the nerve and its branches. If the tumour is superficial to the nerve, its removal is thus accomplished as a *superficial parotidectomy*; however, if the tumour is deep to the nerve, the latter is raised off the deep parotid after superficial parotidectomy and the deep part excised with the tumour — *total parotidectomy*. In either case, if the whole facial nerve and its branches are preserved, the operation is called *conservative;* if one or more branches has to be excised in order to maintain an adequate margin around the tumour, the operation is *semi-conservative;* while if the whole nerve has to be sacrificed, the operation is *radical.*

This policy may require modification. Thus, if the tumour is fixed to bone, any operation to remove the tumour with a wide margin is very deforming and should be preceded by biopsy to clinch the diagnosis of malignancy: it would be disconcerting to do a massive resection of maxilla and mandible with the parotid, only to find that the mass was caused by actinomycosis. Again, if the tumour is growing very rapidly, an immediate attempt at surgical removal probably does more harm than good, and so biopsy followed by radiotherapy, and possibly later by surgery, is the treatment of choice. It is probably not necessary to modify the routine policy, however, for pain or facial nerve involvement.

In all patients, after removal of the tumour with what appeared to be an adequate margin, the histological report may further modify treatment. If the tumour is more malignant than a pleomorphic adenoma or acinic cell tumour — i.e. if it is a mucoepidermoid carcinoma, adenoid cystic carcinoma, or frank carcinoma — then if excision appeared to be complete, radiotherapy is advised, while if the excision appeared to be incomplete an immediate radical parotidectomy should be performed and followed up with radiotherapy.

Lump in the parotid region: an urgent situation

Finally, we revert to a point made earlier in this Chapter. It is most important that any patient with a lump in the parotid region should be *immediately* referred for an expert opinion. This advice is based upon the following facts:

1. The prognosis following the correct treatment of a pleomorphic adenoma of the parotid is excellent.
2. The prognosis following all treatment for a carcinoma of the parotid is very poor: the 5-year survival rate reported in recent series is less than 20 per cent.
3. About one-tenth of all parotid lumps that appear on clinical grounds to be benign are in fact malignant.
4. The common pleomorphic adenoma shows a tendency towards malignant change which increases with the passage of time.
5. In no less than 50 per cent of patients with carcinoma of the parotid, careful histological examination provides evidence that the tumour started as a more benign lesion such as a pleomorphic adenoma.

Parotid surgery has been dominated for too long by fear of damage to the facial nerve. It is particularly noteworthy that the incidence of carcinoma of the parotid, a highly malignant condition notoriously difficult to cure, might be halved if general practitioners adopted the policy of immediate referral of lumps in the parotid region.

Further reading

Conley, J. (1975). *Salivary Glands and the Facial Nerve*. Stuttgart, George Thieme.

Corcoran, M. O., Cook, H. P., Hobsley, M. (1983). Radical surgery following radiotherapy for advanced parotid carcinoma. *British Journal of Surgery* **70,** 261–3.

Hobsley, M. (1973). Salivary tumours. *British Journal of Hospital Medicine* **10,** 553–62.

Patey, D. H. (1971). Recurrent swelling of the parotid gland (recurrent parotitis). In: *Modern Trends in Surgery* **3.** Ed. by W. T. Irvine. London and Boston, Mass., Butterworths.

Thackray, A. C. and Lucas, R. B. (1974). Tumours of the Major Salivary Glands. *Atlas of Tumour Pathology,* Second Series, Fascicle 10. Washington DC, Armed Forces Institute of Pathology.

Watkin, G. T., MacLennan, K. A., Hobsley, M. (1984). Lymphomas presenting as lumps in the parotid region. *British Journal of Surgery* **71,** 701–2.

Chapter 5

The Patient Complains of a Lump in the Breast

The initial decision

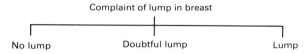

The exact wording of the title of this chapter has been chosen to emphasize that one decision must be made by the patient's medical attendant before he can start consideration of the management of the lump, and that is: does the doctor agree that the patient has a lump in the breast?

Frequently there is no lump. Women are taught by public propaganda to palpate their own breasts in order to achieve an earlier diagnosis of malignant disease, but it is difficult to palpate one's own breast accurately. The female breast consists of soft adipose and glandular tissue arranged between fibrous tissue septa, so that the examining finger prodded into the surface of the breast senses a localized area of resistance which may easily be misconstrued as a lump. For this reason, medical

students are always recommended to examine the breast *with the hand flat,* so that the fingers are not dug in; but it is difficult to educate the public up to this level.

(In passing, it is interesting how many junior medical students seem to think that the palpation should be done with the *flat of the hand.* The palm is of course poorly supplied with tactile sense organs, and many breast lumps would be missed by an examiner who used his palms only.)

So the doctor decides whether he confirms the presence of a lump in the breast, whether he refutes the possibility, or whether he is uncertain whether or not there is a lump. In most cases the practitioner will refer the patient to a surgeon, even if he is sure that there is no lump, because patients demand a specialist opinion in a situation they know might mean cancer.

The rest of this chapter takes the viewpoint of a surgeon in an out-patient clinic.

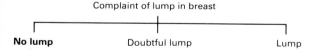

No lump

The management of this situation is deceptively simple: reassurance and discharge. The trouble lies in the severe anxiety to which the patient may have been prey. She wants nothing more than to believe the surgeon, but if after reassurance she still fears that she has cancer she will simply go to another surgeon, and another, until someone is

found to pronounce that an area in the breast is 'doubtful' and should be biopsied. Therefore, reassurance must be very strong, and the most important element in this reassurance is a realization by the patient that the surgeon's examination was very thorough. Time must be taken, and concentration demonstrated.

When the surgeon is absolutely certain that there is no lump in the breast, his reassurance must be complete and whole-hearted. A common mistake is to tell the patient something like this: 'There is nothing to worry about. This area in your breast is the seat of chronic mastitis (or fibroadenosis or benign mammary dysplasia) but there is no cancer.' The patient's attitude to a pronouncement of this sort is: 'So there is *some* disease there. How can he possibly know that it is not cancer?' It is better for the doctor to say: 'You have healthy, normal breasts. You have confused the natural granularity — lumpiness — of normal breast tissue with an actual lump, but your breasts are healthy and normal.'

Two situations now arise: either the patient clearly accepts the reassurance and departs rejoicing, or she does not accept the reassurance and is plainly going to seek another opinion. In the latter circumstance, it is reasonable to say: 'However, I can see that you are still worried about this, so I shall send you for a special investigation of the breast.'

Frankly, one is in this case using the mammogram or ultrasonogram as a placebo. A full consideration of the role of mammography is outside the scope of this book, but it should not be used indis-

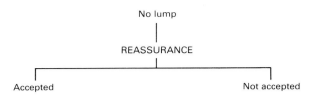

criminately because, at least by most techniques, it exposes the patient to an appreciable dose of x-rays. However, it is more accurate than ultrasound for the breasts of middle-aged and elderly women. On the other hand, ultrasound is safe even when used repeatedly, and very good for examining the dense breasts of young women, but not so useful in older women. In the present circumstances, a negative investigation and its report can be shown to the patient who will usually accept this powerful form of reassurance; if she does not, the problem lies in the patient's mind and she should be referred back to her general practitioner with the comment that the problem is not surgical.

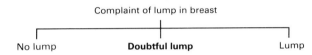

Doubtful lump

This circumstance occurs relatively frequently. There is a wide spectrum in the degree of lumpiness of normal breast tissue, and areas where the irregularity of texture is extreme can be, on first examination, impossible to differentiate clearly from a true dominant swelling. Since the lumpiness of breast tissue seems to depend on the phase of the menstrual cycle, usually being worst during the premenstrual phase of water retention, it is reasonable to ask the patient to return for repeated

examination in 2 weeks' time, i.e. at the opposite phase of her menstrual cycle. Some doctors prescribe an oral diuretic during this fortnight (e.g. frusemide) and some ask for a mammogram or ultrasonogram. Should doubt persist at the time of the second examination, biopsy is indicated and the patient's name should be put on the urgent waiting list for admission. If no doubt persists, the patient falls into the category of 'no lump' (see above) or 'lump confirmed' (see below).

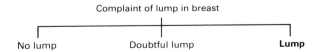

Lump confirmed

There are three pitfalls that need remembering when confirming the presence of a lump in the breast. Firstly, a lump originating in the chest wall

underlying the breast may be mistaken for a lump within the breast, yet it probably requires quite a different line of management. Secondly, the same error may arise with a lump originating in the skin overlying the breast. Thirdly, an error in the opposite sense may arise with a lump originating in *accessory* breast tissue anywhere in the nipple lines that run from axillae through breasts to the groins: the essentially mammary nature of the parent tissue governs the management of such a lesion.

Apart from such problems, the main decision which must be made is whether or not the lump presents the symptoms or signs of acute inflammation. For this purpose, those swellings which present signs and symptoms suggestive of all degrees of activity of chronic inflammation are classified as not presenting with acute inflammation.

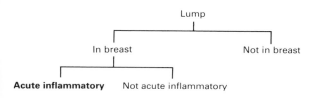

Symptoms and signs of acute inflammation

In general (the major exception is described below), a patient presenting with symptoms and signs of acute inflammation in the breast must be diagnosed as having a breast abscess, and treated accordingly by incision and drainage. Evidence of fluctuation should not be awaited, because usually by the time a focus of inflammation deep within the breast produces reddening and heat of the overlying skin, pus is already present. However, ultrasound can be useful for demonstrating that pus has formed within an inflammatory mass. There is a place for trial of conservative treatment (i.e. antibiotics) in patients in whom the history of pain is very short and the zone of induration does not seem to extend deeply into the breast substance. It must be emphasized that the trial with antibiotics should not be prolonged: a failure to produce a definite response within 48 hours should lead to a decision to operate.

When incision is decided upon, whether or not the patient is admitted depends on several circumstances. In the Western world, most patients with breast abscess are pregnant or in the post-puerperal period. Whether facilities exist for the admission of a baby may decide whether the mother should be admitted. Most patients in the UK are admitted. In developing countries, breast abscess is quite common at times remote from

pregnancy: the reason for this difference is unknown. How good the facilities are for nursing at home, performance of dressings, etc., may decide whether or not the patient should be admitted.

The exception to the general role that inflammatory swellings should be explored is the fairly uncommon condition variously called 'plasma cell mastitis' and 'duct stagnation'. During the decade leading up to the menopause, hormonally induced changes in the breast may result in blocking of the ducts with damming back of inspissated secretions. These changes give rise to an increase in the granularity (lumpiness) of the breast, but if focally accentuated may result in a definite lump. This cannot be distinguished from any other non-inflammatory lump in the breast and will be treated appropriately. Should the pressure within the obstructed ducts rupture the ducts, the extravasation of the duct contents provokes a foreign-body inflammatory response with plasma cells prominent in histological preparations. The clinical picture produced is of an acute inflammatory mass *at the margin of the areola*, triangular in shape with its base extending outwards into the breast, in a woman aged 35–50 years. This picture is sufficiently typical to allow an expectant policy to be adopted. If the provisional diagnosis of plasma cell mastitis is correct, the condition settles down without any definitive treatment within 48 hours. Should it not settle, the mass should be explored.

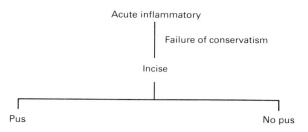

Exploration of acute inflammatory swellings

In most cases, an incision into the swelling demonstrates pus and the operation is completed by ensuring that drainage is adequate by breaking down all loculi to produce a single cavity. Further treatment is as for an abscess anywhere: a specimen of the pus is examined bacteriologically and bacterial sensitivities to various antibodies determined, but in patients without signs of constitutional disturbance (headache, rigors), antibiotics will not be necessary. Dressings are designed to absorb discharge, to prevent secondary infection from outside, and to prevent healing of the skin before the cavity is obliterated by granulation tissue. In some lactating patients it is probably wise to suppress lactation by binding the breasts, although most surgeons arrange for manual expression of the affected breast so that feeding can continue from the opposite breast.

In a few cases, no pus is found. The possible reasons are that the process is basically infective but that pus has not yet formed (unlikely), that it is basically inflammatory but non-pyogenic (plasma cell mastitis, tuberculosis, etc.), or that it is neoplastic. Biopsy with histological and bacteriological examination of the excised tissue is the key to subsequent management; small masses can be excised completely to provide the biopsy. The definitive treatment of carcinoma of the breast is controversial (see Chapter 7), but a very rapidly advancing carcinoma provoking so much host-reaction as to appear inflammatory, does not do well with ablative surgery and is treated with radiotherapy in the first instance.

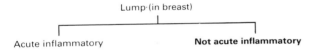

No acute inflammation

In this situation, patients may be divided into one of four categories: gynaecomastia; cyst; fibroadenoma; and all other lumps. The dominant consideration is that all non-inflammatory lumps in the breast should be assumed to be carcinoma unless proved otherwise.

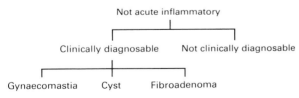

However, *gynaecomastia* presents such a typical clinical picture that a confident clinical diagnosis can be made and accepted as a basis for management. The condition occurs only in the male or the prepubertal female breast, i.e. in breasts in which neoplastic disease is rare. The complaint is that there is a tender swelling deep to the nipple and areola, and on examination the affected breast is more prominent than the contralateral, due to the presence of a firm, tender, discoid mass just larger in diameter than the areola and concentric with the nipple and areola. The mass is the hypertrophied breast tissue, and even in an adult male breast is only about 5 cm in diameter.

Most often, gynaecomastia occurs in infants and at puberty. When it occurs at any other age, a reason for endocrine abnormality should be sought — testicular neoplasms, liver diseases, etc. — and any such cause treated. A common cause is stilboestrol, taken by the patient to control carcinoma of the prostate, but that apart, endocrine abnormalities are rarely found, and the only treatment indicated is reassurance that the condition is not serious and will subside in days or weeks.

A *cyst* can be diagnosed clinically with a fair degree of confidence. Some cysts are fluctuant, but this sign is not essential to the diagnosis because it cannot be elicited from cysts deep in the breast

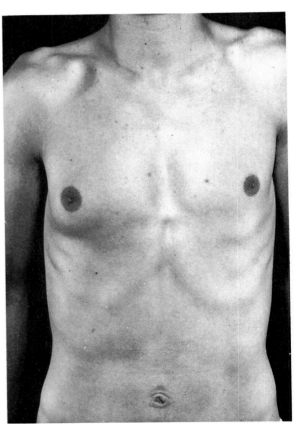

Fig. 5.1   Gynaecomastia in a man aged 22 years. The enlargement of the right breast and enlargement plus deepened pigmentation of the right nipple and areola lasted for about 6 months and then regressed spontaneously. (Photograph by courtesy of Mr David Ralphs)

substance, or those that resist deformation by the examining finger because they contain liquid under considerable pressure, or because their walls are rigid. *The* sign of a cyst is that it is spherical: since pressure in a liquid is transmitted equally in all directions and the breast tissue is homogeneously soft compared with the cyst, the latter as it enlarges must adopt a spherical configuration (p. 10).

A cyst should be treated by aspirating its contents via a syringe and needle in the out-patient clinic at the time of first presentation to the surgeon. The cyst is emptied as completely as possible. Provided that after aspiration the lump completely disappears, *and* that the fluid obtained was typical cyst fluid looking clear and brown by transmitted light or opaque and blue-green-brown by reflected light, and that it does not contain blood, the patient may be reassured that the condition is non-malignant, and discharged. Some surgeons send the cyst liquid for cytological examination for malignant cells but this investigation rarely yields a positive result if the above criteria have been met. If the criteria are not met, the patient should be admitted via the *urgent* waiting list with a working diagnosis of carcinoma.

There are a few protagonists of excision biopsy for breast cysts: they emphasize the undoubted possibility that there is a carcinoma in the wall of the cyst. Protagonists of aspiraton point out that cysts are frequently multiple so that the policy of excision biopsy may result in a series of unsightly scars, and that only a cyst wall carcinoma too small

to be itself palpable will be missed by those who perform aspiration and stick to the rules given in the previous paragraph: this must be a rare occurrence, especially as the overall incidence of carcinoma in the cyst wall is less than 1 per cent. The author subscribes to the school of aspiraton. It is important to remember, however, that simple breast cyst is a safe diagnosis only in the age group from 35 years of age to about 5 years after the menopause, and that rapid recurrence of a cyst in an *identical* position suggests that there is some local cause such as a tumour and demands biopsy.

A *fibroadenoma* can also be diagnosed clinically with a fair degree of accuracy. Traditionally the fibroadenoma is described as a *firm*, almost hard, lump which is particularly *mobile* within the tissues of the breast. About the consistency there is no doubt, but this feature cannot distinguish a fibroadenoma from many other lesions. The mobility is commonly present, but not always — in the early stages of formation of a fibroadenoma it is often not well demarcated from the surrounding breast tissue. Much more typical of a fibroadenoma is the fact that its surface, although smooth in general, nearly always presents in at least one region a linear depression. Such a depression is the groove between two lobulations of what is essentially a *lobulated* swelling. A smooth, firm or hard, lobulated swelling is almost certainly a fibroadenoma. The diagnosis must be confirmed by excision biopsy — under no circumstances can the patient be assured that the lump is definitely benign on a

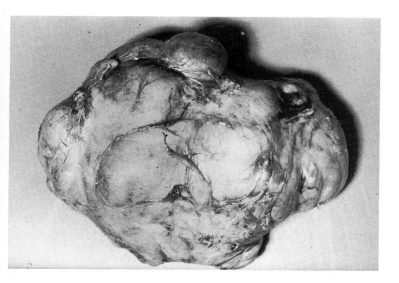

Fig. 5.2 Fibroadenoma of the breast. This is an example of the rather unusual 'giant' variety, measuring 10 cm across. Its surface shows the typical lobulated appearance which, when palpated in a clinical lesion, allows a confident diagnosis of fibroadenoma to be made. (Specimen in the collection of the Bland Sutton Institute of Pathology)

clinical diagnosis only, even if the patient is in the typical age group for the small fibroadenoma (15–25 years). However, the *routine* waiting list would be appropriate for the patient of this age. If the routine waiting list is longer than 6 months, a needle biopsy or aspiration cytology may give confirmation of the clinical diagnosis with reassurance to both patient and surgeon, but it is particularly common in this group for cytology to give equivocal or false positive results. If the patient is older but still menstruating, the diagnosis of fibroadenoma is still possible but the lesions tend to be larger and softer than in the younger age group: usually it is wiser to admit the patient from the *urgent* waiting list. After all, there *is* a fibrosarcoma of the breast (Brodie's tumour) that occurs as a rapidly growing lobulated mass in this age group.

All other lumps in the breast must be assumed to be carcinomatous. Many surgeons perform a needle biopsy or aspiration cytology of the lump in the out-patient clinic, but in any case the patient is admitted urgently.

One should be specially reluctant to diagnose a lipoma in the breast of a woman aged over 70 years, because the atrophic scirrhous carcinoma which occurs in that age group may be as soft as a lipoma. It will be noticed that no mention has been made of whether there are any physical signs present of malignancy — pathological adherence to skin or pectoralis major, peau d'orange, axillary lymph nodes, etc. The reasons are that other lesions (e.g. fat necrosis) may mimic carcinoma and, particularly, that the absence of such signs cannot be taken to indicate that the lesion is benign. The safe rule is that all lumps in the breast which lack symptoms and signs of acute inflammation, and which cannot be confidently diagnosed on clinical grounds as gynaecomastia or a fibroadenoma or proved by aspiration to be a simple cyst, should be admitted *urgently* for a biopsy. After the menopause, very nearly all lumps in the breast are carcinomatous.

Admission for biopsy

If an out-patient needle biopsy or aspiration cytology was positive, treatment can be started as soon as the patient is admitted. In the absence of such evidence, or if the out-patient investigation failed to confirm carcinoma, a biopsy or an excision biopsy is performed — i.e. a small piece of, or the whole lump, is excised. Which is performed depends on the size of the lump and the availability of facilities for an immediate histological examination of the excised tissue, together with the surgeon's opinion of the most likely diagnosis. It is an important principle that if the lump is benign, it should be completely removed at a single operation. There is no point in telling a woman that a piece removed from the lump was benign and therefore she has been left with the rest of the lump. No woman wants a lump in her breast, no matter how innocent, and in any case the question will soon occur to her — even if it does not occur to her surgeon — that the histology of that part of the lump which has been removed may not be identical with the histology of the residue. It follows that, where an immediate histological report is available, the whole lump must be removed. The availability of an immediate histological report permits the surgeon to perform a sample biopsy on a large, probably carcinomatous, lesion, and often such a biopsy is better on technical grounds (i.e.

with regard to any subsequent mastectomy) than an excision biopsy.

Provided the duration of the delay between biopsy or excision biopsy and the performance of any definitive surgical treatment (i.e. some form of mastectomy) is not too great, the available evidence suggests that preliminary biopsy does not worsen the prognosis. Most surgeons feel that 48–72 hours is acceptable, but one should certainly try to prevent the delay exceeding that limit. It follows that, except in the patient with a clinically typical fibroadenoma, all examinations and investigations which might have had a bearing on the definitive treatment should be completed before the biopsy. The most important procedures are those which decide fitness for major surgery and which attempt to establish whether secondary deposits are present. The routine preparation for biopsy therefore includes a careful general physical examination including abdominal and rectal and neurological examination, a haemoglobin estimation and a white blood count (both to establish fitness for withstanding blood loss and to exclude the leucoerythroblastic anaemia of bone secondaries), and a chest x-ray (both to establish general fitness and to exclude metastases in ribs and thoracic spine). How far one goes in the matter of trying to spot secondaries is a matter for the individual

Flow-chart 5.1

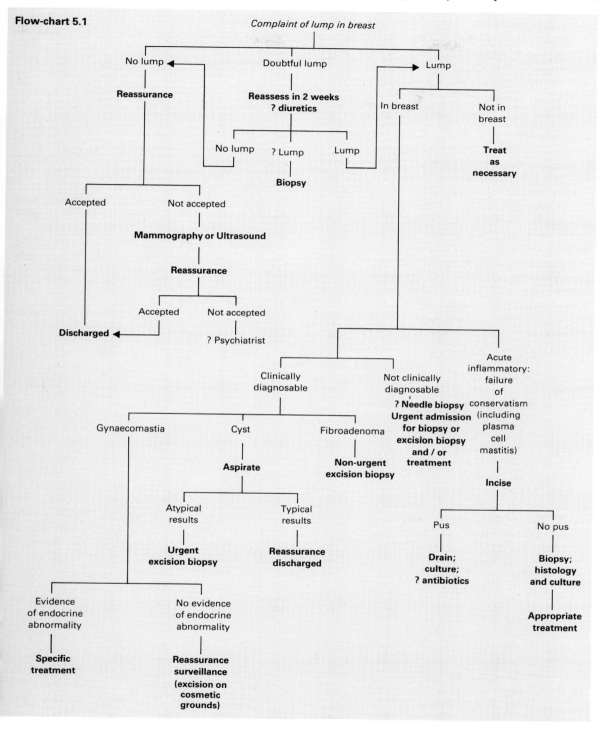

surgeon's choice: the possibilities are an x-ray survey of the whole skeleton, an x-ray mammogram or ultrasonogram of the *opposite* breast, and a scintigram of the whole skeleton. The more complete the survey before biopsy, the less likely any delay in instituting definitive treatment after a positive report of carcinoma on the biopsy specimen is received. The management of carcinoma of the breast is considered separately in Chapter 7.

Further reading

Evans, K. T. and Gravelle, I. H. (1973). *Mammography, Thermography and Ultrasonography in Breast Disease.* London and Boston, Mass., Butterworths.

Haagensen, C. D. (1971). *Diseases of the Breast,* 2nd edn. Philadelphia and Eastbourne, W. B. Saunders.

Hadfield, G. J. (1976). Benign diseases of the breast. In: *Current Surgical Practice,* Vol 1, pp 250–61. Ed. by G. J. Hadfield and M. Hobsley. London, Edward Arnold.

Patey, D. H. and Nurick, A. W. (1953). Natural history of cystic disease of breast treated conservatively. *British Medical Journal* **1,** 15–17.

Rosemond, G. P. (1963). Differentiation between cystic and solid breast mass by needle aspiration. *Surgical Clinics of North America* **43,** 1433–7.

Smallwood, J., Herbert, A., Guyer, P. and Taylor, J. (1985). Accuracy of aspiration cytology in the diagnosis of breast disease. *British Journal of Surgery* **72,** 841–3.

Chapter 6

Discharge from the Nipple

Physiology

Quite apart from the period of lactation, the adult female breast secretes a small quantity of fluid at all times. This fluid passes along the lactiferous ducts to the nipple, and there it emerges on to the surface epithelium to be removed by evaporation and by contact with clothes, or to be washed off in the bath. In normal circumstances a woman is unaware of this secretion. Occasionally, however, the amount of secretion may increase for reasons which basically we do not understand, but are presumably linked with endocrine activity. In such cases the woman will notice a variable amount of moisture appearing at one or both nipples, and she may complain of this phenomenon.

Since this is a physiological phenomenon, it is perfectly safe for the practitioner to reassure his patient that such a discharge is of no serious significance. However, before he does this he must make quite certain that the discharge cannot represent a pathological process within the breast. The twin keys to making a decision about this problem are the nature of the liquid and its site of origin.

Findings on examination

Nature of discharge

To qualify as being possibly physiological in nature, the liquid discharging from the nipple must be clear, colourless or slightly yellow in colour, homogeneous and only slightly sticky in consistency, or else white (i.e., milk). It should be noted that the fact that a discharge can be described in this way does not prove that it is physiological in origin. The converse is certainly true, however, that a discharge which does not fit this description must be assumed to be pathological.

The most important abnormalities of the discharge are staining with frank blood or with a dark colour which suggests altered blood, and turbidity which may amount to particulate matter of a green or blue colour mingled with the liquid.

Exact location

It is of crucial importance to decide whether the discharge arises in all the ducts of the breast or breasts, or whether it is originating in a single duct. It is no exaggeration to say that this is the single most important question that must be answered.

This necessity must be kept clearly in mind by the practitioner, and he should modify his history and his examination so as to take it into account. When a woman is giving a history of having noticed a discharge from the nipple, she very frequently and quite unconsciously gives her breast a squeeze if she has been in the habit of doing this to demonstrate the discharge to herself. She should be warned against doing this. Later, when it comes to the examination, by all means ask her to point to the offending nipple, and even to the area of the nipple if she can localize the discharge to a particular area, but again she should be warned not to touch the breasts at this stage.

For the same reasons, the examination of the breasts starts in the usual way with inspection but does not proceed to the ordinary palpation of the breasts in the search for a lump. Instead, the patient is asked to lie back in a comfortable position, a fine paper tissue is used to wipe away any crusting from each nipple, and then the practitioner presses his index finger on to a single spot at the periphery of the areola just at the commencement of the breast tissue itself. If this pressure produces a bead of discharge at the nipple, the position at which the liquid emerged on to the surface of the nipple is carefully noted, and also the character of this liquid.

Any discharge produced is then wiped carefully away with the tissue, although some authorities advise that it should be collected carefully and sent for clinical detection of haemoglobin, and possibly also for cytological examination. The author has not found these special investigations of help in his own practice although cytological examination is becoming more popular.

Whether or not the manoeuvre produced any discharge, it is now repeated at a neighbouring point around the circumference of the areola, and so on until pressure has been brought to bear at localized points entirely around the margin of the areola. The observer is then in a position to categorize the complaint as a diffuse or a localized nipple discharge.

It often happens that there is only a small quantity of liquid within the duct system, ready to be expressed. Accidental or uncontrolled squeezing of the breast, before the practitioner is concentrating his attention upon the site of origin of the liquid, may result in the breast being empty when he does start his careful examination, and this may prevent a proper diagnosis being made on that occasion. Any delay at this stage can only result in needless anxiety for the patient, and of course it may delay the treatment of any underlying serious disease.

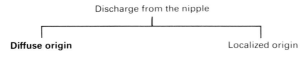

Diffuse origin

Should pressure on all or several of the points at the periphery of the areola produce discharge of the nipple, the condition producing the discharge is clearly a generalized one throughout the breast. There are only two diagnoses compatible with this finding: physiological secretion or duct stagnation.

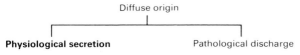

Physiological secretion is diagnosed if the generalized secretion from the breast has the characteristics of physiological secretion as previously described, and if the rest of the examination of the breast shows no abnormality such as a lump. If a confident diagnosis of physiological secretion is made, the patient may be reassured and advised to ignore the secretion. Usually a sensible patient will accept this reassurance, but should it appear that she is reluctant to do so, the practitioner would naturally request a second opinion from a specialist. In passing, it should be noted that though one might expect physiological secretion to be equally prominent in both breasts, this is by no means always so. The fact that the discharge is only from one breast does not rule out physiological secretion.

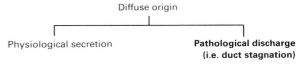

Duct stagnation is a peculiar condition which seems to be due to the hormonal changes that occur in the 5 years or so leading up to the menopause. The secretions from the breast become more viscid, either because of an alteration in the materials dissolved in the liquid or actually because of extra desquamation of cells in the lining of the acini or ducts. Either because there is an actual increase in the amount of secretion, or because there are periods when some ducts become blocked by the viscidity of the secretions and then become unblocked to release a large quantity of pent-up secretions, there is a discharge of sticky liquid containing particulate debris, and expressible from many sectors of the breast. Chronic infection may occur, and give rise to pus with an appropriate change in the colour of the discharge, while blue or green discoloration is probably related to the amount of cholesterol in the discharge. Even blood-staining may occur as a result of infection.

It should be emphasized that discharge from the nipple is not the only manifestation with which duct stagnation may present. The condition may also give rise to a lump in the breast, or to the peculiar type of segmental mastitis referred to on p. 61.

The discharge may give rise to a considerable amount of discomfort in itself, it may raise a suspicion of serious underlying disease such as a carcinoma, and the condition of duct stagnation may give rise to painful inflammation and even abscess formation with the possible production of a fistula between the affected duct and the skin near the edge of the areola, the so-called *mammillary sinus* or *fistula* (Fig. 6.1). For all these reasons, patients in whom the practitioner makes this diagnosis should be referred for a specialist opinion.

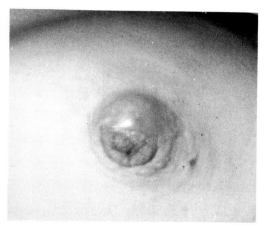

Fig. 6.1 Mammillary fistula. Note the area of inflammatory swelling in the medial half of the nipple (the upper half in this orientation). The opening of the fistula can be seen as a punctum above (to the right) of the nipple.

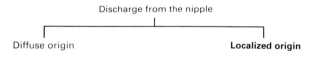

Localized origin

If localized pressure at only one place on the periphery of the areola produces discharge from the nipple, it can be confidently concluded that a single duct is blocked partially. There are only two common causes of this state: *duct papilloma* and *duct carcinoma*. The patient should therefore be referred for an urgent surgical consultation.

In these and all other cases where a surgical opinion is sought, the patient should be reminded to protect her breast against any source of pressure that might empty the breast for at least 48 hours before she sees the surgeon.

Discharge plus

Perhaps it is scarcely necessary to write this, but the demonstration of discharge from the nipple does not complete the examination of the breast. The practitioner should continue with routine palpation of the breasts, axillae, supraclavicular regions and abdomen. Should any other abnormality be found, discharge from the nipple is probably of secondary importance compared with the other condition. The management of a lump in the breast is the dominant consideration, whether or not there happens to be discharge from the nipple.

Other conditions

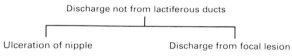

It must not be forgotten that the woman who complains of a discharge from the nipple may be wrong

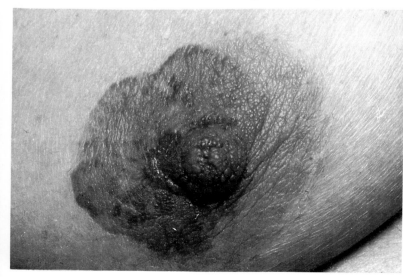

Fig. 6.2 Paget's disease of the nipple. The small area of ulceration with a surrounding region of patchy pigmentation and scaling should arouse suspicion of this lesion. There is always a duct carcinoma in the breast nearby. (Photograph by courtesy of Mr David Ralphs)

in her description. She is usually not a trained observer, and her complaint may be referable to some other condition which might reasonably be confused with a discharge from the nipple. Careful observation at the time of the examination will distinguish these conditions. The common ones are discharge from the surface of the nipple, and discharge from some focus on or near the nipple but not one of the ducts.

Ulceration of the nipple is a condition that must be taken seriously. A diagnosis of eczema was often made in these circumstances, but was usually wrong: eczema of the nipple is very rare. A specialist opinion should be sought. After minor trauma, the commonest condition in an adult is *Paget's disease of the nipple,* in which the external lesion, a slowly spreading erosion of the skin of the nipple and areola, with scaling, is associated with an underlying, often occult, duct carcinoma in the breast nearby (Fig. 6.2).

Discharging foci include the *mammillary sinus (fistula)* previously mentioned, and minor septic lesions due to trauma or infections of local sebaceous glands.

Specialist management

The history and findings are checked. On the basis of these, one or other of the following working diagnoses will be made: physiological secretion, duct stagnation, duct papilloma or duct carcinoma, ulceration of the nipple, mammillary sinus; or else minor traumatic or inflammatory lesions of the nipple which will not be further considered.

Physiological secretion

The patient is given a full explanation of the condition and strongly reassured. Should she accept this reassurance, she is discharged. Occasionally she appears still worried, and mammography or ultrasonography is then useful as a placebo.

Duct stagnation

Management requires a nice judgement. Minor degrees of the condition may respond to reassurance and treatment with hormones to reduce the hormonal lack of the menopause that is approaching in most of these patients. More severe symptoms require Haagensen's operation: through an inferior circumareolar incision, the nipple and areola are elevated and a block of the immediately subjacent tissue excised. This tissue includes the terminal broad portions of the lactiferous ducts. How the operation works is not precisely understood, but the results are good.

Duct papilloma and duct carcinoma

These are histological diagnoses, and it must be emphasized that a distinction between them is not possible on purely clinical grounds. The working diagnosis is that there is a localized obstruction in a single duct. The patient is brought into hopsital via the urgent waiting list. Once she is in hospital, no one is permitted to examine the breast except the surgeon who is to perform the operation. Later, under general anaesthesia, he identifies the orifice of the affected duct by expressing some secretion through it, passes a very fine probe (e.g. a lacrimal duct dilator) along the duct, and gets his assistant to hold the instrument rigidly in position. It is sometimes recommended that the duct should now be dissected out of the nipple and breast tissue, but the author's practice is to excise an oval of skin and the deeper tissues, making sure that the instrument is totally excised with a margin all round it. The specimen is sent for histological examination.

Most pathology services are reluctant to express an opinion as to whether the lesion is a duct papilloma or duct carcinoma on the basis of a frozen-section technique. The duct papilloma is a benign neoplasm: the lesion is a heaping up of the epithelial cells lining the duct in a localized area. In the duct carcinoma there is a similar picture, but some of the cells have taken on maligant properties and are penetrating through the wall of the duct into the stroma of the breast. The incision is closed and the patient returned to the ward. When the definitive histological report is received, a day or two later, the patient is reassured that no further treatment is necessary if the lesion was a papilloma. In about 15 per cent of cases, it turns out that the lesion was a carcinoma. Further treatment then depends on the surgeon's views on the treatment of early carcinoma of the breast (see Chapter 7).

It should be mentioned that blood-staining of the discharge from the nipple is less likely if the lesion is a papilloma rather than a carcinoma, but blood-staining is certainly not proof of malignancy.

Ulceration of the nipple

This should be assumed to be associated with an underlying duct carcinoma (Fig. 6.2) unless there is a clear history of trauma. The patient should therefore be admitted via the urgent waiting list, and the lesion biopsied. Treatment proceeds on the basis of the result of the biopsy. Occasionally, surprising diagnoses will be encountered, such as benign adenoma of the nipple, syphilis, tuberculosis, etc.

Mammillary sinus (fistula)

This is readily diagnosable on clinical grounds as a small opening, discharging pus, at or near the areolar margin. The condition is not very common, and so despite the typical appearance it is often misdiagnosed as infection in a sebaceous gland and mistreated by simple incision and drainage. The typical history is therefore of repeated attacks of inflammation, subsiding spontaneously after the discharge of an abscess or after such incisions, but recurring. The correct treatment is to excise the blocked duct that is the root cause of the fistula. A lacrimal duct dilator is passed through the skin opening, and usually can be introduced to at least some extent into the offending duct. An oval sector of nipple, areola and breast tissue is now excised to include both the sinus track and the duct from which it arises.

Some surgeons use Haagensen's operation for mammillary fistula and for duct papilloma.

Flow-chart 6.1

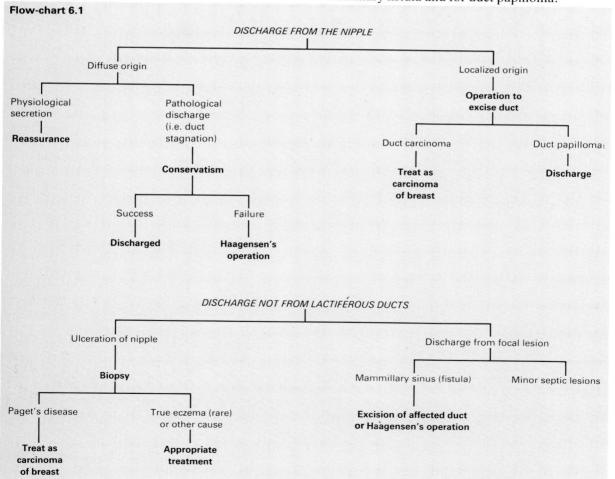

Further reading

Atkins, H. J. B. (1955). Mammillary fistula. *British Medical Journal* **2,** 1473–4.

Atkins, H. J. B. and Wolff, B. (1964). Discharges from the nipple. *British Journal of Surgery* **51,** 602–6.

Haagensen, C. D. (1971). *Diseases of the Breast.* 2nd edn. Philadelphia and Eastbourne, W. B. Saunders.

Hadfield, G. J. (1969). The pathological lesions underlying discharges from the nipple in women. *Annals of the Royal College of Surgeons of England* **44,** 323–33.

Handley, R. S. and Thackray, A. C. (1962). Adenoma of nipple. *British Journal of Cancer* **16,** 187–94.

Sandison, A. T. and Walker, J. C. (1962). Inflammatory mastitis, mammary duct ectasia and mammillary fistula. *British Journal of Surgery* **50,** 57–64.

Stokes, J. F. (1962). Unexpected gynaecomastia. *Lancet* **ii.** 911–13.

Chapter 7

Management of Carcinoma of the Breast

Philosophy

At some point a clinician makes a firm diagnosis of carcinoma of the breast, and the question then arises of how the patient should be managed in the light of this decision. Carcinoma of the breast is a very common disease with a poor prognosis, and it presents in a bewildering variety of forms and clinical situations. Moreover, the best treatment for any particular form of the disease is usually uncertain, and all forms of treatment have a high failure rate. In these circumstances, it might appear to the student that it would be impossible to develop a theme of management to which the majority of doctors would subscribe. Nevertheless, there is an underlying basis for agreement in what may be termed a philosophical approach to the nature of the problem.

The simple concept

Carcinoma of the breast starts at a single focus, possibly within a single cell, within the breast. As the malignant cells multiply, they form by accretion, the *primary* lesion. At some time during the process of formation of the primary lesion, malignant cells show a tendency to disseminate (*metastasize*) via the lymphatic channels and/or via the veins. Some of the malignant cells disseminated in this way are arrested in lymph nodes or in other tissues or organs, and multiply at those sites to produce aggregations of tumour tissue that are discontinuous with the primary lesion and are called *metastases*. Tumour cells shed by desquamation into the lumen of a hollow viscus or into a large serous cavity such as the peritoneum may remain viable and implant on a distant area of the space involved, having moved to the new site under the influence of mechanical forces such as peristalsis or pressure differentials. This form of spread is called, for example, 'transcoelomic' when it occurs across a serous cavity, and 'im-

plantation' when a hollow viscus is involved. An uncommon form of spread that bridges the gap between direct spread and discontinuous dissemination is *lymphatic permeation*: tumour cells grow as a solid cord along a lymph channel, perhaps because the next lymph gland is blocked.

Tumour versus host

A tumour cell has, at least to some extent, gained autonomy and is therefore no longer completely subject to the host's natural mechanisms for coordinating the growth of individual cells, tissues and organs. Like invading micro-organisms, tumour cells may be thought of as having an individual degree of virulence or invasiveness, while the host may be credited with an individual degree of resistance. In the case of any particular patient, the balance between these two factors of virulence and resistance varies with time, and also with the host tissue. These hypotheses are necessary to explain the continuous gradation between entirely innocent and very malignant tumours, the fact that some tumours which on histological examination look very malignant may yet progress very slowly or remain static, that tumours which have been steadily progressive for a time may very occasionally regress or even vanish, and that secondary deposits are very common in some tissues and organs but very rare in others.

Factors modifying the tumour/host relationship

Non-specific factors

While there is no proof, many experts believe that the resistance of a host to malignant disease is related to his general state of health. Unfavourable factors include a debilitating disease, a surgical operation or other severe trauma, and exposure to ionizing radiations. Such non-specific factors may act in some unexplained fashion on the host as a whole, or on a specific region of the host. An example of the latter phenomenon is the crop of metastases that may occur in a sharply demarcated area of skin which has been exposed to x-rays.

Specific factors

There is increasing evidence that, at least in certain kinds of tumour, part of the mechanism of the host's resistance is immunity. The tumour cells behave as a foreign antigen and provoke an immune response from the host. Occasionally this response is expressed by circulating antibodies, but more often in the case of human tumours the response is of the fixed type in the local lymph nodes. This mechanism is, of course, entirely specific to the tumour in question.

Endocrine factors

Tumours of organs that secrete, or are under the control of, hormones, may to a variable extent be influenced in their rate of growth by the concentration of the appropriate or related hormones. One-third of patients with human breast cancer are sensitive to the level of oestrogens in the tissues, but the effect of altering the level is only temporary.

Chemotherapy

Many chemical agents have been discovered which attack neoplastic tissue more vigorously than normal tissue. Since the difference in their destructiveness for the two types of cells is a matter of degree, they all have unpleasant and dangerous side-effects. A decision to use them needs particularly careful consideration. They may be used for a generalized effect upon the whole patient, or by infusion of a local area via the local blood vessels so as to achieve a maximum response locally with a minimum of overall toxic effects.

Rationale of treatment

Cure

Naturally one's first thought is to rid the patient of his disease, so that it no longer affects his life-span. To achieve this goal it may be necessary to inflict pain and other suffering which may be temporary

or even permanent. All doctors agree about the goal, but the dividing line between justifiable and non-justifiable suffering varies somewhat with the individual practitioner, and also with the individual patient.

There is also general agreement about how this aim should be tackled: if possible, all the diseased cells must be removed or destroyed. Local disease is most efficiently treated by local measures, such as surgical excision or radiotherapy. Widespread disease (i.e. metastases) or neoplasia affecting circulating tissues such as erythrocytes and leucocytes, require generalized modes of treatment such as immunotherapy, hormone therapy and chemotherapy.

The question arises, what if the practitioner thinks it very likely that the removal of neoplastic tissue will be incomplete? Until recent years, there was practically complete agreement on the answer to this question: as much neoplastic tissue as possible should be removed or destroyed, so that the body's defences were as strong as possible in relation to the dose of tumour cells left for them to deal with. Because of this philosophy, it has been common practice to include the regional lymph nodes, where practicable, in any surgical or radiotherapeutic attack on a primary tumour. Recently, however, the idea has been mooted that local lymph nodes have an important immunological role in attacking the primary tumour, and should be preserved even at the risk of leaving tumour cells within them. Supporters of this idea, a diminishing band, remove the primary tumour but leave the lymph nodes.

Palliation

The doctor's role, however, is not limited to cure. At some stage in the progress of the disease it may become wise to accept that, short of some rare event such as spontaneous regression, the tumour is bound to kill the patient. This is the most difficult stage for the doctor to treat. A nice judgement is required to hold in balance the treatments that are available to slow down the progress of the disease, and the ill-consequences of those treatments. The important principle that local manifestations respond best to local measures, generalized to generalized measures, holds good. It is crucial to bear in mind that when purely palliative treatment is being considered, there must be something requiring palliation. The mere presence of metastases is thus not in itself an indication for treatment. Metastases require treatment only if they threaten life or serious illness (e.g. intracranial and spinal lesions), cause symptoms, or show by their rate of progress that the patient will soon die unless that rate can be reduced.

Applications to breast carcinoma

Breast carcinoma most often presents as the primary lesion, usually as a lump in the breast but occasionally as a discharge from the nipple or in rarer forms. At the time of presentation there may be no clincal evidence of spread of the disease. Even in the absence of clinical evidence, special methods of investigation reveal that a considerable proportion of patients, possibly the majority, have deposits of disease in the local lymph nodes, or more distant blood-borne deposits, or both. Local lymph node deposits are more common than the more remote lesions, and the axillary lymph nodes are involved more often than the internal mammary glands. In patients with extensive axillary involvement, extension of the disease to the supraclavicular lymph nodes can sometimes be demonstrated. Any tissue or organ in the body can be the site of metastases, but the common sites of early metastatic involvement are the marrow cavity of the bones, the lungs and the liver.

The most important decision in management is where to draw the line between the curative and the palliative situation. There is general agreement that, apart from any improvements which may result from the exploration of recent advances in chemotherapy, patients with lymphatic deposits in the internal mammary and supraclavicular regions are very likely to have succumbed to their disease within 5 years, and the same applies to patients with deposits in any site more remote than the regional lymph nodes. The axillary lymph nodes occupy borderline territory. Patients who undergo radical mastectomy — which may be defined as the removal of the breast together with the axillary lymph nodes in a single block of tissue — fall into two different prognostic groups according to whether or not histological examination of the axillary glands demonstrates tumour cells. If there are no deposits, the 5-year survival rate approximates to 80 per cent; if there are deposits, to 45 per cent. There is even some evidence that the height in the axilla to which the disease has progressed has a demonstrable effect on the prognosis. The significance of the highest axillary gland being invaded seems to be much the same as invasion of the supraclavicular glands.

The possible ways of dealing with the primary lesion are surgical excision and local radiotherapy. There are controlled series that suggest that wide local removal of the tumour combined with radiotherapy is as effective as removal of the whole breast. The exception to this statement is that cases in which the primary is progressing rapidly (e.g. carcinomatous mastitis) are often aggravated by surgery, and are therefore better treated by radiotherapy, at least in the first instance.

There is good evidence that surgery and radiotherapy give equally good results in dealing with the axilla, when performed as an adjunct to removal of the breast.

Finally, where the primary in the breast is the only manifestation of the disease, it is not known whether the destruction of the axillary lymph nodes by surgery or radiotherapy improves the chance of cure.

We are now in a position to discuss the management of patients with carcinoma of the breast, according to the manner in which they present. The cardinal feature to be decided is whether the case is an early one, so that one may aim for a cure, or whether it is advanced, so that palliation is the only object.

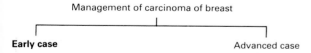

The early case

Clinical definition

In most cases there is a primary tumour in the breast. The primary mass should be small in relation to the size of the breast, not growing rapidly, and without inflammatory signs, while any area of skin involvement as shown by tethering, dimpling or oedema (*peau d'orange*) should not be much larger than the lump. With regard to secondary spread, the question of palpable axillary lymph nodes is considered in a separate section below. However, no supraclavicular lymph nodes should be palpable, nor hepatic nodules on abdominal examination, nor peritoneal deposits on rectal examination.

The less common situation of a patient presenting with axillary metastases following previous surgical removal of the primary tumour is considered on page 79.

Special investigations

There should be no evidence of pulmonary metastases on a chest x-ray, or of bone marrow metastases in a blood count (anaemia or leucopenia). Many clinicians also insist on x-rays of the skeleton, scintiscanning of the skeleton, or both, in order to reduce the risk of missing osseous metastases, but the accuracy of these investigations has not been completely established. At presentation, scintiscanning gives as many false positive as true positive for positive results is less than 5 per cent. The technique is becoming recognized as of more value during follow-up.

Palpable axillary lymph nodes

Lymph nodes palpable in the ipsilateral axilla do not constitute evidence of axillary node invasion by the tumour. The glands may be invaded, but they may also be the seat simply of reactive hyperplasia. Indeed, should histological examination subsequently prove that the axilla was not invaded, the patient is likely to do better than if the glands had not been palpable. This is one piece of evidence to suggest that carcinoma of the breast may provoke a beneficial immune response. Palpability of axillary lymph nodes should therefore not affect the choice of operative procedure: the surgeon is entitled to hope that the case is still early. Sometimes, however, the palpable nodes are so large and fixed as to suggest that excision will be technically very difficult or impossible. In this event the patient should be considered an advanced case.

Granted that by all these criteria the case is early, then once histological evidence is obtained that the lesion is a carcinoma the primary is treated by excision rather than by radiotherapy.

Timing of the biopsy

There are two approaches, which might be termed the orthodox and the modern.

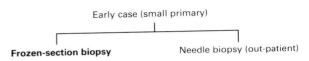

Orthodox: use of frozen section

In order to save the patient from having two separate anaesthetics in quick succession, the biopsy and the definitive operation are performed under the same anaesthetic. A rapid technique of histological examination, such as by frozen section, is therefore necessary. The patient must be fully informed about the circumstances beforehand, and permission obtained to proceed to the definitive operation — usually some form of mastectomy. The patient therefore submits herself to the anaesthetic not knowing whether she will wake with two breasts or one. The patient's full and comprehending consent is vital. Quite apart from the medicolegal implications, a woman who did not realize that she might be about to lose her breast never adjusts to the loss, and this is a source of much mental and emotional disturbance thereafter.

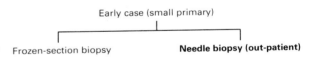

Modern: use of needle biopsy

Various forms of needle biopsy, yielding tissue for cytological or histological examination, are now available and can be performed under local anaesthesia as an out-patient. There is no evidence that such techniques disseminate malignant cells, or in any other way worsen the prognosis, at least as long as the definitive procedure is carried out within a few days. The advantage of this approach is that if the result is positive the patient is spared uncertainty before the main operation. However, these techniques are not as accurate as open biopsy, and a negative result should not be trusted, so for these the orthodox approach is still necessary.

Scope of excision

The aim is to remove the primary completely, so that the tumour does not recur locally. It is the nature of carcinoma to spread through the tissues beyond the visible or palpable limits of the tumour, and therefore a wide margin of excision must be achieved. Exactly how wide, is a question on which there are many shades of opinion. It has been shown that the greater the area of skin excised, the smaller the incidence of recurrent nodules in the skin. Some surgeons routinely take so much skin that they have to use a skin graft to close the subsequent defect. The majority view is to excise a margin of 5 cm all round the tumour, a procedure which is associated with an acceptably low, though not zero, skin recurrence rate. With regard to breast tissue itself, the classical (Halsted) mastectomy excises not only the whole breast but the subcutaneous tissues of the chest wall upwards to the clavicle and medially to the mid-line as well. Less radical is the Patey type of mastectomy, in which just the whole breast is removed. Recently, interest has revived in a more localized excision of the lump, preserving enough of the breast if possible to give a good cosmetic result. This procedure clearly risks a higher rate of local recurrence, especially as the occasional case with a clinically solitary tumour can be demonstrated to have multiple foci of carcinoma. The author's personal preference is for the Patey type of resection, particularly as a local resection of a tumour of some bulk rarely gives a cosmetically satisfactory result. However, local excision is combined with radiotherapy by many experts. Perhaps the patient should be offered a choice: some women cannot get rid of the affected breast soon enough, others cannot bear the prospect of the ablation of an important secondary sexual organ.

Attitude to the lymph glands

Here there is a particularly wide spectrum of opinion, polarized about two different attitudes. One pole is the view that as much as possible of the tumour tissue must be removed so as to give the host's defences the best chance of dealing with the remainder. The most extreme adherents of this view are prepared to excise the supraclavicular and internal mammary lymph nodes as well as the axillary nodes, in continuity with the breast (Urban's masteetomy). Halsted removed the axillary nodes only, and certainly they are much more often invaded than the internal mammary, while one might argue that if the invasion has reached the supraclavicular nodes, the patient should be categorized a late case. Halsted also removed the pectoralis major muscle on the mistaken grounds

that some of the lymphatic vessels draining the breast passed through this muscle on the way to the axilla. Patey preserved the pectoralis major, but also dissected the axilla. Handley demonstrated that if the tumour was in the medial part of the breast or in the region of the nipple, there was a high incidence of involvement of the internal mammary lymph nodes. He therefore biopsied these nodes, and if they were involved he removed the breast only; otherwise he performed a Patey procedure. Haagensen advised biopsying not only the internal mammary but also the apical axillary lymph nodes. Only if none of these was involved did he proceed with radical mastectomy. McWhirter showed that the results of mastectomy plus radiotherapy to the axilla were as good as radical mastectomy.

The opposite pole is the attitude that the body's best defence mechanism against the tumour is the local barrier of lymph nodes, and that therefore these should not be removed. Adherents remove the primary by mastectomy or local excision, and make no effort to deal with the lymph nodes. It should be stressed that there is no direct evidence in favour of this view: it remains an interesting hypothesis.

The author's personal preference is for a Patey type of radical mastectomy.

After operation

Even in those cases where the operation on the primary has shown no evidence of spread to the lymph nodes, and the local excision has been apparently adequate since no local recurrence has ensued, there is a steady incidence of metastatic recurrence and eventual death from the disease. This phenomenon is presumably due to the fact that occult early metastasis has occurred in many patients who appear to be in an early stage. In an effort to reduce the frequency of this progression, various forms of treatment have been tried as prophylaxis immediately after the definitive operation. Prophylactic radiotherapy to the axilla, supraclavicular region and chest wall does not appear to improve the results of radical mastectomy alone, a finding first demonstrated by Paterson. Prophylactic oöphorectomy makes a statistically doubtful improvement which in practical terms is clearly not worth while. At present the effect of prophylactic chemotherapy in a series of short courses for 6 months after the operation is being tried. It would appear that some regimes can prolong the recurrence-free interval, but whether this effect is worthwhile in comparison with the side-effects of the chemotherapy is still debatable. Perhaps more definite is the retardation of growth of metastases produced by the anti-oestrogenic agent, tamoxifen. Tamoxifen works better after the menopause, chemotherapy before it.

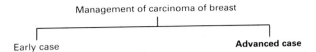

Management of carcinoma of breast

Early case   **Advanced case**

The advanced case

Advanced cases may be considered under three headings: patients with a primary breast tumour; patients with local recurrences after excision of a primary tumour; and patients with metastases. Many patients fall into both the first and third categories, but the management of the primary lesion can be considered separately from the management of metastases.

In the locally advanced case, radiotherapy may produce an excellent result: all the local manifestations of the disease may disappear. Many authorities recommend mastectomy a few weeks later as the best insurance against local recurrence. Should radiotherapy fail, one is forced to try the more generalized forms of treatment as described later with the management of metastases.

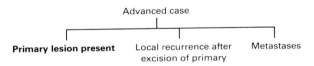

Advanced case

Primary lesion present   Local recurrence after   Metastases
                              excision of primary

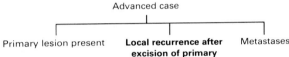

Advanced case

Primary lesion present   **Local recurrence after**   Metastases
                          excision of primary

The breast lump

The patient may be considered to be an advanced case either because the primary tumour is associated with lymph node or widespread metastases, or because the primary tumour is itself in the advanced category. The principle for dealing with the breast lump remains that all reasonable efforts should be made to prevent local recurrence. With a primary that is small in relation to the size of the breast, not advancing rapidly and without inflammatory signs, the surgeon will employ excision, either of the whole breast or of the lump and its local surroundings, according to his personal views as previously discussed. Should, however, any of the unfavourable features mentioned be present, radiotherapy is indicated in the first instance.

The late results of a neglected primary breast tumour can be extremely distressing. The growth erupts through the skin to produce a malignant ulcer; the latter becomes infected, and to the patient's pain is added a malodorous discharge. Spread of tumour through the neighbouring skin produces a hard plaque of tissue, the *cancer en cuirasse*, which may increase pain and even restrict breathing.

Local recurrence

The incomplete removal of a primary breast tumour may result in the appearance of one or more nodules of tumour in the skin flaps, near the scar of the incision. A solitary nodule should be excised and its histological nature confirmed. If there are several nodules, an excision biopsy is done of one of these, and when the diagnosis is confirmed radiotherapy is used.

Local recurrence does not in itself constitute proof that the carcinoma is incurable, and many patients go on to do well after the excision of a recurrent nodule. Nevertheless, the prognosis is adversely affected in statistical terms, and so this situation has been included under the heading of the advanced case. Again, should surgery and radiotherapy fail, one goes on to consider other forms of treatment.

Regional lymph nodes

It is worth gathering together here the various factors governing the management of the regional lymph nodes.

The patient with a primary breast tumour and palpable axillary lymph nodes that are large and fixed will probably be treated by some form of resection of the primary and biopsy of, followed by radiotherapy to, the affected lymph nodes. The same applies to patients with a primary breast tumour and supraclavicular lymph node involvement. Clinical involvement of the internal mammary lymph nodes at the time that the patient presents is very rare.

After previous treatment for a primary breast tumour, the appearance of nodules in the primary lymph drainage areas is an indication for treatment along the lines of the previous paragraph, with one exception: if the treatment of the primary breast tumour has been some form of resection without any treatment to the axilla, then the appearance of unfixed nodules in the axilla is an indication for surgical axillary clearance (or radiotherapy) on the assumption that the situation is still curable. Thus this is an unusual presentation of the early case (see the management scheme, p. 81).

Occasionally a patient presents with a primary breast tumour and clinically palpable nodes in the *opposite* axilla. This is far from being a necessarily bad prognostic sign, because biopsy usually reveals that the enlargement of the nodes is due to reactive hyperplasia. Indeed, such patients do better than the average, and this is another fact which suggests that the local lymph nodes may be conferring some measure of protection.

A rare presentation is the patient with a palpable axillary lymph node which, after the usual diagnostic measures have culminated in a biopsy, turns out to be due to invasion with carcinoma which on histological grounds is likely to have originated in the breast. In the absence of physical signs in the breast, amputation of that organ requires great courage on the part of the surgeon and faith on the part of the patient, but this step, together with some form of treatment to the axilla, is the classical advice. With the advent of mammography and ultrasonography, it is now most unlikely that a small primary tumour in the breast would be missed, and it is wiser, if imaging were negative, to wait and re-examine frequently.

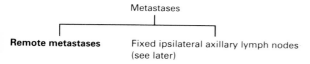

Remote metastases

Principles

These follow directly from the discussion in earlier parts of this Chapter. First, the management of distant metastases must not be allowed to overshadow the management of the primary tumour, because the symptoms produced by an uncontrolled primary loom large in the wide spectrum of morbidity produced by the disease. Secondly, the presence of distant metastases does not in itself constitute an indication for treatment. The correct indications are symptoms and a rapid rate of growth that must cause early death unless the rate can be reduced. Thirdly, if the metastases requiring treatment are solitary, or localized in a small group, then local methods of treatment are used in the first instance because they have a higher success rate than generalized methods.

Local methods

The most obvious example is radiotherapy. A common situation demanding its use is backache. It has been said that the chance of a patient with carcinoma of the breast developing osseous metastases is so high that if such a patient complains of backache the diagnosis can be accepted even in the absence of radiographic or scanning evidence. Radiotherapy localized to the affected area is very efficient in relieving pain. Another important indication for radiotherapy is pathological fractures, which heal well following radiotherapy and the appropriate orthopaedic measures. Even mild backache must be viewed as a possible emergency and investigated immediately, as collapse of vertebrae can threaten the integrity of the spinal cord so that paraplegia may be imminent.

Chemotherapy can be a local form of treatment. Localized arterial infusions are rarely indicated; for example, metastases confined to a single limb, and therefore suitable for treatment by temporary isolation of the limb and local arterial infusion, practically never occur. However, peritoneal deposits presenting as ascites or pleural deposits presenting as an effusion are common, and may respond well to the injection of chemotherapeutic agents into the affected serous cavity after the effusion has been tapped.

Generalized methods

Immunotherapy has made little progress in this field. Chemotherapy may be beginning to find a place as an adjunct to surgery in the treatment of the early case. It is the most effective (but most toxic) form of treatment. Otherwise, its role is not clearly defined. This leaves for consideration hormone therapy.

The hormones that may affect the progress of carcinoma of the breast are oestrogens and androgens, progesterones and possibly prolactin. The most useful agents seem to be synthetic anti-oestrogens (e.g. tamoxifen). The effect of a change in the pattern of the sex hormones is beneficial in only about one-third of cases. In another third of patients the hormones have no effect on the course of the disease. It is often not appreciated that in the final third of patients, the disease is actually accelerated by the treatment. This phenomenon reinforces the view already discussed that precise indications are needed for starting this form of treatment. One approach to this problem is to examine the tumour cells, growing in artificial culture, for oestrogen receptor sites that specifically take up oestrogens added to the culture medium. The situation is not clear: there is no clear subdivision between some cells with no receptors and others with many. Nevertheless, if the tumour has a higher than average concentration of oestrogen receptors, it is statistically more likely to respond to hormone therapy than one with a low concentration.

The remission that may be produced by hormones is never permanent: after a pause in which there may be improvement, or even disappearance, of the clinical manifestations, progress recommences. A remarkable feature of hormone treatment is that when one method of applying it has had some success, the inevitable relapse may still respond to some other method of changing the sex hormone environment. It also seems that the duration of any remission, usually a matter of a few months or even a year or so, is not dependent on the stage which the disease has reached. In other words, there appears to be some advantage in holding off the hormone treatment for as long as feasible.

Menopausal status has an important influence on hormone therapy. Before the menopause, and for 5 years after it, oestrogens are likely to make the disease worse rather than better, and so only androgens or methods that reduce oestrogen levels should be employed. After this age, oestrogens and androgens both have their place in treatment.

The methods of applying hormone treatment are to give the patient oestrogens, to give her androgens or antioestrogens, or to reduce oestrogen production by destroying the ovaries (by surgical excision or radiotherapy; preferably the former which is more efficient), and by the further measure of either hypophysectomy or bilateral adrenalectomy which are no longer in common use.

All methods have their disadvantages. Oestrogens may produce vaginal bleeding and increase nipple pigmentation, and the patient should be warned accordingly. More seriously, these compounds tend to result in retention of water, with headache, nausea, hypertension and congestive cardiac failure as possible sequelae. Androgens cause masculinization, with deepening of the voice, hypertrophy of clitoris, hirsutism, etc. They are therefore no longer used. Instead, the anti-oestrogen tamoxifen is used with good effect in the treatment of the elderly, a perhaps surprising result in view of the natural fall in oestrogen levels after the menopause. The menopausal symptoms produced by oöphorectomy can be particularly devastating in the younger woman. Aminoglutethamide is the most recent of the agents blocking adrenal steroid formation. Adrenalectomy results in the patient being entirely dependent on substitution therapy for her adrenocorticosteroids, with all the attendant risks, particularly if she is exposed to sudden stress. Similar treatment is needed after hypophysectomy, together with antidiuretic hormone temporarily and thyroxine long term; nevertheless, despite these multiple deficiencies, the patient's condition after hypophysectomy is usually more stable and more easily controlled than after adrenalectomy which has now by and large been given up.

The choice between adrenalectomy and hypophysectomy depends upon a number of factors. The remission rate achieved by both is similar. Adrenalectomy can be performed by a general surgeon. Hypophysectomy requires the services of a specially trained neurosurgeon or otolaryngologist. The old dangerous transfrontal craniotomy approach has been abandoned, and the new procedures are either the implantation of radioactive yttrium into the pituitary fossa by stereotactic techniques via the nose, or a direct surgical approach to the fossa via the ethmoid sinus. Since the postoperative course is smoother after hypophysectomy, it is probably the procedure of choice, if available.

There remains the question, how should patients be selected for these formidable operative procedures? A few simple guidelines are available. If the patient has responded well to oral hormone therapy previously, she is more likely to respond well to hormone surgery. A long gap between the time of definitive treatment of the primary and the

Flow-chart 7.1

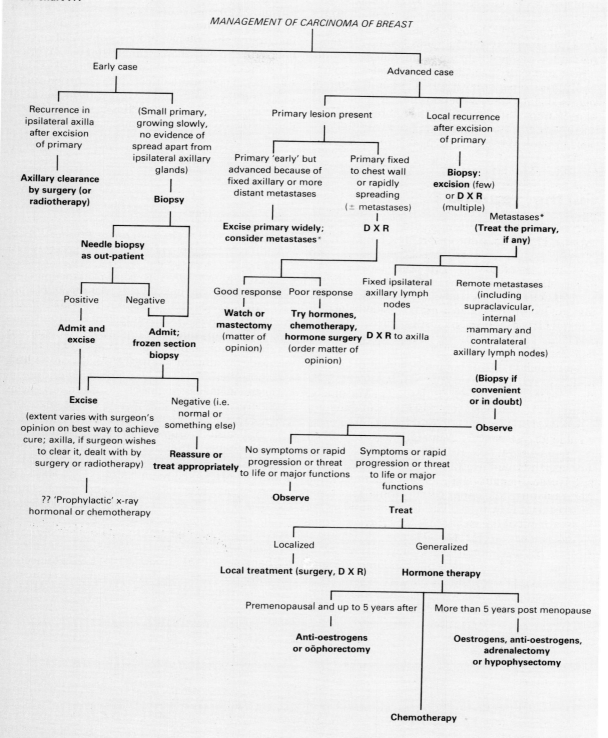

MANAGEMENT OF CARCINOMA OF BREAST

Early case

Recurrence in ipsilateral axilla after excision of primary

Axillary clearance by surgery (or radiotherapy)

(Small primary, growing slowly, no evidence of spread apart from ipsilateral axillary glands)

Biopsy

Needle biopsy as out-patient

Positive

Admit and excise

Negative

Admit; frozen section biopsy

Excise

(extent varies with surgeon's opinion on best way to achieve cure; axilla, if surgeon wishes to clear it, dealt with by surgery or radiotherapy)

?? 'Prophylactic' x-ray hormonal or chemotherapy

Negative (i.e. normal or something else)

Reassure or treat appropriately

Advanced case

Primary lesion present

Primary 'early' but advanced because of fixed axillary or more distant metastases

Excise primary widely; consider metastases*

Good response

Watch or mastectomy (matter of opinion)

Poor response

Try hormones, chemotherapy, hormone surgery (order matter of opinion)

Primary fixed to chest wall or rapidly spreading (± metastases)

D X R

Fixed ipsilateral axillary lymph nodes

D X R to axilla

Remote metastases (including supraclavicular, internal mammary and contralateral axillary lymph nodes)

(Biopsy if convenient or in doubt)

Observe

Local recurrence after excision of primary

Biopsy: excision (few) or **D X R** (multiple)

Metastases* **(Treat the primary, if any)**

No symptoms or rapid progression or threat to life or major functions

Observe

Symptoms or rapid progression or threat to life or major functions

Treat

Localized

Local treatment (surgery, D X R)

Generalized

Hormone therapy

Premenopausal and up to 5 years after

Anti-oestrogens or oöphorectomy

More than 5 years post menopause

Oestrogens, anti-oestrogens, adrenalectomy or hypophysectomy

Chemotherapy

* Indicates a continuance of flow.

appearance of recurrent tumour has a similar significance. Metastases in bone are more likely to respond than visceral deposits. Positive oestrogen receptor status is encouraging. None of these methods is of much help in the individual case, and a host of factors need to be taken into account: how old is the patient, what are her family commitments, what is her general state of health and expectation of life apart from the tumour, and how severe are her symptoms compared with the possible or likely side-effects of the operation. There is still room in clinical medicine for judgement, opinion and common sense.

What of the future? The view seems to be gaining ground that we need to know more about the nature of the *individual* primary tumour. Work is in progress with recombinant cDNA to try to identify specific abnormalities at the chromosomal level and there is related work with monoclonal antibodies. Knowledge like this may enable us to choose the best treatment for each individual patient.

Further reading

Atkins, H. J. B., Bulbrook, R. D., Falconer, M. A., Hayward, J. L., MacLean, K. S. and Schurr, P. N. (1968). Ten years experience of steroid assays in management of breast cancer. *Lancet* ii, 1255–60.

Bloom, H. J. G., Richardson, W. W. and Harries, E. J. (1962). Natural history of untreated breast cancer (1805–1933). *British Medical Journal* 2, 213–21.

Bonadonna, G., Brusamolino, E., Valagussa, P., Ross, A., Brugnatelli, L., Brambilla, C., de Lena, M., Tancini, G., Bajetta, E., Musumeci, R. and Veronesi, U. (1976). Combination chemotherapy as an adjuvant treatment in operable breast cancer. *New England Journal of Medicine* 294, 405–10.

Fisher, B., Bauer, M., Margolese, R. *et al.* (1985). Five year results of a randomized clinical trial comparing total mastectomy and segmental mastectomy with or without radiation in the treatment of breast cancer. *New England Journal of Medicine* 312, 665–73.

Fisher, B., Redmond, C., Fisher, E. R., *et al.* (1985). Ten-year results of a randomized clinical trial comparing radical mastectomy and total mastectomy with or without radiation. *New England Journal of Medicine* 312, 674–8.

Haagensen, C. D. (1971). *Diseases of the Breast*, 2nd edn. Philadelphia and Eastbourne, W. B. Saunders.

Hawkins, R. A. (1985). Receptors in the management of breast cancer. *British Journal of Hospital Medicine* 34, 160–64.

McWhirter, R. (1955). Simple mastectomy and radiotherapy in the treatment of breast cancer. *British Journal of Radiology* 28, 128–39.

Nolvadex Adjuvant Trial Organisation (1985). Controlled trial of Tamoxifen as single adjuvant agent in management of early breast cancer. *Lancet* i, 836–39.

Palmer, M. K. and Ribiero, G. G. (1985). Thirty four year follow up of patients with breast cancer in clinical trial of postoperative radiotherapy. *British Medical Journal* 291, 1088–91.

Patey, D. H. and Dyson, W. I. H. (1948). The prognosis of carcinoma of the breast in relation to the type of operation performed. *British Journal of Cancer* 2, 7–13.

Rayner, C. R. (1983). Breast implants. *British Journal of Hospital Medicine* 32, 243–7.

Urban, J. and Castro, E. B. (1971). Selecting variations in extent of surgical procedure for breast cancer. *Cancer* 28, 1615–23.

Chapter 8

Dysphagia

Dysphagia means difficulty in swallowing. The symptom may be very mild — a momentary spasm — or complete. In some conditions it may result from pain.

The complaint of dysphagia must always be taken seriously because patients usually have an organic basis for the complaint. When the symptom is severe and swallowing becomes impossible, there may be nutritional problems unless the condition is acute and shortly remits. Furthermore, the causes underlying dysphagia include a number of important diseases with a highly lethal potential, so early diagnosis is mandatory.

One must be careful to distinguish dysphagia from disturbances resulting from neuromuscular incoordination during swallowing. If the nasopharynx and larynx are not shut off from the oropharynx by the normal reflex mechanisms activating the sphincters that protect these regions, the act of swallowing causes part of the pharyngeal contents to regurgitate into the nose or spill into the larynx. The consequent choking sensation, coughing, bronchospasm, etc., may be misinterpreted by the patient as difficulty on swallowing. In any case that is at all difficult to interpret from the history, it is worth asking the patient to drink or eat something under observation. Palatal paralysis should then become easy to diagnose. Immediate and severe overspill into the respiratory passages is usually evidence of neuromuscular abnormality, but may simply mean that a truly dysphagic patient is very weak. This arises in adults with a long history of dysphagia with consequent starvation, or in neonates with congenital deformities preventing swallowing. It is also true that even in reasonably fit adults, the presence of stagnant oesophageal contents above an obstruction favours overspill into the respiratory passages, especially at night when the patient is lying flat and his guarding reflexes are depressed by sleep. The resultant clinical picture is one of recurrent attacks of chest pain, fever and cough, in association with the clinical and radiological signs of areas of collapse and consolidation in the lungs.

Apart from the presentation in neonates, which is considered briefly below, cases may be divided into the acute and the chronic.

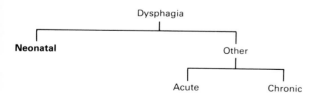

Neonatal oesophageal obstruction

The important thing for the practitioner to remember is that a baby who will not accept his bottle, and in whom attempts to feed produce coughing attacks and cyanosis, is very likely to have an oesophageal obstruction. In some infants other congenital anomalies coexist, but there may well be no external abnormalities, so no matter how normal the baby seems he should be referred immediately for specialist advice from a paediatric unit. Details of the further management are beyond the scope of this book. The commonest cause of obstruction is some form of oesophageal atresia; in one variety of this condition the upper segment of the oesophagus, instead of ending blindly at the site of atresia, opens into the trachea, and infants with this malformation are of course particularly prone to respiratory distress during attempted feeding. The other likely cause of oesophageal obstruction is a stricture, resulting from reflux oesophagitis and usually associated with a hiatus hernia, just as in adults (p. 90).

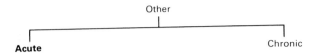

Acute dysphagia

A person presenting with severe acute dysphagia has either drunk a corrosive liquid or swallowed a foreign body, or else he suffers from a local acute inflammatory process.

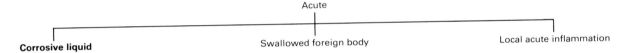

Corrosive liquids

Strong acids and alkalis when swallowed naturally produce a very severe inflammation of the oesophagus and pharynx, and no doubt, to some extent, of the stomach as well if sufficient has been ingested. The patient complains of intense pain in the mouth, throat and retrosternal area, present all the time but aggravated by the least attempt to swallow. The history is usually clear-cut — drinking from a mislabelled bottle or a suicide attempt. The most important feature of the immediate management is pain relief, and this requires large doses of opiates. When the patient is calmer, it should be possible to attempt to wash away some of the corrosive agent by washing out the mouth, and even possibly by persuading the patient to swallow some water. If it is known that the liquid swallowed was a strong acid, it is logical to use a dilute solution of an alkali for this wash, and vice versa.

The important short-term problem is to be able to recognize oesophageal perforation at an early stage, should this rather rare complication occur. Oesophageal perforation results in mediastinitis. If the perforation is small, any leak of oesophageal contents may be very gradual and the pain involved minor by comparison with the pain of severe oesophagitis. A careful watch must therefore be kept for other evidence, such as pyrexia, abnormal pulmonary signs, or a widening of the medias-

tinum in a chest x-ray. Particularly valuable is a routine of performing haemoglobin or haematocrit estimations at frequent intervals, even 4-hourly at first, since mediastinitis is associated with a large exudation of plasma-like material and results in a proportionately large haemoconcentration (p. 269). By the same token, the infusion of plasma or plasma substitute is an important part of the treatment of the shock that is produced.

The preservation of nutrition needs careful consideration. During the stage of acute symptoms, fluid and electrolyte balance is maintained intravenously. When the pain abates, the oesophagus should still be rested as far as possible to promote healing. One has a choice between an indwelling nasogastric tube, a temporary gastrostomy, and the intravenous route for feeding the patient. In ideal circumstances, the choice lies between the second and third possibilities. Once the most severe symptoms have subsided, a stricture may form surprisingly rapidly. As soon as possible, therefore, the patient should swallow a very fine tube, or even a weighted thread, so that this may act as a guide for any subsequent endoscopic dilatation. The long and often tortuous stricture that ensures may be very difficult to negotiate with an oesophagoscope unless this precaution has been taken.

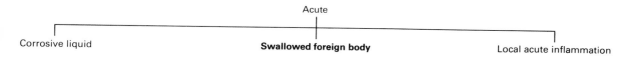

Acute

Corrosive liquid   **Swallowed foreign body**   Local acute inflammation

Swallowed foreign body

The history usually makes the diagnosis obvious. During a meal, the patient suddenly feels something stick as he swallows. There may be immediate severe pain, or only mild discomfort at first which gradually increases. Even the attempt to swallow saliva produces agony.

If the symptoms persist unchanged, or worsen for more than a few minutes, the patient should be referred to hospital for immediate admission.

In hospital baseline observations are made in the hope that if mediastinitis occurs it will be de-tected at an early stage (see p. 84). A plain x-ray is taken in case the foreign body is radio-opaque. However, if the history is convincing, oesophagos-copy is required even if the x-ray is negative. The patient is anaesthetized as soon as practicable, and an oesophagoscope passed so that the offending object can be seen and removed. After this has been accomplished, the patient should be watched carefully for at least 24 hours since delayed per-foration of the oesophagus may occur during that time, either from the foreign body itself or from trauma inflicted by its removal.

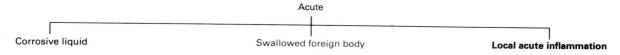

Acute

Corrosive liquid   Swallowed foreign body   **Local acute inflammation**

Local acute conditions

Any acute inflammatory process affecting the pharynx, oesophagus, or contiguous structures renders swallowing uncomfortable. These conditions, such as tonsillitis and pharyngitis, are usually self-limiting or readily curable by medical measures. Occasionally, an abscess forms and requires incision and drainage; e.g. a peritonsillar abscess or quinsy, or a retropharyngeal abscess. The diagnosis is readily made on inspection of the affected area, and if medical treatment does not suffice, the patient should be referred to an oto-laryngologist.

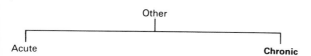

Other

Acute   **Chronic**

Chronic dysphagia

Pointers from the history

Only rarely can the cause of long-standing dysphagia be elucidated from the history. If the patient says that a lump appears in the lower neck (usually but not always on the left side) as the meal proceeds and that this is associated with increasing difficulty in swallowing, or that there is gurgling on swallowing, then there is almost certainly a pharyngeal diverticulum present. If pressure over the mass produces gurgling and regurgitation of food then that confirms the diagnosis beyond doubt. Some features of the history are helpful in assigning the case to a particular group of conditions. A slow, unrelenting progression of the symptom from mild difficulty with tough solids only, at first, to a final stage in which even clear liquids become impossible, is very suggestive of a malignant stricture, intrinsic to the oesophagus or extrinsic. A concomitant or preceding symptom of severe heartburn points towards peptic oesophagitis as the cause of a benign stricture. Dysphagia that is variable in severity may be due to neuromuscular incoordination or diseases of the nervous system.

These pointers are not specific, however, and should not be permitted to affect the management of the case. All patients with chronic dysphagia should be assumed to have malignant disease even if certain features of the history suggest a benign origin. They should therefore be referred immediately for a specialist opinion.

The examination

The practitioner's examination of the patient may be relevant to the decision that he sends him to one specialist rather than another; for example, an otolaryngologist, a neurologist, or a thoracic surgeon. The general surgeon must, however, be prepared to deal with all forms of the general problem in the first instance, and the following discussion relates to his point of view.

The examination basically divides the patients into two groups: those where the general surgeon is sure that the case lies in the province of some other specialist, and those in which the cause lies definitely or possibly in his own province.

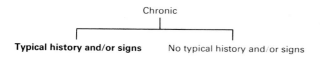

Cases for referral

If there is sufficient clinical information to make a confident diagnosis of neurological or neuromuscular disease, such as bulbar palsy or myasthenia gravis, the patient should be referred to the appropriate medical specialist. A lesion in the mouth or oropharynx is likely to be malignant, and the patient is referred to the otolaryngologist. There may be clear evidence of carcinoma of the bronchus, in which case the dysphagia is presumably due to pressure of invaded lymph glands in the mediastinum, and the patient is referred to the thoracic surgeon. Pharyngeal pouch has already been mentioned.

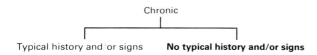

Cases not for referral

Most cases in fact seem to fall into this category. In most of these there are no relevant physical signs to assist with the diagnosis. In a few there are physical signs which may be relevant to the cause of the dysphagia. For example, the patient may have palpable cervical lymph nodes, suggesting secondary spread from a neoplasm of the oesophagus or cardia, or a woman may be frankly anaemic, a combination which suggests the Paterson–Brown–Kelly syndrome (sideropenic dysphagia, p. 89). No matter what the exact clinical picture, the pattern of management is essentially identical — prompt and thorough special investigation. Patients already suffering severely from malnutrition should be admitted immediately, but the investigation of all cases should be considered urgent.

Special investigations

The twin foundations for the diagnosis of most cases of dysphagia are radiology and endoscopy.

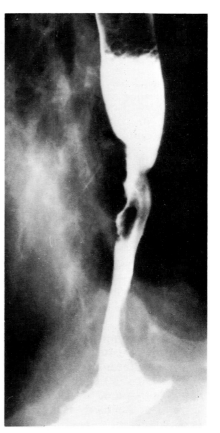

Fig. 8.1   Barium swallow in a patient with carcinoma of the oesophagus. There is a long stricture of the lower end of the oesophagus with moderate dilatation proximal to the stricture. Note the appearance of 'shoulders' at the ends of the stricture: this is practically pathognomonic of malignancy.

Radiology

The barium swallow and meal (Fig. 8.1) demonstrates the site and length of any stricture or other lesion narrowing the oesophagus, the degree of dilatation of the oesophagus proximal to the obstruction, and the presence or absence of a hiatus hernia, or of gastro-oesophageal reflux. The evidence of this investigation, particularly the observations on screening, can suggest but not decide the answers to two further questions: is the narrowing due to extrinsic disease of neighbouring structures? and if intrinsic, is the lesion benign or malignant? Neuromuscular incoordination can also be hinted at by abnormalities of the contractions of the oesophagus as seen during screening.

Endoscopy

The endoscopist also demonstrates the site of any narrowing of the lumen, and takes tissue from the lesion for histological examination. He can attempt to dilate a stricture, and pass his instrument beyond it to determine the exact relation of the lower border of the lesion to the cardia. He can comment on the appearance of the oesophageal mucous membrane, drawing attention to oesophagitis, and can see whether gastric juice regurgitates into the lower oesophagus.

Oesophagoscopy may be performed with the rigid instrument, or with a modern flexible instrument using the fibre-optic principle. The latter has certain advantages in some patients, especially those with severe kyphosis, but does not give as adequate a view or allow large biopsies or the removal of foreign bodies. Whichever is used, a risk of perforation is present, and the patient should always be admitted for the investigation and observed closely for 24 hours afterwards.

Other investigations

In special centres more specialized techniques are available. Pressure measurements in the region of the lower end of the oesophagus are useful in achalasia (p. 89), luminal pH can be monitored continuously for 24 hours with a pH-sensitive electrode swallowed at the end of a fine catheter, while a single swallow of a radiolabelled liquid followed during its progress down the oesophagus with an external gamma camera can help with the quantification of gastro-oesophageal reflux and oesophageal incoordination (p. 89).

Following the investigations, the diagnosis may have been established or remain in doubt. The management of patients with established diagnoses is now described.

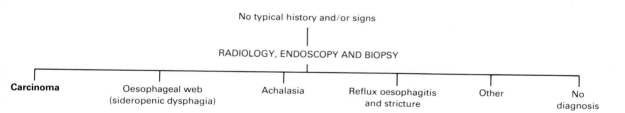

Carcinoma of the oesophagus

This is probably the commonest of the diagnoses established by radiology and endoscopy. Cancer of the oesophagus is a disease of old age, although it also occurs in younger adults. Predisposing factors include achalasia of the oesophagus (p. 89), long-standing benign strictures, especially those due to corrosives, and the Paterson–Brown–Kelly syndrome (p. 89). Most cases are epitheliomas that arise from the stratified squamous epithelium lining most of the oesophagus. At the lower end, adenocarcinomas also occur, arising from the gastric mucous membrane itself or from islets of gas-

tric mucosa that may sometimes be found in the lower oesophagus.

The prognosis is grave: in many series the 5-year survival rate is less than 10 per cent. One reason is that the lesion tends to spread submucosally upwards and downwards along the oesophagus, so that the length of oesophagus involved may be far greater than it appears to investigation or to the naked eye. Another is that spread outwards from the oesophagus, whether by direct extension or by the lymphatics, rapidly involves vital structures such as the heart, the root of the lungs, the tracheal bifurcation and the arch of the aorta. From the lower end of the oesophagus, the lymphatic pathways lead via the left gastric pedicle to the lymph nodes in the region of the coeliac axis.

For this reason, the present trend is to assume that treatment is going to be palliative even if there is no definite sign of spread such as palpable supraclavicular nodes or a phrenic nerve paralysis. Exceptions occur, but the main aim is palliation, which in this context means the ability to swallow in comfort till the patient dies. Note that the simple procedure of gastrostomy unfortunately does not meet this requirement: it provides a route for feeding the patient, but does not allow him to swallow his own saliva.

Cancer of the lower third

The adenocarcinoma is resistant to radiotherapy, and surgery is the only treatment practicable. The conventional operation is abdominothoracic oesophagogastrectomy. The upper abdomen is opened, and the tumour, which lies at the junction of oesophagus and stomach, is assessed for mobility. If the surgeon decides that removal is possible, he extends the incision along the left eighth rib and enters the chest. The lower third of the oesophagus is excised from below the arch of the aorta, together with the upper half of the stomach. The digestive tract is reconstituted by mobilizing the rest of the stomach and anastomosing it to the cut end of the oesophagus in the chest, or by preparing a Roux loop of jejunum and bringing it up to the oesophagus. Should excision prove impossible, the usual procedure is to pass a special, tough plastic tube through the growth so that its lower end lies in the stomach. The tube maintains the patency of the channel despite continued growth of the tumour. One such pattern of tube (Mousseau—Barbin) ends below in a long rat-tail that can be manipulated through even a tight stricture, while its top end is shouldered so that it impacts in the growth when the tube is pulled downwards from the stomach.

The squamous celled carcinoma of the lower third of the oesophagus may be treated in the same way, or by radiotherapy with or without intubation.

Cancer of the mid-third

The alternatives are radiotherapy and surgery. The surgery here involves opening the abdomen and mobilizing the stomach, then turning the patient on his left side and performing a right thor-

acotomy. Division of the azygos vein gives access to the oesophagus throughout its thoracic course, and excision of the tumour with a wide margin of oesophagus above and the whole of the lower oesophagus performed. The mobilized stomach is pulled upwards into the chest for an anastomosis above the arch of the aorta. This is the Ivor Lewis operation.

Cancer of the upper third

This is an unusual site, except for the very topmost segment of the oesophagus, where the so-called postcricoid carcinoma occurs. The initial treatment is by radiotherapy, and the results with postcricoid carcinoma are better than in other parts of the oesophagus. Cure rather than simple palliation is the aim. Should the tumour recur, very extensive surgery is necessary. The lower pharynx, larynx and the whole of the oesophagus are excised, together with block dissection of the cervical lymph nodes on one or both sides are indicated by the presence of palpable lymph nodes. The cut end of the trachea is brought out on the skin as a permanent tracheostomy, through which the patient breathes; the stomach or colon is mobilized by a second surgical team and passed up to the neck through the posterior mediastinum, along the bed from which the oesophagus has been enucleated by blind dissection from the neck downwards and from the abdomen upwards. Phonation is of course lost, but a number of the patients develop pharyngeal speech and swallowing is excellent.

Modern trends

The success of this extensive procedure of pharyngolaryngo-oesophagectomy has been one factor leading to a reappraisal of the treatment of carcinoma of the oesophagus. The results of radiotherapy are not very good; the results of the standard operations are probably better, but their drawback is that these operations have a high incidence of serious complications and death. The reasons for this are: that oesophageal anastomoses do not heal well, probably for anatomical reasons connected with their blood supply and arrangement of muscle fibres, and lack of a peritoneal coat; and that a leak at the anastomosis, if the latter lies within the chest, is likely to produce a grave disturbance of the function of respiration by such complications as empyema and massive collapse of the lung. Pharyngeal anastomoses, however, seem to heal better, and an anastomotic leak has less serious consequences in the neck than in the chest.

For these reasons there is a trend towards bypassing tumours of the middle third by taking mobilized stomach or colon up to the cervical oesophagus via a substernal tunnel. If the stomach is used, the oesophagus may be drained into the small intestine via a Roux loop, although it appears safe just to close the lower end of the oesophagus instead. A similar approach is beginning to be used for upper and lower third tumours. Indeed, in many centres the treatment of carcinoma of the lower third is now mobilization of the lower third from the abdomen under direct vision (the oesophageal hiatus in the diaphragm is split forwards and a good view can then be obtained), the rest of the oesophagus is blindly mobilized from the abdomen and neck, the whole oesophagus excised and the mobilized stomach taken up through the oesophageal bed to be anastomosed to the cervical oesophagus.

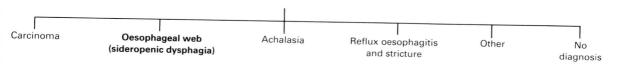

Sideropenic dysphagia

The barium swallow shows a delicate mucosal fold arising from the anterior wall of the upper oesophagus and the blood count shows iron-deficiency (sideropenic) anaemia and/or a reduced serum iron. This combination is seen in middle-aged females, and is often referred to as the Paterson–Brown–Kelly syndrome or, erroneously, as the Plummer–Vinson syndrome.

The nature of the oesophageal web is not clearly understood. In many patients the web persists for a while even though dysphagia may have been relieved by correction of the anaemia.

These patients should be carefully followed up, because there is an increased incidence of subsequent postcricoid carcinoma.

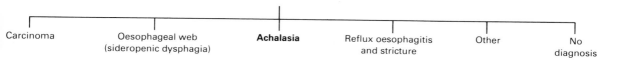

Achalasia of the oesophagus

The barium swallow shows a hold-up at the lower end of the oesophagus, apparently due to a stricture. The lower oesophagus tapers smoothly, and there are no irregularities or shoulder-defects such as are common in carcinoma. The condition may progress particularly slowly over a number of years, so that the oesophagus has the chance to dilate to an enormous size and elongate until it is frankly S-shaped. These features are well demonstrated in the barium meal, and a preliminary plain chest x-ray often shows the shadow of the distended oesophagus with a broad air/fluid level wider than the mediastinum.

Oesophagoscopy confirms the distended oesophagus, containing stagnant food residues and with a marked inflammation of its wall, but demonstrates that there is no stricture. The instrument passes without obstruction through the lower end into the stomach. Histology of mucosal biopsies shows no evidence of malignancy.

These findings are diagnostic of achalasia of the oesophagus. The condition used to be called 'achalasia of the cardia' until it was appreciated as a result of manometric studies of the lower oesophageal sphincter that the abnormality arises in a variable length of the lowermost portion of the oesophagus rather than at the stomach opening itself. The abnormality consists in this segment of the gullet failing to relax as a wave of peristalsis reaches it from the proximal oesophagus. Histology of the muscle in the lower oesophagus shows a paucity of the ganglion cells of the myenteric plexuses of nerves. The analogy with Hirschsprung's disease of the colon (p. 320) is obvious. The radiographic appearance suggesting a stricture is due to the contrast between the narrow terminal segment of the oesophagus and the distended reaches above this.

Achalasia usually starts in young adult life, and its course is very variable and erratic. The mildest degrees require reassurance only. Many patients can be taught to pass bougies on themselves regularly so as to keep the lower end of the oesophagus dilated, thereby encouraging the oesophagus to empty into the stomach by gravity. Severe dys-

phagia demands forcible balloon dilatation of the lower oesophagus via an endoscope, or Heller's operation: a longitudinal incision is made along the lower 10 cm of oesophagus. The incision is through the muscle coats but leaves the mucosa intact, and the latter can then bulge freely through the muscular split, thereby enlarging the lumen. There is a definite incidence of gastro-oesophageal reflux after this operation, particularly if the muscular split is carried down on to the stomach wall.

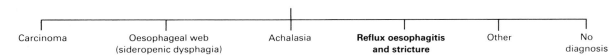

Carcinoma | Oesophageal web (sideropenic dysphagia) | Achalasia | **Reflux oesophagitis and stricture** | Other | No diagnosis

Stricture with peptic oesophagitis

Typically, the barium swallow shows a ragged stricture at the lower end of the oesophagus without any of the hallmarks of malignancy, and free reflux of stomach contents into the oesophagus when the patient is tilted head downwards and his abdomen gently compressed.

The endoscopist confirms the stricture and the reflux, and observes the changes of oesophagitis affecting the mucosa of the lower oesophagus. He takes several portions of tissue for biopsy, and these show only oesophagitis and fibrosis without any evidence of malignancy. Another important reason for taking these biopsies is that they might confirm oesophagitis despite the *absence* of typical naked eye appearances.

There is a diagnostic trap here. Gastro-oesophageal reflux is a common condition which may coexist with carcinoma of the lower oesopha-

gus: hence the insistence on several biopsy specimens. If there is any shadow of doubt, the endoscopy and biopsies should be repeated. The author remembers one patient in whom the diagnosis of carcinoma was clinched only at the seventh examination. Clearly that was unusual, but it emphasizes the point that negative evidence is not as reliable as positive evidence.

The management of a stricture with peptic oesophagitis can be very difficult. Dilatation by bougies relieves the dysphagia, but may increase reflux and set the stage for further stenosis. Conservative measures to reduce reflux and oesophagitis (p. 96) plus H_2-antagonists to reduce gastric acid and pepsin secretion may suffice in mild cases, but if bouginage is necessary then surgical measures to reduce reflux, and probably to reduce gastric secretion as well, are mandatory (p. 104).

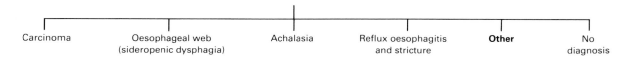

Carcinoma | Oesophageal web (sideropenic dysphagia) | Achalasia | Reflux oesophagitis and stricture | **Other** | No diagnosis

Other established diagnoses

There are many possible diagnoses, although this group is only a small proportion of all the cases of dysphagia that are investigated. A representative sample will be mentioned.

The treatment of a pharyngeal pouch is discussed elsewhere (p. 85). Benign tumours of the

oesophagus are very rare: they can sometimes be excised as well as simply biopsied by the endoscopist. Diverticula of the oesophagus may require excision, followed by repair of the oesophageal wall plus any treatment necessary for the cause of the diverticulum such as tuberculous lymph nodes. Extrinsic pressure on the oesophagus may have been shown to be due to a retrosternal goitre, carcinoma of the bronchus, or enlarged lymph nodes at the hilum of the lung. Further investigation may be called for to decide the correct management of these lesions. The cause for indentation of the wall of the oesophagus may be unclear at this stage, and require further investigation — for example, an aortic arch angiogram to demonstrate an aneursym, or an anomalous pattern of the great vessels. Finally, the characteristic constriction ring of the type described by Schatzki may have been observed (Fig. 8.2). But there are many other patterns of neuromuscular incoordination and they will probably need to be sorted out with the radiolabelled swallow technique for quantifying oesophageal transit rates at various sites as the bolus travels down the oesophagus.

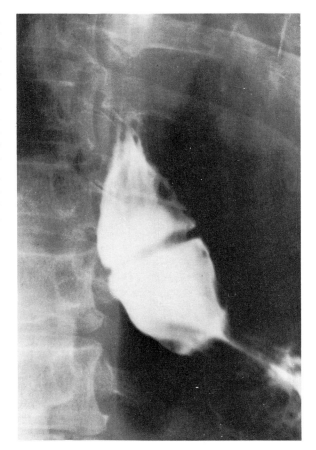

Fig. 8.2 Barium swallow, showing the circumferential indentation of·a Schatzki ring near the lower end of the oesophagus. The patient was a 70-year-old male who complained of mild dysphagia, which responded to reassurance.

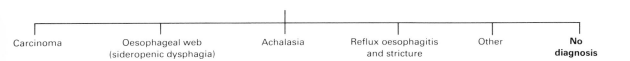

| Carcinoma | Oesophageal web (sideropenic dysphagia) | Achalasia | Reflux oesophagitis and stricture | Other | **No diagnosis** |

The undiagnosed remnant

Where routine investigation fails to establish a diagnosis, further management depends upon whether any abnormality was noted during the examinations. If the findings were absolutely normal, and there are no clinical features to suggest any of the possibilities mentioned below, it is reasonable to conclude for the moment that the patient is hysterical, and reassure him accordingly. Dysphagia without apparent organic cause frequently improves under these circumstances.

Before this reassurance is given, however, one should bear in mind the following possibilities: scleroderma, oesophageal Crohn's disease, neuro-muscular diseases such as bulbar palsy and alcoholic neuritis. The histological appearances of biopsy material in the first two diseases may be difficult to interpret. Neuromuscular disease is unlikely if the radiologist screening the barium swallow was satisfied that propulsive waves in the oesophagus looked normal. However, more refined studies with the radiolabelled swallow technique help to elucidate the really difficult case.

Flow-chart 8.1

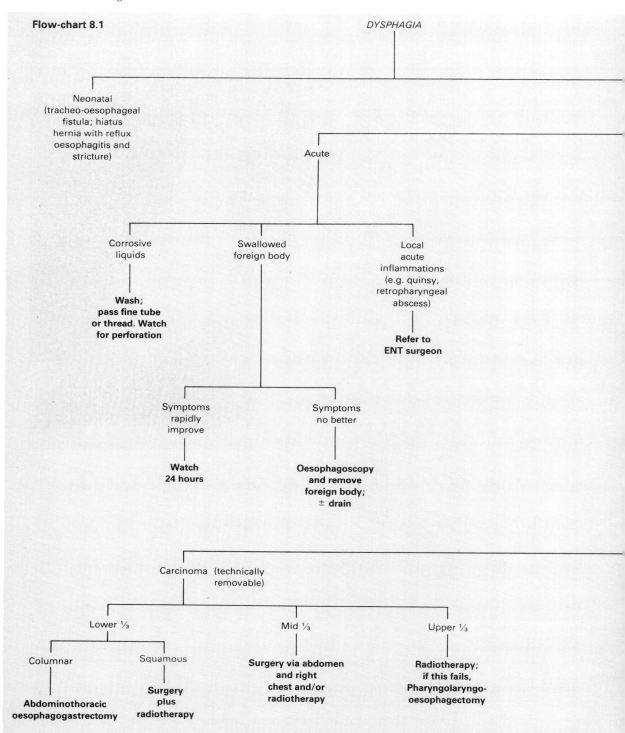

DYSPHAGIA

Neonatal (tracheo-oesophageal fistula; hiatus hernia with reflux oesophagitis and stricture)

Acute

Corrosive liquids

Wash; pass fine tube or thread. Watch for perforation

Swallowed foreign body

Local acute inflammations (e.g. quinsy, retropharyngeal abscess)

Refer to ENT surgeon

Symptoms rapidly improve

Watch 24 hours

Symptoms no better

Oesophagoscopy and remove foreign body; ± drain

Carcinoma (technically removable)

Lower ⅓

Mid ⅓

Upper ⅓

Columnar

Abdominothoracic oesophagogastrectomy

Squamous

Surgery plus radiotherapy

Surgery via abdomen and right chest and/or radiotherapy

Radiotherapy; if this fails, Pharyngolaryngo-oesophagectomy

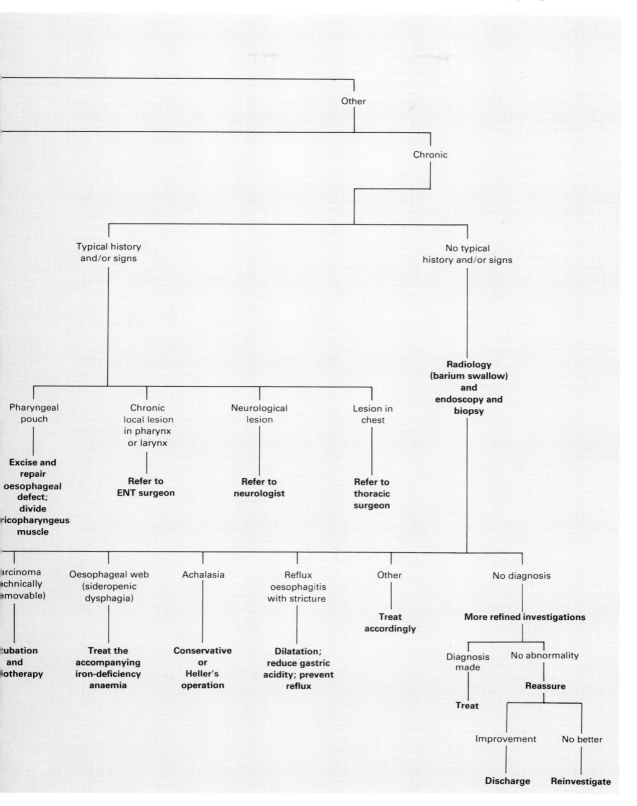

Other

Chronic

Typical history
and/or signs

No typical
history and/or signs

**Radiology
(barium swallow)
and
endoscopy and
biopsy**

Pharyngeal
pouch

Chronic
local lesion
in pharynx
or larynx

Neurological
lesion

Lesion in
chest

**Excise and
repair
oesophageal
defect;
divide
cricopharyngeus
muscle**

**Refer to
ENT surgeon**

**Refer to
neurologist**

**Refer to
thoracic
surgeon**

arcinoma
echnically
emovable)

Oesophageal web
(sideropenic
dysphagia)

Achalasia

Reflux
oesophagitis
with stricture

Other

No diagnosis

**Treat
accordingly**

More refined investigations

tubation
and
iotherapy

**Treat the
accompanying
iron-deficiency
anaemia**

**Conservative
or
Heller's
operation**

**Dilatation;
reduce gastric
acidity; prevent
reflux**

Diagnosis
made

No abnormality

Reassure

Treat

Improvement

No better

Discharge

Reinvestigate

Further reading

Carcona, J. C. and Daly, J. F. (1971). Current management of corrosive oesophagitis. *Annals of Otology, Rhinology and Laryngology* **80**, 522–7.

Deverall, P. B. (1968). Smooth-muscle tumours of the oesophagus. *British Journal of Surgery* **55**, 457–61.

Earlam, R. J. (1975). *Clinical Tests of Oesophageal Function*. London, Crosby, Lockwood & Staples.

Editorial (1969). The Paterson–Kelly lesion. *British Medical Journal* **2**, 530.

Le Quesne, L. P. and Ranger, D. (1966). Pharyngo-laryngectomy with immediate pharyngogastric anastomosis. *British Journal of Surgery* **53**, 105–9.

McKeown, K. C. (1972). Trends in oesophageal resection for carcinoma. *Annals of the Royal College of Surgeons of England* **51**, 213–39.

MacMahon, H. E., Schatzki, R. and Gary, J. E. (1958). Pathology of a lower oesophageal ring. *New England Journal of Medicine* **259**, 1–12.

Polk, H. C. Jr. and Zeppa, R. (1971). Hiatal hernia and esophagitis: a survey of indications for operation and technique and results of fundoplication. *Annals of Surgery* **173**, 775–81.

Smith, B. (1970). The neurological lesion in achalasia of the cardia. *Gut* **11**, 388–91.

Vantrappen, G., Hellemans, J., Deloof, W., Valembois, P. and Vandebroucke, J. (1971). Treatment of achalasia with pneumatic dilatations. *Gut* **12**, 268–75.

Walker, W. S., Cameron, E. W. J., and Walbaum, P. R. (1985). Diagnosis and management of spontaneous transmural rupture of the oesophagus (Boerhaave's syndrome). *British Journal of Surgery* **72**, 204–8.

Watson, A. (1984). Carcinoma of the oesophagus. *Surgery* (Oxford) **1**, 292–5.

Watson, A. and Celestin, L. R. (eds) (1984). *Disorders of the Oesophagus. Advances and Controversies*. Pitman, London.

Chapter 9

Chronic or Recurrent Upper Abdominal Pain

The practitioner's problem

Chronic upper abdominal pain is one of the commonest problems to be brought to the general practitioner's surgery. The cause of such a complaint may be one of a large number of serious diseases, of which only six are at all common. On the other hand, even if the symptoms are severe at the time, one knows that the majority of patients who present with this complaint will recover spontaneously in a few days and have no further trouble for years. Another very common pattern is of very mild symptoms which recur from time to time but never become worse and never really interfere with the patient's enjoyment of life, and even on detailed investigation can never be shown to be due to a definite organic abnormality.

The snag is that the small minority of remaining patients may have similar symptoms to the others, yet harbour serious underlying disease which may ultimately give rise to life-threatening complications, or may steadily get worse until the patient is a chronic invalid.

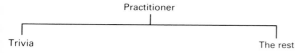

The practitioner's problem is how to weed out from the mass of trivia those patients who should be referred for a specialist opinion. Naturally, he must refer all those who ask for a second opinion, or who have severe symptoms that do not respond to simple medical treatment with antacids, antispasmodics, etc. Continuous symptoms in the sense that the patient has some pain every day for several weeks is another clear indication. So is pain that is severe enough to cause absence from work, especially if more than one such episode has occur-

red. Housewives who do not go out to work are notoriously difficult to assess.

Apart from these general considerations, any patient in whom the practitioner feels there is a real possibility of serious underlying disease should be referred unless the practitioner has direct access to such investigations as gastro-intestinal endoscopy, ultrasound, sigmoidoscopy and barium enemas. The conclusion that this is a real possibility will probably have been determined by the patient's history, since in most cases there are no abnormal physical signs.

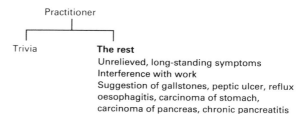

Pointers from the history

In descending order of frequency, the six common diseases are gallstones, peptic ulcer, reflux oesophagitis, carcinoma of the stomach, carcinoma of the pancreas and chronic pancreatitis. (This statement is true for the United Kingdom. In many countries where alcoholism is a more serious problem, chronic pancreatitis is further up the order, while in many developing countries peptic ulcer is more common than gallstones.)

Gallstones

The pain comes in attacks lasting a few hours to a

few days. During an attack the pain may vary in intensity, but the patient is never free from pain. There is no consistent relationship between the onset of an attack and a meal, and once the pain starts there may be associated nausea and vomiting. Attacks occur in random fashion, with pain-free intervals of several weeks or months. The pain is mid-line epigastric, or in the right upper quadrant, but occasionally even in the left upper quadrant. There may be radiation of this pain round the (right) ribs to the back, or through to the back, or to the right shoulder-tip.

These features are, of course, those of acute cholecystitis (p. 324), and diagnosis is considerably easier if the patient is examined during the attack. Nevertheless, a history alone of such episodes should be confidently diagnosed as gallstones, and the patient referred to a surgical clinic.

There is a much more vague clinical presentation which is traditionally said to suggest gallstones. The patient has mild epigastric discomfort at random times, associated with abdominal distension and eructations, and sometimes heartburn. Such a patient, especially if female, fat, fertile (the mother of several children), and in her forties, and complaining that fatty foods are particularly likely to bring on the symptoms, is usually considered almost certain to have gallstones. The truth of this assertion has been challenged. There is no doubt that true fat intolerance is very rare, if the investigator searching for it makes sure that the subject cannot recognize any fat in the food he is given; and gallstones may be as common in patients without the overall picture as in patients with it. It is probably safer to err on the side of caution and send such patients for investigation, recognizing that many will not be found to have gallstones.

Peptic ulcer

For practical purposes, the less common gastric ulcer cannot be distinguished, on clinical grounds, from the much commoner duodenal variety, and both types will be discussed together as a peptic ulcer. The characteristic features are epigastric pain that comes on shortly after a meal, radiation in some cases through to the back, a burning or gnawing character, usually much less intensity than the pain of acute cholecystitis, relief by food or alkalis, and periodicity. This last point is most important because if present it is almost pathognomonic, and it is present in a high proportion of cases. The patient may go weeks or months without symptoms, and then develops pain after meals

every day for a few weeks. This bout of symptoms then settles, and he has a further remission for weeks or months.

It may take skilful questioning to elicit the relation of the pain to food. Some patients say they are scared to eat because it brings on the pain: they mean that half an hour after the meal severe symptoms develop. Other patients say they have to eat to avoid symptoms: the remission produced by the food lasts much longer in their case. In both types, pain during the taking of food is very rare, and most patients have found that, at least in the early stages of the disease, a glass of milk gives relief. In other words, the relation is not so much to food as to an empty stomach, and this explains why it is quite common for the pain to wake the patient in the early hours of the morning.

When a clinical diagnosis of a probable peptic ulcer has been made, it is good practice to get confirmation by special investigation. If the practitioner has access to suitable facilities, he can request an upper gastrointestinal tract endoscopy (a barium meal is very inferior in its power of diagnosis for peptic ulcer); otherwise, he will refer the patient to a medical out-patient clinic. If the diagnosis is confirmed, the management is either conservative or surgical as discussed later. If only a barium study was available and showed no abnormality, he has the choice of waiting to see how things go with symptomatic remedies such as antacids and antispasmodics, or referring the patient for a specialist opinion.

Reflux oesophagitis

The cardinal feature of this condition is postural heartburn; that is, a burning sensation starting in the epigastrium and radiating upwards for a variable distance behind the sternum, brought on or aggravated by stooping or lying flat. Odynophagia, i.e. pain on swallowing, is also a very important symptom.

Heartburn itself, without the postural link, is common in many patients with peptic ulcer or gallstones, or indeed with no serious underlying disease. Heartburn related to posture suggests very strongly that the mechanism at the cardia for preventing reflux of stomach contents into the oesophagus is incompetent.

If the symptom is isolated — that is, there is no suggestion of any of the other diseases discussed in this chapter — simple remedial measures are advised. The most important of these is to correct the obesity which is nearly always present. Obesity, and of course such obvious factors as tight belts and corsets, raise the intra-abdominal pressure and increase the tendency to reflux. Meals late in the evening should be avoided. The symptoms are usually severe at night, and the patient is advised to raise the head of his bed at least 12 cm. It is useless to recommend sleeping propped up on pillows, because sleepers always fall sideways off pillows during the night, and the postural symptoms start again. It is also worth reminding the patient that if his bed stands on castors, it will tend to roll forwards off the supports used to raise the head end so the castors at the foot should be wedged immobile. The patient should be strongly advised to give up smoking. Finally, antacids, particularly the kind presented as a mucilage which can be expected to coat the oesophagus with a protective lining, can be most effective in relieving acute symptoms while long-term treatment with the newer antisecretory agents, cimetidine and ranitidine, has a favourable influence.

If the symptoms fail to respond to these simple methods, or if there is a recurrence despite adequate weight reduction, the patient should be referred for specialist opinion.

Carcinoma of the stomach

This disease does not always produce pain; when it does, the pain may be similar to that of a peptic ulcer, or it may have no recognizable pattern. From the viewpoint of this Chapter, a patient who complains of epigastric pain in association with marked anorexia and weight loss should be assumed to have carcinoma of the stomach and referred for urgent specialist opinion. Many such patients will, in the event, prove to have a benign gastric ulcer, but the distinction cannot be made clinically. It must be stressed that anorexia and weight loss, without the pain, constitute sufficient grounds for a presumptive diagnosis of carcinoma of the stomach.

Carcinoma of the pancreas

This neoplasm seems to be increasing in incidence. Some reports suggested an aetiological link with a high consumption of coffee, but have received no confirmation. Like carcinoma of the stomach, it may unfortunately remain symptomless until far too advanced to cure. Also like carcinoma of the stomach, weight loss may be a prominent feature. Pain, when it occurs, is typically felt in the back, worse when the patient lies down, and relieved particularly by his adopting a squatting position.

Chronic pancreatitis

The pain of chronic pancreatitis is epigastric, it may be exacerbated by lying down and by the ingestion of alcohol, and radiation through to the back is common. However, these features are not constant, and the severity of the pain may vary widely and without any recognizable pattern. The diagnosis is suggested by such features as a history of chronic alcohol abuse, of steatorrhoea, or of diabetes mellitus. Specialist opinion is needed for such patients: both the diagnosis and the treatment of this condition may be very difficult.

The practitioner's task of making a diagnosis of one (or more) of these six conditions may be simplified by the finding of abnormal physical signs, but these will be considered in conjunction with the specialist's approach to these problems. See in particular the comment on mid-line epigastric hernia, p. 110.

An important pitfall

This Chapter has so far discussed the problem of epigastric pain, even when it is clearly related to food, without the use of the words *dyspepsia* or *indigestion*. The reason is that these words have no precise meaning, and tend to mean different things to different people. Patients may use these terms to describe any symptom related in their mind to the digestive tract, from headache to constipation. Acceptance by the doctor of these terms without probing into what the patient really means can result in serious misunderstandings and therefore misdiagnoses.

The specialist's problem

The foregoing discussion has avoided, except in one instance, defining whether the specialist to whom the case is referred should be a physician or a surgeon. On the whole the distinction is of little

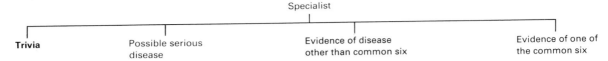

importance: it is much more important that, whether he is a physician or surgeon, he should have a special interest in gastroenterology.

If the practitioner has had access to special investigations, the diagnosis may have already been made. Otherwise, the specialist proceeds with the usual history and examination. First, with the perspective of time since the patient last consulted the practitioner, and with the benefit of special experience, the specialist sorts a group of patients who in his opinion have trivial complaints that do not warrant further investigation, and for whom reassurance and symptomatic remedies will be adequate. Anyone can make a mistake, and if he is wise he adds, in his letter to the practitioner, a rider to the effect that if the symptoms recur or persist he would be very happy to see the patient again.

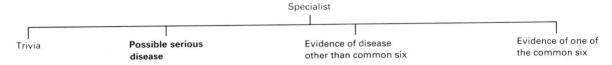

Secondly, there is a group of patients in whom the history and examination suggest that there is a serious underlying disease, but do not give a strong lead on its most likely nature. A good way of dealing with this situation is to ask the imaging department to perform an ultrasound examination, and to view the oesophagus, stomach and duodenum (if this has not already been done) with an endoscope.

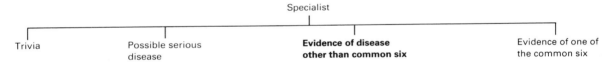

Thirdly, in a small number of patients a diagnosis will be reached different from the main group, and it is even possible that the disease diagnosed originates far from the upper abdomen. Of a wide range of possibilities, one may single out four. In the mid-line of the upper abdomen, a very localized point of tenderness that becomes more, rather than less, tender when the patient contracts his recti muscles, signifies a herniation of extraperitoneal fat through a small defect in the linea alba. A routine operation to reduce the tag of fat and repair the defect readily cures the symptoms. Epigastric pain and tenderness may be due to an abdominal aortic aneurysm (p. 114), or to tension in the capsule of a liver enlarging rapidly due to congestive cardiac failure, or inflammatory, cystic or neoplastic disease. Finally, it is important to remember that pain related to meals can result from organic disease of the large bowel, because eating a meal activates the gastrocolic reflex and the resultant peristaltic rushes in the colon may aggravate symptoms due to inflammation or partial obstruction (Chapter 12), and that the functional disorder known as 'irritable colon' can also give epigastric or right upper quadrant pain.

Further management of patients in this third group proceeds according to the individual condition diagnosed or suspected. Many of the situations are discussed elsewhere.

Finally, there is a group where the history alone, or taken in conjunction with abnormal physical findings, directs attention to either the gall bladder or the stomach and duodenum. It should be noted that a suspicion of pancreatic disease requires both ultrasound and endoscopy, because both may show features relevant to the management of the case.

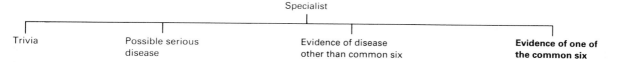

Specialist

| Trivia | Possible serious disease | Evidence of disease other than common six | **Evidence of one of the common six** |

Relevant physical signs

Signs pointing to the gall bladder include jaundice, a palpable gall bladder (p. 111), abdominal tenderness in the right upper quadrant and exacerbation of this tenderness when the subject takes a deep breath (Murphy's sign).

A palpable supraclavicular lymph node suggests a secondary deposit from a carcinoma of the stomach. Localized tenderness in the mid-line of the epigastrium also points to the stomach and duodenum rather than to the gall bladder. A gastric mass may be palpable (p. 111). Finally, there may be the signs of pyloric obstruction: visible peristalsis from left to right, often at a surprisingly low level in the abdomen; a succussion splash, a gurgling sound from the stomach contents when the patient's abdomen is gently shaken (in order to be significant, the patient should not have eaten or drunk within the previous 2 hours); and in advanced cases the signs of extracellular depletion (p. 269).

There are no relevant physical signs in patients with reflux oesophagitis, and few in patients with pancreatic disease although a pancreatic mass may very occasionally be palpable. Finally, liver palpably containing secondary deposits (p. 112) is, in the present context, most likely to have resulted from carcinoma of the pancreas or stomach, although many other primary sites are possible.

A jaundiced patient, one with severe pyloric stenosis, and anyone who looks ill, should be admitted as soon as possible. In patients with pyloric stenosis, endoscopy is hazardous because of the risk of the patient aspirating stomach contents into his respiratory passages. The stomach must be thoroughly washed out and emptied before the procedure is undertaken. The remaining patients are sent for the appropriate examinations on an outpatient basis.

Ultrasonography

This is a most valuable investigation to look for disease of the biliary apparatus and pancreas. Stones in the gall bladder, dilatation of the extrahepatic bile ducts, and masses in the region including within the pancreas itself are reliably visualized. Even a small stone in the common bile duct may be detected. Oedema of the gall bladder wall in acute cholecystitis and swelling of the pancreas in acute pancreatitis can also be demonstrated.

Oesophagogastroduodenoscopy

Examination and biopsy of the lower oesophagus to diagnose reflux oesophagitis has already been mentioned. The position of the oesophagogastric junction in relation to distance from the incisor teeth is noted. A short oesophagus implies a sliding hiatal hernia. In the stomach, the endoscopist pays particular attention first to the lesser curvature where most peptic ulcers (and many carcinomas) lie. A typical peptic ulcer has a sharp vertical ('punched out') edge, while a carcinoma has heaped edges. Several biopsy specimens are taken of the edge of any lesion: while the commonest diagnoses revealed are peptic ulcer and carcinoma of the stomach, others less common include lymphomas and benign polypoid tumours of the smooth muscle of the gastric wall, leiomyomas. Of particular importance to the surgeon is that the endoscopist can give him some idea of the extent of spread of a carcinoma, thereby enabling him to plan his operation more accurately. A well-known pitfall, however, is that there may be submucous spread of the tumour beyond its visible margins, and a stiffness of the wall of the stomach may be apparent due to deep neoplastic infiltration (linitis plastica or leather-bottle stomach).

If the gastric mucosal folds are particularly coarse, the Zollinger—Ellison syndrome is suspected (p. 104). Multiple polyposis (Menetrier's disease) may be found.

In the duodenum, an ulcer is almost certainly peptic — carcinoma of the duodenum is very rare. A distal site for the ulcer, i.e., beyond the 'duodenal bulb' region, the 2–4 cm immediately beyond the pylorus, or multiple ulcers also suggest the Z–E syndrome. However, a pair of 'kissing' ulcers, one each on anterior and posterior walls of the first part of the duodenum, are common and do not have this connotation. A diverticulum from the inner border of the curve of the second part of the duodenum is very rarely of clinical significance. The papilla of Vater is inspected and any associated abnormality biopsied.

Status of cholecystography and barium meal

Cholecystography is an obsolete investigation for the gall bladder and biliary tract. Where reliable ultrasonography is available, the test is not performed. However, it is still useful if ultrasonography is not available. The principle is that an organic iodine compound (iopanoic acid; Telepaque) is swallowed, absorbed from the gastrointestinal tract, excretred by the liver, and stored and concentrated by the gall bladder, thereby opacifying the latter to x-rays. Gallstones may be visible on the preliminary plain x-ray, typically as ring shadows because calcium salts tend to be adsorbed in high concentration on to a calcium-free nucleus. Radiolucent gallstones appear as filling defects in the opacified gall bladder.

Barium meal is an obsolescent investigation where facilities exist for upper gastrointestinal endoscopy. Its value at present lies in elucidating the anatomy of the gastric remnant and various attached loops of the intestine if the patient has undergone gastric resection elsewhere and there is inadequate information about the exact operation performed; and in delineating a hiatal hernia of the rolling or mixed type. The common *sliding* variety consists of a sliding of the cardia and upper stomach upwards through the hiatus. Much less common is the *rolling* variety, in which the stomach twists to permit a segment of the greater curve to herniate upwards through the hiatus alongside the oesophagus but the cardia maintains its position below the diaphragm. A *combined* form is also described.

After the investigations

The patients return to the out-patient clinic with the results of their endoscopy and ultrasound.

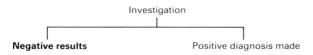

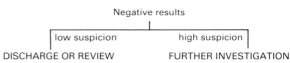

The negative results group

The specialist has the chance to reassess the patient. If his level of suspicion of serious disease was not very high anyway and the further interview yields no new information, he tries the effect of reassurance. If the patient readily accepts that there is unlikely to be anything serious amiss, he is returned to his practitioner with the usual proviso about re-referral if necessary. On the other hand, if the specialist still feels that there is a chance that serious disease is present he has the choice of asking the patient to return in perhaps a month for reappraisal and repeated investigations. The accuracy of cholecystogram and barium meals in excluding serious disease is less than 80 per cent. The choice between reappraisal and different investigations depends on whether there is any evidence suggesting a particular line of attack, and whether the facilities are available for more searching tests of the possibilities.

If the stomach and duodenum are particularly in question, gastroduodenoscopy is a powerful tool. The barium meal is not 100 per cent efficient at demonstrating peptic ulcers, and the ability to get a direct view of the whole of the inside of the stomach and the first part of the duodenum has added greatly to the accuracy of diagnosis. Oesophagoscopy and biopsy have already been discussed in the diagnosis of reflux oesophagitis, but if they fail to clinch the diagnosis further evidence may be provided by pressure measurements obtained via an open-tipped catheter swallowed by the subject. The catheter first measures the pressure in the stomach, and is then gradually withdrawn. The physiological sphincter at the lower end of the oesophagus can be recognized as a zone of high pressure, and the relationship of this zone to the level of the diaphragm can confirm the presence of a suspected hiatus hernia which radiography failed to reveal. The Bernstein test can also be useful: decinormal hydrochloric acid instilled into the mid-oesophagus via a swallowed tube may reproduce the symptoms of a patient complaining of heartburn even though a control instillation of normal saline does not. The 24-hour measurement of lower oesophageal pH is beginning to prove a valuable tool, and so is the oesophageal transit study with a radio-labelled liquid bolus.

The pancreas presents a particularly interesting problem. Clinical clues may include disturbance of pancreatic exocrine or endocrine function. With regard to exocrine function, the serum amylase level is rarely raised in chronic, as distinct from acute, pancreatic disease. Steatorrhoea — the passage of pale, greasy-looking stools with a high fat content — can be confirmed by collecting the stools for 3 days on a normal ward diet: the upper limit for normal fat excretion is 5 g/day. However, there are many causes for steatorrhoea other than pancreatic disease, and many patients with pancreatitis do not have steatorrhoea. The presence of undigested muscle fibres in the stools, recognized microscopically, is good evidence that pancreatic exocrine function is below normal. With regard to endocrine function, tests for diabetes mellitus such as the glucose tolerance test may be abnormal. At present, however, a policy of looking for anatomical rather than physiological abnormalities pays better dividends. Ultrasound and CT-scanning are equally good at demonstrating such lesions as swelling of the whole gland, a focal mass in one area, or a pseudocyst. Ultrasound is far cheaper, but more operator-dependent. Should imaging procedures indicate an abnormality, further information can be obtained with the help of endoscopy. Duodenoscopes are now available which give a direct view of the ampulla of Vater, and in the majority of patients it is possible for the endoscopist to cannulate separately the common bile duct (p. 123) and the pancreatic duct. Radiographic contrast material can then be injected along the pancreatic duct and x-rays taken: these give an accurate diagnosis of anatomical abnormalities of the pancreas such as strictures of the duct.

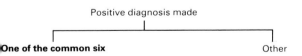

The positive results group

On the one hand, the positive results may point to an unexpected disease as being the cause of the symptoms; for example, aneurysm of the aorta or carcinoma of the colon, as already discussed. In this event the management follows the lines for those conditions, as described in other Chapters. On the other hand, it is much more likely that the diagnosis will be made of one of the six conditions emphasized in this Chapter. These are now described in order.

Gallstones

The problem with this condition is not to make the diagnosis but to decide whether to do anything about it! On the one hand there are patients who, while symptomless most of the time, have clear-cut attacks of epigastric pain lasting several hours at a time and requiring opiates for the relief of pain. On the other, there are patients with vague, chronic symptoms of flatulence, fat intolerance and epigastric discomfort, without any obvious pattern in relation to time or to external factors. The case for treatment is much stronger in the former group, where there is little doubt that the gallstones are the cause of the symptoms, than in the latter, where the gallstones are probably an incidental finding. Provided that there are no overwhelming contraindications, such as severe aortic stenosis that might unacceptably increase the risk of a general anaesthetic, patients in the former group should be advised to undergo cholecystectomy and admitted from the routine waiting list unless any features such as severe persistent pain or a recent episode of jaundice demand more urgent admission. Moreover, gall bladder calculi are liable to proceed to painful and dangerous complications: acute cholecystitis, perforation of the gall bladder with generalized peritonitis, migration of stones into the common duct with the consequent possibilities of obstructive jaundice and ascending cholangitis.

The operation of cholecystectomy is routine, although it can technically be very difficult for reasons of anatomical anomalies or the blurring of anatomy produced by fibrosis following inflammation. The crux of the operation is the demonstration of the junction of the cystic, hepatic and common ducts, so that the latter two cannot be inadvertently damaged by being mistaken for the cystic duct and therefore ligated. The cystic artery can also be awkward to secure, or the right hepatic artery mistaken for it. The major conceptual problem of the operation, however, is to decide the indications for exploration of the common bile duct. It is axiomatic that such common duct stones should be removed at the time of cholecystectomy because they are unlikely to pass the sphincter of Oddi spontaneously and because any subsequent operation to remove them is likely to be much more difficult. Stones left in the duct are a real threat to health as they may impact in the sphincter to produce obstructive jaundice, or, as foreign bodies, predispose to infection (ascending cholangitis). The classical teaching is that the duct should be explored if a stone is palpable within it, if the duct looks dilated, if the gall bladder is full of small stones, or if there has been jaundice. Experience with the technique of per-operative cholangiography during the last 20 years has proved that it is of considerable assistance in this area, since if it is properly performed and the x-rays are properly interpreted, it can accurately diagnose that the common duct does not contain stones and hence avoid many unnecessary explorations. For further details, see Hand, 1976.

The above has been a conventional account. Evidence is accumulating that an alternative approach — sphincterotomy of the papilla of Vater via the endoscopic route — has merit in selected cases. Sphincterotomy permits access to the common bile duct for endoscopic instruments with which common duct stones can be removed. Even if the stones cannot be thus removed, an adequate sphincterotomy allows them to pass spontaneously into the duodenum. Such an approach arguably does less damage to the delicate lower end of the duct than operative removal. Indeed, in the poor-risk elderly patient it might be justifiable to avoid open operation altogether, and simply to perform endoscopic sphincterotomy, although this plan does nothing to reduce the risk of acute cholecystitis itself: it simply reduces the risk of choledochal calculous complications — cholangitis and obstructive jaundice.

Peptic ulcer

Peptic ulcers, whether of stomach or duodenum, never occur in the complete absence of hydrochloric acid—*achlorhydria*. In a sense, it is difficult to understand why the acid-pepsin mixture secreted by the stomach does not digest the lining wall of the stomach and first part of the duodenum. There must be defence mechanisms that protect the wall, and a peptic ulcer probably results from any shift in the balance between acid attack and mucosal defence.

The most reliable treatment for peptic ulceration is via the reduction of acid/pepsin secretion. The H_2-receptor antagonists, e.g., cimetidine, ranitidine, can be used orally to reduce maximally stimulated gastric secretion by respectively 70 per cent, 90 per cent. On a regime of twice-daily (or even just once, in the evening) of an H_2-

antagonist, 80 per cent of patients with duodenal ulcer lose their symptoms and heal their ulcer by 4–6 weeks. The snag is that the relapse-rate is high if the antagonist is stopped. In most patients there have been recurrent symptoms by the time two years have passed.

Recurrence can usually be successfully treated again with H_2-antagonists. Thus some doctors prescribe them to be taken 'on demand', i.e., when symptoms recur. The only alternative is to take them continuously, and for an indefinite period. This raises the problem of complications of long-term medication. Cimetidine in particular can cause depression and various sex-hormone effects such as impotence and testicular atrophy.

Apart from reducing acid secretion, the only measures that have been shown to accelerate the rate of healing of a peptic ulcer are bed-rest, stopping smoking, and certain drugs such as carbenoxolone and sucralfate that are considered to increase mucosal resistance. However, surgery is the only form of treatment known to be able to cure peptic ulcer, i.e., to produce a permanent effect without a subsequent relapse. The diagnosis of peptic ulcer does not constitute, in itself, an indication for surgery. There are no precise figures available to describe what happens to a large group of patients in whom the diagnosis is made. Obviously, much depends on how ready the patients are to seek advice for their symptoms. It is generally accepted, however, that probably the majority of patients have symptoms so mild, or so transient and self-limiting, that they do not require surgery. For many others, perhaps the majority, H_2-antagonists either on demand or continuously will give adequate control.

The indications for surgery are the presence of pyloric stenosis, a history of the other serious complications of perforation and bleeding, and severe symptoms unresponsive to medical measures. It is the last category that is difficult to assess, and a sharp distinction must be made between gastric ulcer and duodenal ulcer. In practice, the possibility that a duodenal ulcer may become malignant is so remote that it can be ignored. The differentiation between a benign and a malignant gastric ulcer can be very difficult to make by gastroscopy and radiology and even by biopsy, since there is undoubtedly the possibility that a benign ulcer becomes malignant in one part of its crater, and carcinoma of the stomach is very common. A patient with a supposedly benign gastric ulcer should therefore be given the benefit of one good course of medical treatment (6 weeks of stopping smoking, and either bed-rest or a course of carbenoxolone or cimetidine) and the stomach then reassessed gastroscopically. If the ulcer persists, or later recurs, surgery should be advised.

The duodenal ulcer can be left much longer, and one cannot lay down rules for deciding when the patient should be offered surgery. Until recently it was often considered necessary to wait until the patient had so much pain that he asked for an operation, but nowadays surgery is often advised at a much earlier stage. Time off work is a good index of the severity of symptoms. A long history does not in itself constitute an indication if the symptoms are very mild, but one can at least deduce that an ulcer which has been present for 5 years is very likely to go on giving symptoms at least as severe as at the present unless surgery is undertaken.

Surgery relies on the reduction of the ability of the stomach to produce acid-pepsin when maximally stimulated, and a variety of operations have been used. The first commonly employed was gastroenterostomy, which probably worked by diluting and neutralizing the gastric contents with alkaline liquid from the duodenum, that refluxed into the stomach via the artificial stoma. This operation gave good results in the short term, but as the years passed it became clear that the incidence of recurrent ulceration was at least 40 per cent. Partial gastrectomy then became popular: in this operation the distal half to two-thirds of the stomach, including the whole of the pyloric antrum, is resected (Fig. 9.1). This removes a considerable portion of the parietal cell mass from the body of the stomach, while the sacrifice of the antrum destroys the chemical stimulatory effect upon the rest of the parietel cell mass of the antral gastrin. Partial gastrectomy gives excellent results in terms of a low recurrence rate of peptic ulceration, but it is technically difficult and is associated with a definite mortality rate around 1 per cent and unpleasant sequelae may be encountered. For these reasons the search for a better operation continued and the present fashion in many parts of the world favours some form of vagotomy.

The theoretical basis of vagotomy is that the destruction of the vagal nerve supply to the stomach prevents the stomach responding to secretory stimuli which normally follow the vagal pathway (sight and smell of food and direct contact of food with the stomach wall), and also diminishes the response of the intact parietal cell mass to chemical stimulation via the gastrin mechanism. The operation of truncal vagotomy divides the two main trunks of the vagus nerves as they lie in front of and behind the abdominal oesophagus. Early experience with this operation suggested that it produced gastric stasis with unacceptable frequency, and so it is usual to combine the operation with some procedure meant to increase the rate of gastric emptying such as gastroenterostomy or pyloroplasty.

Total truncal vagotomy denervates not only the stomach but also the intestines down to the transverse colon and the liver, gall bladder and pancreas. Since the widespread parasympathetic denervation was considered by some to be a possible cause of certain postvagotomy complications such as diarrhoea, attempts have been made to restrict the effect of a vagotomy to the whole stomach (selective vagotomy) or to the

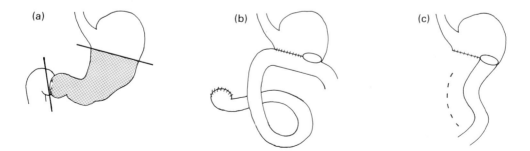

Fig. 9.1 Partial gastrectomy. (a) The shaded section, consisting of the distal two-thirds of the stomach and the proximal centimetre of the duodenum, is the average amount excised. (b) Gastrojejunal reconstruction (Billroth II or Polya). The duodenal stump is closed and a loop of jejunum anastomosed to the stomach remnant. (c) Gastroduodenal reconstruction (Billroth I). The duodenum is mobilized by incising the peritoneum lateral to its second part (Kocher's manoeuvre) and anastomosed to the cut end of the stomach.

parietel cell mass itself with preservation of the vagal innervation of the pylorus and antrum (proximal gastric or highly selective vagotomy). Since the antrum and pylorus are denervated in selective vagotomy, it is usually presumed that the same disturbance of stomach emptying noted after truncal vagotomy may occur after this operation, so it is combined with a drainage procedure. After proximal gastric vagotomy, however, it seems quite clear that no drainage procedure is necessary.

The technique of the restricted vagotomies is well worked out, but their introduction has been too recent to assess their results in terms of recurrent ulceration. For the moment it may be safest to class them as under examination.

The choice of operation in any individual with a peptic ulcer is to some extent a matter of the preference of the individual surgeon. For benign gastric ulcer, the popular procedure is a partial gastrectomy of the Billroth I type, i.e. with a gastroduodenal reconstitution. Vagotomy is used by some surgeons, but the problem of possible malignancy and the necessity of excising the ulcer completely if a negative biopsy is to be relied on to exclude carcinoma, deter most surgeons. For benign duodenal ulcer, the standard operations are: partial gastrectomy of the Billroth II type (with a gastrojejunal anastomosis), because the risk of recurrent ulceration with the Billroth I type has been found to be unacceptably high; or truncal vagotomy with a drainage procedure. The latter operation is the more common in the United Kingdom at present, but in many parts of the world partial gastrectomy still holds sway. The commonest drainage procedure used with a vagotomy is the Heineke–Mikulicz pyloroplasty, which widens the pylorus through the sewing up transversely of a longitudinal incision along the first part of a duodenum and the pyloric antrum.

A particularly intractable form of peptic ulcer diathesis, the Zollinger–Ellison syndrome, results from gastric hypersecretion in response to hypergastrinaemia produced by a tumour of gastrin-secreting cells in the pancreas. Nothing short of **total** gastrectomy prevents recurrent peptic ulceration.

Reflux oesophagitis

The simple medical measures that control most cases of reflux oesophagitis have already been described, but when these fail to control symptoms an operation should be advised if a sliding hiatus hernia has been demonstrated. There is no satisfactory treatment available if no hernia can be demonstrated, but good results are usually achieved if a sliding hernia can be repaired. The snag is that while operation is nearly always successful for a time, recurrence is very common. A large number of operations to repair a hiatus hernia have been described, a sure sign that none is very satisfactory. There is no agreement whether the operation should be done through the chest or through the abdomen. As performed by a general surgeon, the operation usually consists of reducing the hernia by pulling down the stomach; some procedure to maintain the reduced position, for example by sewing the crura together tightly around the oesophagus; and some procedure aimed at increasing the strength of the valve-like mechanism at the cardia for preventing reflux, for example fixing the fundus of the stomach in a position wrapped around the lower end of the oesophagus.

One of the problems of the assessment of the results of these operations is that the correlation between the symptoms of oesophagitis, the presence of reflux, and the presence or absence of a hiatus hernia is by no means precise. Another is that the diagnosis of recurrence of the hernia is radiologically not easy because the complex curved shape of the dome of the diaphragm is seen as a single curve on a flat x-ray plate, and it may be impossible to decide with confidence whether the stomach shadow projects above the diaphragm. This is not one of the most satisfactory fields of operative surgery.

Carcinoma of the stomach

Treatment depends greatly on the details of the anatomical position and extent of the carcinoma, signs of spread of the disease, the patient's general fitness and expectation of life apart from his cancer, his social circumstances, and so on. A few rules of general applicability can be laid down. If technical considerations permit removal of the tumour with reasonable ease and safety, this should be done even if there is no chance of cure. The relief of symptoms such as anorexia and nausea is more likely to be achieved if an ulcerated, infected mass in the stomach can be excised. Even in a palliative resection, the lines of section should be as far as feasible from the visible and palpable borders of the growth to reduce the risk of recurrence at the anastomosis because the consequent obstruction produces very distressing symptoms which may be difficult to relieve. By the same token, the anastomosis should be as wide as possible, and this excludes the Billroth I type of reconstruction which is limited by the small calibre of the duodenum. If obstruction has already occurred and the growth is irremovable, then palliation may call for a complicated bypass procedure. Finally, the tendency towards spread by the lymphatics is marked, and such spread reaches at an early stage lymph glands in vital areas such as around the coeliac axis and aorta, in the pancreas, and in the porta hepatis. For these reasons earlier enthusiasm for attempts at curative surgery have waned. It may be considered reasonable to excise the greater omentum en bloc with the stomach resection and to divide the left gastric artery far back on the posterior abdominal wall, close to its origin from the coeliac axis; but few surgeons now remove the spleen and the tail of the pancreas as a routine.

The prognosis of carcinoma of the stomach is in general bad, because this is a highly malignant tumour. However, the prognosis in the individual case is remarkably uncertain, and a few patients live for many years despite features that seem to herald a poor prognosis. Experience in Japan suggests that very early diagnosis resulting from endoscopic screening of the population may improve prognosis.

Carcinoma of the pancreas and chronic pancreatitis

It is best to consider these two diseases under a single heading, both because they can coexist and because a mass in the pancreas may be due to either and the diagnosis may remain unclear even after laparotomy.

There are five main situations.

Focal pancreatic mass
A mass in the pancreas is usually demonstrated by ultrasound or ERCP (p. 123). The diagnosis is often achieved without operation by aspiration biopsy under ultrasound control, a long slender needle being inserted through the abdominal wall and into the lesion. The needle must often on occasion traverse the bowel, but no harm seems to ensue so any leak of bowel contents into the peritoneal cavity must be very small and self-limiting. Seeding of malignant cells along the tumour track to produce tumour deposits in the abdominal wall does occur, but only infrequently, though this freedom from implantation may be due to the highly

and rapidly lethal nature of carcinoma of the pancreas so that the patient dies before the seedlings have a chance to develop.

If the cytologist is experienced, a diagnosis of carcinoma is reliable. Modern experience suggests that, except in the special case of carcinoma in the region of the papilla of Vater (these tend to be diagnosed early because they draw attention to themselves by producing obstructive jaundice and are readily diagnosed by ERCP and endoscopy) carcinoma of the pancreas is very unlikely to be curable by resection. Operations to prevent incipient jaundice (cholecystenterostomy, choledochoenterostomy) or pyloric obstruction (gastroenterostomy) may be advisable.

When the cytology does not confirm carcinoma, the situation is more difficult, but most surgeons tend towards conservatism.
Strictures, dilatations of main pancreatic ducts
Ultrasound can demonstrate dilatations of the pancreatic duct, in the best hands: otherwise, ERCP may be necessary. This picture indicates chronic pancreatitis.

There are two main aetiological factors, gallstones and alcohol abuse. In most parts of the United Kingdom, the former is much the more common, but in many countries, e.g., France, the United States, the latter dominates.

If either of these factors is present, then the first and most important line of therapy is to deal with these. Cholecystectomy is performed and stones removed from the common bile duct: the patient who abuses alcohol is advised to stop drinking. Such measures are usually successful. Even if they are not, and the symptoms continue, a conservative approach is maintained for as long as possible. Operations on these patients are not usually very rewarding. The surgeon forced to operate has a variety of procedures, though none gives reliable results.

In the subgroup of patients with familial calcific chronic pancreatitis (widespread calcification is seen in the pancreatic region in plain x-ray films), the popular procedure seems to be Puestow's: an incision is made along the whole length of the pancreas from the front, opening into the main duct, and the split pancreas is anastomosed to a long length of jejunum similarly split open. If there is a stricture near the tail end of the gland, the left part of the gland, including the stricture, is excised. For a narrowing nearer the head of the gland, the tail is excised and the remaining stump implanted into small intestine via a Roux loop. These operations are dangerous and have a high morbidity:

Flow-chart 9.1

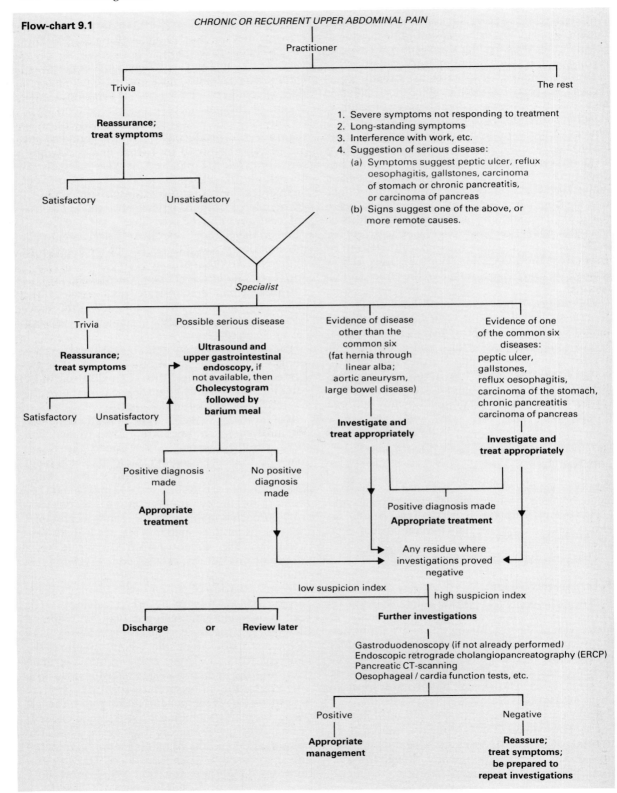

CHRONIC OR RECURRENT UPPER ABDOMINAL PAIN

Practitioner

Trivia

The rest

**Reassurance;
treat symptoms**

1. Severe symptoms not responding to treatment
2. Long-standing symptoms
3. Interference with work, etc.
4. Suggestion of serious disease:
   (a) Symptoms suggest peptic ulcer, reflux
       oesophagitis, gallstones, carcinoma
       of stomach or chronic pancreatitis,
       or carcinoma of pancreas
   (b) Signs suggest one of the above, or
       more remote causes.

Satisfactory   Unsatisfactory

Specialist

Trivia

**Reassurance;
treat symptoms**

Satisfactory   Unsatisfactory

Possible serious disease

**Ultrasound and
upper gastrointestinal
endoscopy,** if
not available, then
**Cholecystogram
followed by
barium meal**

Positive diagnosis
made

**Appropriate
treatment**

No positive
diagnosis
made

Evidence of disease
other than the
common six
(fat hernia through
linear alba;
aortic aneurysm,
large bowel disease)

**Investigate and
treat appropriately**

Evidence of one
of the common six
diseases:
peptic ulcer,
gallstones,
reflux oesophagitis,
carcinoma of the stomach,
chronic pancreatitis
carcinoma of pancreas

**Investigate and
treat appropriately**

Positive diagnosis made
Appropriate treatment

Any residue where
investigations proved
negative

low suspicion index   high suspicion index

Discharge   or   Review later

Further investigations

Gastroduodenoscopy (if not already performed)
Endoscopic retrograde cholangiopancreatography (ERCP)
Pancreatic CT-scanning
Oesophageal / cardia function tests, etc.

Positive

**Appropriate
management**

Negative

**Reassure;
treat symptoms;
be prepared to
repeat investigations**

they should be performed only in specially selected cases with strong indications, and by a surgeon with special interest in and experience of these situations. Very occasionally the whole pancreas seems to be disorganized, and if symptoms are severe enough it may be necessary to resort to the extreme step of total pancreatectomy. The patient can thereafter be maintained in a reasonable state of nutrition by very careful replacement therapy with the enzymes of pancreatic exocrine secretion together with insulin for the ensuing diabetes mellitus, but the problems of the operation and the aftercare are formidable. A recent development attacks the problem that the routine operation for resection of the head of the pancreas, whether as part of a total pancreatectomy or of the head only, say for carcinoma of the head, also removes the curve of the duodenum and the pylorus and pyloric antrum so that the tribulations of the patient after the operation are exacerbated by the dumping syndrome. It has, however, been shown to be technically feasible to remove the head of the pancreas leaving stomach and duodenum *in situ*, the so-called pylorus-preserving pancreatectomy.

Pancreas divisum
A special case of pancreatic duct stricture is when ERCP of the main pancreatic duct proves to be impossible, or can be cannulated only for a very short distance. This raises the possibility of the congenital abnormality known as pancreas divisum. The dorsal and ventral buds of the pancreas have failed to fuse, and most of the pancreas drains through the accessory pancreatic duct (of Santorini) which emerges at the duodenum at a separate accessory papilla. It seems that the drainage through Santorini's duct is often inadequate, and some of the resultant cases of chronic pancreatitis (especially if the clinical picture is one of recurrent attacks of acute pancreatitis) respond favourably to an open operation at which the opening of the accessory duct is enlarged (sphincteroplasty).

Obstructive jaundice
This presentation is discussed in Chapter 11.

Pancreatic pseudocyst

A pancreatic pseudocyst is a mass of tissue of chronic inflammatory nature containing a cavity that communicates, at the surface of the pancreas, with the pancreatic duct system. Presumably it results from rupture of a duct through the surface of the pancreas, and containment of the resultant slow leak of pancreatic exocrine secretion by reactionary tissue. It usually follows an attack of acute pancreatitis (p. 324). It may present clinically as a mass, or be diagnosed only by ultrasound or CT-scan.

The best way of dealing with this lesion, at its usual site posterior to the body of the stomach, is to anastomose it to the stomach so that the pancreatic secretions drain via the alimentary tract.

Further reading

Bainton, D., Davies, G. T., Evans, K. T. and Gravelle, I. H. (1976). Gallbladder disease: prevalence in a South Wales industrial town. *New England Journal of Medicine* **204**, 1147–9.

Cooper, M. J. and Williamson, R. C. N. (1984). Drainage operation in chronic pancreatitis. *British Journal of Surgery* **71**, 761–6.

Cotton, P. B. (1984). Endoscopic management of bile duct stones; (apples and oranges). *Gut* **25**, 587–97.

DeVries, B. C., Schattenkerk, M. E., Smith, E. E. J., Spencer, J., Jackson, D. S., Alexander-Williams, J. and Dorricott, N. J. (1983). Prospective randomized multi-centre trial of proximal gastric vagotomy or truncal vagotomy and antrectomy for chronic duodenal ulcer; results after 5–7 years. *British Journal of Surgery* **70**, 701–3.

Earlam, R. J. (1975). *Clinical Tests of Oesophageal Function*. London, Crosby, Lockwood & Staples.

Gilbertson, V. A. (1969). Results of treatment of stomach cancer. An appraisal of efforts for extensive surgery and a report of 1983 cases. *Cancer* **23**, 1305–8.

Hand, B. H. (1976). Presentation and management of stones in the common bile duct. In: *Current Surgical Practice*, Vol. 1, pp. 114–31. Ed. by G. J. Hadfield and M. Hobsley. London, Edward Arnold.

Hobsley, M. (1978). Problems after gastric surgery. In: *Current Surgical Practice,* Vol. 2, pp 20–38. Ed by G. J. Hadfield and M. Hobsley. London, Edward Arnold.

Hobsley, M. (1981). Dumping and diarrhoea. *British Journal of Surgery* **68,** 681–4.

Johnston, D. (1976). Modern surgical attitudes to peptic ulceration. In: *Current Surgical Practice,* Vol. 1, pp. 73–114. Ed. by G. J. Hadfield and M. Hobsley. London, Edward Arnold.

Lundh, G., Burn, J. I. and Kolig, G. (1974). A cooperative international study of gastric cancer. *Annals of the Royal College of Surgeons of England* **54,** 219–28.

Price, W. H. (1963). Gallbladder dyspepsia. *British Medical Journal* **2,** 138–41.

Rogers, I. M., Moule, B., Sokhi, G. S., Joffe, S. N. and Blumgart, L. H. (1976). Endoscopy and routine and double-contrast barium meal in diagnosis of gastric and duodenal disorders. *Lancet* **i,** 901–2.

Russell, R. C. G., Wong, N. W. and Cotton, P. B. (1984) Accessory sphincterotomy (endoscopic and surgical) in patients with pancreas divisum. *British Journal of Surgery* **71,** 954–7.

Trapnell, J. E. (1976). Pancreatitis: acute and chronic. In: *Current Surgical Practice,* Vol. 1, pp. 132–48. Ed. by G. J. Hadfield and M. Hobsley. London, Edward Arnold.

Chapter 10

Palpable Abdominal Mass

A palpable abdominal mass must be presumed to be due to serious abdominal disease unless the doctor is certain that the mass is a normal abdominal viscus.

General considerations

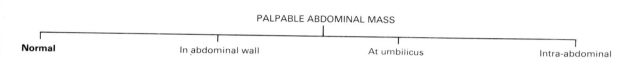

PALPABLE ABDOMINAL MASS

Normal   In abdominal wall   At umbilicus   Intra-abdominal

Normal abdominal masses

The normal bladder becomes palpable in everyone if it is sufficiently distended by retained urine. The lower pole of the right kidney is sometimes, of the left kidney rarely, palpable. In a thin person with ill-developed musculature, the abdominal aorta is palpable in the epigastrium. In infants, for a variable period of a few days or weeks after birth, the normal liver is palpable in the upper abdomen. In complete health the intestines cannot be felt direct, but pressure over a loop that happens to be distended with gas and liquid gives a typical squashy sensation and a squelching noise, while faeces in a loop may be palpable in a thin and costive patient. In no other circumstances (apart from pregnancy) should a palpable abdominal mass be assumed to be normal.

Status of the liver

Except in neonates, the list above did not include normal liver. This omisson is contrary to standard teaching. It is often taught that the normal liver is quite often palpable, 'depending upon how far it happens to project downwards below the costal margin'. Every abdominal surgeon knows from the experience of laparotomy that, in the patient lying supine, the liver projects well below the costal margin in the vast majority of patients, so that this projection in itself is unlikely to be the cause of the palpability of the normal liver in the small minority claimed by the standard view. In terms of physical science, the reason for being able to feel structure B through structure A is that B is firmer than A: the mere presence of B deep to A is not sufficient. Doubters are advised to experiment, with the aid of a friendly butcher, a slice of liver and a portion of steak.

The explanation for the error in the standard teaching is the presence of a fibrous intersection running transversely through the rectus muscle at about the level of the tip of the ninth costal cartilage. This may be mistaken for the edge of the liver, especially as it will tend to become more prominent as the rectus contracts during deep inspiration. If in doubt, one should feel in the symmetrical position over the *left* rectus sheath. It will then become obvious that the 'liver edge' is a horizontal line running between the two costal margins.

Normal liver is palpable in the neonate probably because of the high proportion of firmer reticuloendothelial tissue in the neonate compared with the adult.

Site

Most palpable abdominal swellings can be classified according to their site into one of the following categories: hernial orifices including the umbilicus, right upper quadrant, left upper quadrant, mid-line epigastric, right lower quadrant, left lower quadrant and suprapubic. A minority cannot be assigned to any one of these sites and must remain unclassified.

Before dealing with each site in turn, the significance of two important physical signs must be discussed. A third, the equally important sign of cough impulse, is discussed on p. 10.

Abdominal wall or intra-abdominal?

The importance of making this decision is frequently overlooked, with consequent stupid misdiagnoses. When the patient contracts his abdominal muscles, an intra-abdominal swelling becomes less prominent or disappears while a mass in the abdominal wall becomes firmer and more obvious.

For approximately mid-line swellings, the patient is asked to lift his head off the bed without the aid of propping himself up on his elbows: this causes maximal contraction in the recti. For more lateral masses, all the muscles of the anterior abdominal wall should be brought into play by asking the patient to strain.

Movement with respiratory excursions

The patient is asked to take deep breaths in and out, and the lower margin of the swelling is carefully observed and palpated to determine whether it moves downwards during inspiration and upwards with expiration. This sign is easy to elicit but often more difficult to interpret. The simple interpretation is that the mass is, or arises in, some abdominal viscus that is in contact with the diaphgram, so that it is constrained to move with the excursions of the latter. This statement must be modified by the considerations that the part of the organ connecting the mass with the under-surface of the diaphragm must be rigid enough to transmit the thrust, and that the mass will move with ventilation if it is in indirect contact with the diaphragm via another interposed organ which is rigid enough to transmit the thrust. The relevance of these considerations will be discussed under various upper abdominal swellings. Those which move with respiration are more likely to be diagnosable from clinical signs than those which do not.

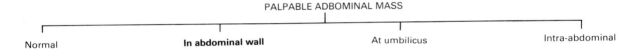

PALPABLE ADBOMINAL MASS

Normal   **In abdominal wall**   At umbilicus   Intra-abdominal

Lumps of the anterior abdominal wall

Lumps superficial to the muscles, i.e. in the skin and subcutaneous tissues, may be of the same nature as lesions occurring in the skin and subcutaneous tissues elsewhere (p. 16), i.e. lipoma, fibroma, etc. Most are demonstrably free of the underlying muscle, and their management is straightforward along the lines of biopsy and excision in the first instance. There are also some lesions which are specific to the anterior abdominal wall, and for the most part these show evidence of attachment to the muscle layer. These consist of hernias and certain umbilical lesions.

Hernias

These occur when the scar of an abdominal incision is weak (incisional hernia), or at specific hernial orifices — that is, places where the musculature of the abdominal wall is normally defective and the gap is closed only by fibrous tissue. The common groin hernias are discussed in Chapter 13. The mid-line raphe of the linea alba may stretch, especially in obese elderly patients with poorly developed muscles, resulting in the lesion known as divarication of the recti. The lateral border of the rectus musucle is also a point of potential weakness, especially in the lower third of the abdomen where it has no posterior sheath, and a hernia coming through between the rectus and the lateral abdominal muscles is called a Spigelian hernia, a rare entity. The very rare lumbar hernia protrudes through the space between the quadratus lumborum and the transversus abdominis muscles. The umbilicus is an obvious site of weakness, and two different kinds of hernia occur. One is a persistence of the fetal prolongation of the peritoneum through the umbilical scar. This true umbilical hernia is common in infants at birth as a relatively small bulge, and requires no treatment except reassurance of the mother, because it is a self-limiting condition that always undergoes spontaneous cure, usually by the age of 2 years and certainly by 5. (In the negro race spontaneous resolution does not always occur and an operation may become necessary). There is a much more severe form of this defect, exomphalos, in which the neonate's whole abdominal contents may lie outside the umbilicus. This rare situation demands difficult surgery to achieve skin cover for the viscera. The second form of hernia at the umbilicus protrudes through a defect in the linea alba very close to, but not actually through, the umbilical scar. This is the paraumbilical hernia, common in the elderly obese subject, and it requires formal operation for its cure.

These hernias are easy to diagnose when there is no question of strangulation, by means of their expansile cough impulse. Those with a narrow neck, such as the paraumbilical, are much more likely to become strangulated than those with a broad neck, such as a divarication of the recti. All (except the true umbilical) are best managed by surgical repair, but an abdominal supportive belt may be reasonable treatment for a broad-necked hernia in a patient in whom there are medical contraindications to operation.

See p. 98 for the fatty hernia of the linea alba.

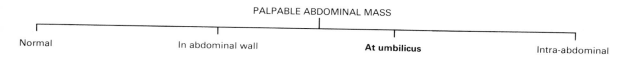

Umbilical nodules

Apart from hernias, umbilical nodules include a granuloma in the neonate resulting from low-grade infection of the stump of the umbilical cord, a primary tumour, or secondary deposit from an intra-abdominal neoplasm. Faulty toilet may result in a nodule of foreign material that can give rise to mistakes in diagnosis.

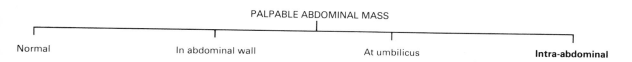

Intra-abdominal masses

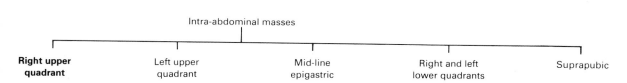

Right upper quadrant

If the mass moves with ventilation, the likely possibilities are liver, kidney, and gall bladder. The liver and kidney are rigid organs in contact with the diaphragm. The gall bladder is normally soft and supple, but distension of this organ as a result of obstruction of the biliary passages results in sufficient enlargement for it to come into contact with the abdominal wall, sufficient firmness for it to become palpable through the muscles, and sufficient rigidity for its lower border to be forced downwards as the liver itself descends. A mass in the region of the pylorus or the porta hepatis — for example, a carcinoma of the antrum or a mass of secondary carcinoma in the lymph nodes of the free edge of the lesser omentum — may also be sufficiently mobile and sufficiently in contact with the under-surface of the liver to move.

The characteristic feature of the liver is its thin, sharp, inferior border, where its anterior and inferoposterior surfaces meet: this margin may be blurred by the disease affecting the liver, but it is nearly always sufficiently distinct to aid the diagnosis. By contrast, the gall bladder and the lower pole of the kidney have no definite edge; their lower aspect is a smooth hemisphere. The kidney is always palpable in the loin, and can be ballotted between two hands, one on the anterior abdominal wall and the other behind the patient in contact with the loin. The gall bladder is an anterior structure and therefore not palpable in the loin. The liver and gall bladder are dull to percussion, but the kidney is resonant. The mass in the gastric antrum or nearby is rarely recognized as such on physical examination. The conclusion is usually reached that it is a prominent nodule of secondary neoplasm in the lower border of the liver because this is a commoner explanation of these physical findings, the rest of the liver being normal and therefore impalpable.

Masses in the right upper quadrant that do not move with respiration may arise in the hepatic flexure and neighbouring segments of the large bowel, the duodenum or head of pancreas, the small bowel and its mesentery, or in structures such as lymph nodes on the posterior abdominal wall. Of these possibilities, masses arising in the small bowel and mesentery are likely to be mobile, but the others are retroperitoneal structures that are bound down to the posterior abdominal wall and therefore fixed. It should be added here that fixity can be a secondary phenomenon: a mass with the general characteristics of an enlarged kidney may be fixed because the carcinoma of the kidney has spread to involve the posterior abdominal wall. Apart from the guide given by overall mobility, it is unlikely that physical examination will help further in the diagnosis of the masses that do not move on respiration.

The further management of masses diagnosed as hepatic, cholecystic or renal follows. The obscure case is discussed at the end of this Chapter.

Liver

A smooth and uniformly palpable liver suggests that it is engorged with blood or bile, or diffusely infiltrated with new growth. An increased content of blood may arise from congestive cardiac failure, in which case the usual symptoms and signs of that condition, including a raised jugular venous pressure, should be identifiable, or from portal hypertension (p. 277). Engorgement with bile implies jaundice (p. 122). Infiltrations include reticuloses and some unusual diseases of unknown aetiology such as Hand—Schüller—Christian disease in which granulomatous lesions develop with a proliferation of histiocytes. The diagnosis of these conditions depends upon liver biopsy, and this may be obtained by aspiration needle or at laparotomy, depending upon whether such features as enlarged lymph nodes or spleen, an abnormal leucocyte count or bone marrow findings suggest a generalized reticulosis.

A finely nodular liver suggests biliary cirrhosis, but the patient is then jaundiced. A coarsely nodular liver suggests Laennec's cirrhosis (hobnail liver; alcoholic cirrhosis) or multiple secondary deposits. A history of chronic alcoholism or the stigmata of liver failure point to the former; replacement of liver tissue by malignant deposits has to proceed almost to completion before hepatic failure results. If secondaries are suspected, a careful search is made for a primary in the statistically likely areas: breast in women, bronchus in men, and stomach and colon in both sexes. The clinching of the diagnosis will be by biopsy, probably by aspiration for the likely cirrhotic, by laparotomy (or laparoscopy with needle biopsy) for the case with a possible intra-abdominal carcinoma.

A palpable solitary mass in the liver is either basically inflammatory, in which case the patient is usually gravely ill, or neoplastic. The inflammatory type of lesion includes pyogenic abscess and amoebic abscess, while the well patient group includes primary neoplasm (hepatoma), secondary neoplasm, a congenital cyst or a hydatid cyst. In an ill patient who has at any time been in a country where amoebic disease is endemic, it is worth trying a course of antiamoeba treatment while the bacteriologists are trying to grow pyogenic organisms from venous blood samples. A suspected liver abscess must be explored and drained. It is worth mentioning that there is often a septic source such as an appendix or subphrenic abscess which needs to be drained as well. In a well patient, evidence of hydatid disease should always be sought by the Casoni or the complement fixation test or both. If these tests are negative, neoplasia becomes the most likely diagnosis. Primary hepatoma is rare in Britain, although common in certain parts of the world such as China, South Africa and Malaysia, where it is associated with hepatitis B. Moreover, when it does occur in Britain, it is nearly always in a cirrhotic liver and multicentric, and therefore unlikely to be amenable to treatment by surgery. The distribution of the branches of the hepatic artery, visualized by aortography, may give information prior to laparotomy about whether a resection is likely to be feasible. Radioactive scanning, CT-scanning and ultrasonography do not seem to be very helpful techniques in the investigation of hepatic masses, and the final diagnosis of all these cases usually requires laparotomy.

Gall bladder

If the patient is not jaundiced, the cystic duct is obstructed by a stone and cholecystectomy is indicated (p. 101). Usually, but not always, there has been a history of acute cholecystitis, and when the gall bladder is removed it is found to contain pus (empyema of the gall bladder) or mucus (mucocele). If the patient shows the features of obstructive jaundice, the likely cause of the obstruction is a carcinoma at the lower end of the bile duct, arising from the ampulla of Vater or the head of the pancreas (p. 123). For investigations and management, see Chapter 12.

Kidney

Remember that the normal right kidney may be palpable. However, if there is a history of any symptom referable to the urinary tract, or any feature of the lump that seems abnormal (e.g. tenderness, size or irregularity), further investigation is necessary. In the first instance this comprises a blood count and haemoglobin estimation, blood urea, ultrasonography and an intravenous pyelogram. The possible diagnoses may be categorized as obstructive, neoplastic or congenital, and considerable help may be derived from whether or not the other kidney is also palpable. Bilateral abnormalities suggest congenital anomalies such as polycystic kidneys or horseshoe kidney, or else obstruction of the lower urinary tract (bladder and below) where a single locus of obstruction produces back-pressure in both upper renal tracts. If the abnormality is confined to one side, any obstructive lesion must be in the upper tract on that side and neoplasia becomes a possibility. The blood count may show an iron-deficiency anaemia due to a bleeding lesion, but it may also show the polycythaemia which may sometimes be produced by excessive secretion of erythropoietin by a renal carcinoma. The blood urea is important as a reasonably accurate index of renal function.

Often these investigations result in a diagnosis that is sufficiently accurate to decide treatment. Sometimes further investigations are necessary, and the commonly useful ones are the aortogram (with examination of the renal arteries and their distribution), renal isotope scanning, and cystoscopy and retrograde pyelography. Further details of the management of the conditions diagnosed are given in Chapter 15.

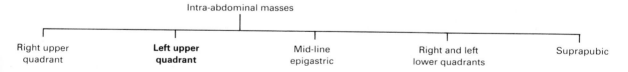

Intra-abdominal masses — Right upper quadrant — **Left upper quadrant** — Mid-line epigastric — Right and left lower quadrants — Suprapubic

Left upper quadrant

In this quadrant a mass that moves with respiration arises from liver, kidney or spleen, while one that does not probably arises from colon, small bowel, mesentery, or lymph nodes, etc., of the posterior abdominal wall.

Compared with the characteristics of the liver and kidney, which have already been detailed, the spleen has a fairly sharp inferior border and is dull to percussion, so that it is unlikely to be confused with the kidney. More difficulty may arise in distinguishing spleen from liver. If the liver is palpable in the right upper quadrant as well as in the left, one can usually follow its lower border across the mid-line of the abdomen to demonstrate that what is palpable to the left of the mid-line is one and the same swelling as that to the right. Occasionally, a mass in the left lobe of the liver projects downwards and is palpable only to the left of the mid-line while the right upper quadrant feels normal, and in these circumstances liver may easily be mistaken for spleen. The spleen is said to move downwards and to the right on deep inspiration, rather than just downwards, and if one can feel the characteristic notch halfway along the inferior border there can be no doubt but that the mass is spleen. Particular difficulty may be experienced when the spleen and liver are simultaneously palpable, a not uncommon event in the reticuloses and portal hypertension.

Further management if the lump is kidney or liver has already been described. In cases of splenic enlargement, one proceeds by examining the peripheral blood for evidence of excessive haemolysis, of infections, including such parasitic ones as malaria, or of reticulosis, by looking for evidence of portal hypertension (p. 277), and if necessary by further investigation of the reticuloendothelial system by biopsy of any palpable lymph nodes and by lymphangiography.

Management of reticuloses

The pathology of these conditions is complex, and most aspects of their management lie in the province of the radiotherapist or the physician with a special interest in oncology. The surgeon is not usually an expert in the pathological niceties or the details of radio- or chemotherapy, but in recent years his importance in the therapeutic team has increased. The main reason is the realization that, with effective and thorough treatment, the prognosis of many of the diseases in the general group of reticuloses is not as bad as used to be thought. Many respond excellently to either or both of the available forms of treatment: radiotherapy or chemotherapy. Recent advances in the latter include triple therapy — the use of three different agents in combined courses may be dramatically more effective than each one given separately. It seems to be important, however, that the whole area involved in the disease is accurately mapped out from the beginning and treated. It used not to be appreci-

ated that a patient presenting with a solitary palpable lymph node, say in the neck, might have demonstrable intra-abdominal disease of the same type without any symptoms or signs. The surgeon's services are therefore in demand to remove lymph nodes from various peripheral sites (i.e. neck, axilla, groin) and to perform laparotomy, splenectomy, and biopsy of the liver and of the lymph nodes on the posterior abdominal wall. This aggressive policy has been found to pay dividends, especially for example in Hodgkin's disease. When the exact extent of spread of the disease is accurately known, the precise details of radiotherapy or chemotherapy, or of a combination of the two, can be decided. Where a good imaging service is available (ultrasound and particularly CT-scanning), the surgeon's rôle is much less important.

Excessive haemolysis

Evidence of this condition is provided by a low haemoglobin concentration, a raised reticulocyte count, and an increased concentration of prehepatic bilirubin in the plasma. Excessive destruction of erythrocytes may be due to excessive haemolytic activity by the spleen or to abnormally fragile red cells. In the situation we are discussing of an enlarged spleen, it is probable that the spleen is at fault (hypersplenism), and the aetiology may be any of the diseases which can cause an enlargement of the spleen. However, the possibility that the red cells are abnormal may need investigation by direct measurement of their fragility when exposed to saline of various concentrations, and by seeking any antibody coating the cells by the Coombs' test. Expert haematological advice should always be sought.

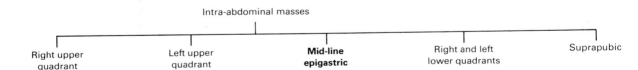

Mid-line epigastric

Masses in the mid-line of the epigastrium that move with respiration are either spleen, liver or, occasionally, a mass in the pyloric region of the stomach, and all these have received consideration. Of the important epigastric masses that do not move with respiration, only one can be di-

agnosed confidently from its clinical characteristics — the aneurysm of the abdominal aorta. This presents as a vertical longitudinal mass extending downwards from the costal margin to about the region of the umbilicus, and exhibiting expansile pulsation in time with the pulse beat elsewhere. It is important to emphasize that the pulsation must be demonstrably expansile: that is, while the anterior surface moves forwards, the right margin of the mass moves to the right and the left margin to the left. Any epigastric mass may conduct the impulse of the underlying aorta to the examiner's hand as a thrust which moves forwards over the whole area (transmitted pulsation). Only from the aorta itself will expansile pulsation be received. Remember that it is normal to be able to feel the pulsation of the aorta in the epigastrium, and that in a thin subject it is normal to be able to feel the aorta itself. The dividing line between a normally palpable aorta and an aneurysm is usually set at a width of 5 cm, but the clinical decision can be difficult.

Help with this decision is obtained by looking at a lateral view of the abdomen in a plan x-ray. An aneurysm of the abdominal aorta is always visible as the calcified shadow of its anterior and posterior walls (Fig. 10.1). Aortography is practically never necessary in making the diagnosis, and indeed may be misleading because much of the lumen may be obliterated by clot. Ultrasound is an excellent technique for demonstrating the precise anatomy of the lesion.

The management of an abdominal aortic aneurysm depends upon a number of features.

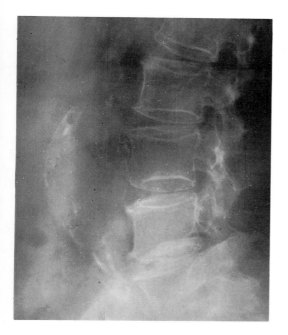

Fig. 10.1 Lateral plain radiograph of the abdomen, showing calcification in the wall of an aneurysm of the abdominal aorta, anterior to the lumbar vertebrae. (Radiograph kindly provided by Mr Adrian Marston)

First, has the patient had any symptoms suggestive of impending rupture? Central abdominal pain or backache or both must be taken seriously, and are likely to outweigh most contraindications. Embolic episodes affecting the lower limits have a similar significance. Acute symptoms (pain, shock, etc.; p. 273) indicate urgent laparotomy, without time for further investigations. In non-urgent cases, as accurate an estimate of the risk of surgery as possible must be obtained; it is here that it may become necessary to delineate the exact anatomy of the aneurysm by ultrasonography.

The most important evidence to be gained from ultrasonography is the upper limit of the aneurysm. If this lies above the level of the renal arteries, the aneurysm must, under ordinary circumstances, be considered inoperable. During the operation to excise an aneurysm of the abdominal aorta, that vessel must be clamped above and below the lesion while the latter is excised and a prosthesis sewn into place. A clamp above the renal arteries stops the blood supply to the kidneys, and fatal ischaemia would result during the length of time needed for the operation. Special techniques, such as bypassing the clamp with an artificial circulation to the kidneys, is occasionally possible, but such a technique adds considerably to the already appreciable risks of this sort of major vascular surgery. Dacron grafts for replacing the renal arteries are available, but very expensive. Alternatively, the renal arteries can be preserved after division from the aneurysm, and reimplanted into the dacron aortic prosthesis.

The lower extent of the aneurysm is much less important, since prostheses are available which terminate below in a bifurcation into two cylinders, the 'trousers' graft, for ready anastomosis to the common iliac arteries should the aneurysm involve the bifurcation of the aorta. However, aortography also helps to quantify the risk of operating by showing whether the arterial tree remote from the aneurysm is heavily affected by atheroma. This point has a bearing on the likelihood of successfully suturing the prosthesis into place, and also warns if the disease is generalized, and if therefore the patient's prognosis from the viewpoint of other manifestations of arterial disease such as cardiac infarction is very poor. An assessment of cardiac function, with ECG and chest x-ray, is mandatory and then other more complicated investigations may be required, such as coronary angiography and the so-called muga-scan — a radiolabel technique that measures the ejection-fraction of the left ventricle. Evidence of cerebral

Flow-chart 10.1   *PALPABLE ABDOMINAL MASS*

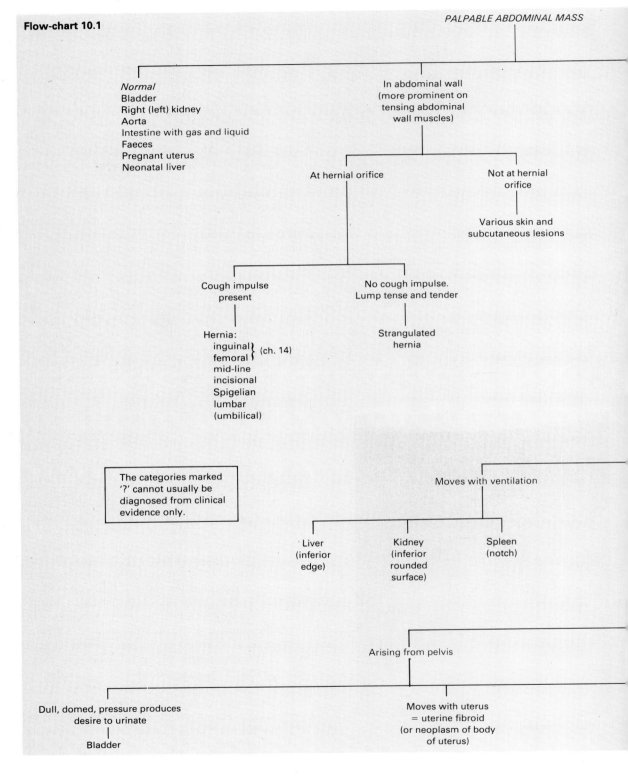

Normal
Bladder
Right (left) kidney
Aorta
Intestine with gas and liquid
Faeces
Pregnant uterus
Neonatal liver

In abdominal wall
(more prominent on
tensing abdominal
wall muscles)

At hernial orifice

Not at hernial
orifice

Various skin and
subcutaneous lesions

Cough impulse
present

No cough impulse.
Lump tense and tender

Hernia:
  inguinal ⎫ (ch. 14)
  femoral ⎭
  mid-line
  incisional
  Spigelian
  lumbar
  (umbilical)

Strangulated
hernia

The categories marked
'?' cannot usually be
diagnosed from clinical
evidence only.

Moves with ventilation

Liver
(inferior
edge)

Kidney
(inferior
rounded
surface)

Spleen
(notch)

Arising from pelvis

Dull, domed, pressure produces
desire to urinate

Bladder

Moves with uterus
= uterine fibroid
(or neoplasm of body
of uterus)

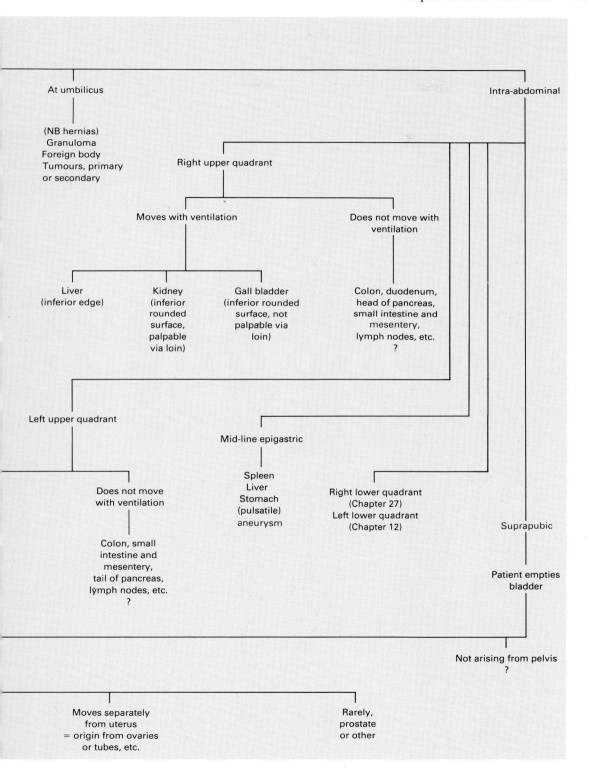

At umbilicus

(NB hernias)
Granuloma
Foreign body
Tumours, primary
or secondary

Right upper quadrant

Intra-abdominal

Moves with ventilation

Does not move with
ventilation

Liver
(inferior edge)

Kidney
(inferior
rounded
surface,
palpable
via loin)

Gall bladder
(inferior rounded
surface, not
palpable via
loin)

Colon, duodenum,
head of pancreas,
small intestine and
mesentery,
lymph nodes, etc.
?

Left upper quadrant

Mid-line epigastric

Does not move
with ventilation

Spleen
Liver
Stomach
(pulsatile)
aneurysm

Right lower quadrant
(Chapter 27)
Left lower quadrant
(Chapter 12)

Suprapubic

Colon, small
intestine and
mesentery,
tail of pancreas,
lymph nodes, etc.
?

Patient empties
bladder

Not arising from pelvis
?

Moves separately
from uterus
= origin from ovaries
or tubes, etc.

Rarely,
prostate
or other

ischaemia or carotid obstruction must also be carefully sought. The natural history of an aneurysm of the abdominal aorta is that it gradually grows, with an increasing threat of rupture, so that there is a good case for operation. However, it is only after all the evidence has been collected that a rational decision can be made.

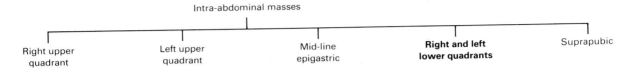

Intra-abdominal masses

| Right upper quadrant | Left upper quadrant | Mid-line epigastric | **Right and left lower quadrants** | Suprapubic |

Both lower quadrants

Masses in the right lower quadrant are considered on p. 331. Masses in the left lower quadrant are considered in Chapter 12.

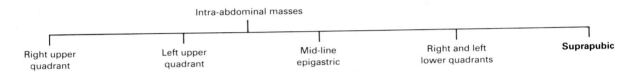

Intra-abdominal masses

| Right upper quadrant | Left upper quadrant | Mid-line epigastric | Right and left lower quadrants | **Suprapubic** |

Suprapubic

One situation relatively easy to assess is that the mass arises from the pubic bone. Radiology followed by biopsy usually indicates that the lesion is neoplastic, although the non-specific inflammatory condition called osteitis pubis may occasionally present in this way. An orthopaedic opinion is usually advisable in this group of cases.

If the lump is not attached to bone, the next question to ask is, can one get below the swelling or does it arise from the pelvis? Masses emerging from the pelvis are likely to be the urinary bladder, an ovarian cyst, a uterine fibroid or, much less commonly, an enlargement of other pelvic structures such as the prostate or rectum. The bladder is usually recognized as dull to percussion, of a typical domed shape, and as arousing in the patient the desire to micturate when the examiner presses gently on the overlying anterior abdominal wall. If there have been no symptoms referable to micturition, the patient is asked to pass his water and the lump should then have disappeared. Note, however, that a large diverticulum of the bladder may be still palpable, because the wall of such a diverticulum contains no muscle so that the act of micturition may even make it larger by transferring urine from the contracting bladder to the diverticulum!

Whether or not one thinks the mass is a bladder, it is wise to ask the patient to micturate before completing the examination. The physical signs may seem very different afterwards.

Pelvic examination via the rectum, vagina, or both is required for differentiating the other masses arising from the pelvis. Bimanual palpation determines whether the mass moves with the uterus, and is therefore likely to be a fibroid or, less commonly, a neoplasm of the body of the uterus, or whether it moves independently of the uterus and therefore is likely to originate in the ovaries, tubes or related structures. Other rarer sites of origin are also identified during this examination.

The ovarian cyst requires two other comments. First, students often find it difficult to understand how an ovary, which is one of a pair of bilaterally disposed structures, can give rise to the mid-line swelling of an ovarian cyst. The answer lies in the fact that each ovary only lies a few centimetres from the mid-line, and that as the organ enlarges it can only emerge from the pelvis to become palpable through the abdomen when it is so large that all evidence of its unilateral origin is obscured, especially as the brim of the pelvis through which the tumour emerges lies symmetrically about the mid-line. Secondly, an ovarian cyst may grow to such a large size, and be so soft in consistency, that its physical signs can be confused with the fluid thrill and shifting dullness of ascites. In the difficult case a plain x-ray of the abdomen reveals whether the gas shadows of the small bowel are displaced to the upper abdomen by a huge tumour, or whether they are disposed as usual all over the abdominal cavity, but rather separated from one another by the ascitic fluid. Ultrasound is also valuable here.

The management of lesions of the female reproductive organs is the province of the gynaecologist, while the enlarged bladder is discussed elsewhere (pp. 174 and 228).

The difficult case

Essentially this section comprises masses in the upper or mid-abdomen that do not move on respiration, and masses in the suprapubic region that do not arise from the pelvis. All such lesions have in common the fact that physical signs are most unlikely to be sufficient to enable a firm diagnosis to be reached. In these circumstances the history may be invaluable in directing attention to the organ of origin, but failing a lead from the history one proceeds by bearing the following considerations in mind.

First, if the mass is mobile it is likely to arise from structures which normally possess a mesentery; i.e. the gastrointestinal tract, excluding the duodenum, the ascending and descending colon, and the hepatic and splenic flexures of the colon. If the mass is fixed, the possibilities are that it was originally mobile but has become secondarily attached by inflammation or tumour growth, or that it arises in retroperitoneal parts of the gastrointestinal tract, including the pancreas, or other structures fixed to the posterior abdominal wall such as lymph nodes.

Secondly, ultrasonography is the investigation statistically most likely to give diagnostic information if the nature of the swelling cannot be deduced from physical examination. Next in importance are endoscopy of the alimentary tract and then opaque meal radiology.

Thirdly, it is difficult to get a view of the whole of both kidneys during the laparotomy, and therefore an exploratory laparotomy should always be preceded by an ultrasound examination and if necessary an intravenous pyelogram to exonerate the kidneys.

Fourthly, ultrasonography and CT-scanning of such organs as the pancreas are very helpful, but angiograms of the major abdominal visceral arteries such as the hepatic, coeliac, and superior and inferior mesenteric may yield valuable clues in expert hands.

Finally, preliminary investigations should not be prolonged indefinitely; an undiagnosed intra-abdominal swelling must be subjected to diagnostic laparotomy at some time, and preferably while it is still amenable to treatment!

Further reading

Bearn, J. G. and Pilkington, T. R. E. (1959). Organs palpable in the normal adult abdomen. *Lancet* **ii**, 212–13.

Ralphs, D. N. L., Venn, G., Palmer, G. J., Cameron, D. E. and Hobsley, M. (1983). Is the undeniably palpable liver ever 'normal'? *Annals of the Royal College of Surgeons of England* **65**, 160–61.

Chapter 11

Jaundice

Jaundice is defined as a yellow discoloration of the skin and mucous membranes due to staining with bilirubin in the presence of a plasma concentration greater than 18 μmol/litre (1 mg/100 ml).

Adult jaundice

Physiology of bilirubin

The management of a patient with jaundice hinges upon a clear understanding of the physiology of the excretion of bilirubin.

Aged erythrocytes are broken down in the reticuloendothelial system, particularly the spleen, and their haemoglobin is converted into bilirubin. This unconjugated bilirubin is insoluble in water, and is transported in the plasma by being bound to albumin. On reaching the liver, the unconjugated bilirubin is taken up by two proteins, Y and Z, and transported through the liver cell. In the cell, bilirubin is conjugated to form bilirubin diglucuronide, a reaction catalysed by the enzyme bilirubin UDP glucuronyl transferase. Conjugated bilirubin is water-soluble.

The conjugated bilirubin passes into the biliary canaliculi and thence via the biliary tree into the duodenum. In the lumen of the small intestine the conjugation is split by bacterial glucuronidases, the unconjugated bilirubin is reduced to urobilinogen, and some of this is reabsorbed but the remainder is excreted in the faeces. The reabsorbed urobilinogen is partly re-excreted via the liver and partly excreted by the kidneys. Urine therefore normally contains a little urobilinogen, but no bilirubin because unconjugated (prehepatic) bilirubin is bound to albumin and insoluble in water. Faeces likewise normally contain a small quantity of urobilinogen (usually called stercobilinogen in faeces).

Disturbances of the excretion may occur at any point along the pathway described. The main subdivision of cases of adult jaundice, because the easiest to make, depends upon whether the bilirubin present in the plasma in excess of 18 μmol/litre (1 mg/100 ml) is unconjugated, or whether an appreciable proportion is conjugated. In the former case, either the load of bilirubin being presented to the liver in unconjugated form is excessive, or the processes of transport through the liver cell or conjugation are deficient. There is no bilirubin in the urine, and this group is therefore called acholuric jaundice. On the other hand, if there is much conjugated bilirubin in the plasma, the reason must be some interference with the mechanism of passage from the liver cells along the bile ducts, and such cases are called cholestatic jaundice. The conjugated bilirubin formed within the liver cells regurgitates back into the plasma and, since it is water-soluble, appears in the urine. The examination of the urine for bilirubin and the identification of unconjugated and conjugated forms of bilirubin in the plasma are therefore the important observations needed to divide the patients into these two groups.

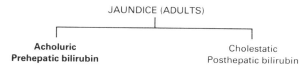

JAUNDICE (ADULTS)

Acholuric
Prehepatic bilirubin

Cholestatic
Posthepatic bilirubin

Acholuric jaundice

Haematological investigations are the key to management of this group of patients. If there is excessive haemolysis, it may be possible to demonstrate an excess of free haem pigment in the plasma or a reduced life-span of the erythrocytes. Usually these refinements are unnecessary: a low haemoglobin concentration and an increased reticulocyte count are sufficient evidence if a reason for increased haemolysis can be demonstrated. Such conditions include abnormalities of the red cell, such as the spherocytes of congenital spherocytic jaundice and the erythrocytes containing abnormal haemoglobins in the thalassaemias, the megaloblasts of pernicious anaemia, and the antibody-coated cells of acquired haemolytic anaemias demonstrated by the Coombs' test. If there is no obvious cause for haemolysis, the red cell fragility test can be tried: cells are suspended in various concentrations of sodium chloride, and the limits of concentration outside which haemolysis occurs are compared with normal cells.

If the erythrocytes are entirely normal, it may be that abnormally marked haemolysis is due to overactivity of the spleen in the conditions grouped as hypersplenism (p. 114). If the spleen is not palpable, however, this is an unlikely possibility. There may still occur rare conditions in which sources other than mature circulating red cells are responsible for the excess of plasma bilirubin, but usually the fault lies with the processes of uptake in the liver cells or conjugation within them. In the adult, the commonest possibility is Gilbert's syndrome, due partly to a defect of transport of unconjugated bilirubin into the liver cell and partly to a reduced concentration of the enzyme bilirubin UDP glucuronyl transferase. This condition is genetically determined, and is one of the causes of neonatal jaundice (p. 127), but it is very mild so a young adult usually presents with this condition without a clear-cut history of jaundice since birth; for reasons that are not clear the jaundice is usually only intermittent. If the story is typical, the hyper-

bilirubinaemia is definitely of the unconjugated variety and the clinical condition very mild, there is no need to investigate further, but in cases of doubt a needle biopsy of the liver and appropriate staining methods confirm the diagnosis.

The importance to a surgeon of assigning a patient with jaundice to the acholuric group is that he does not need to consider surgical measures for relieving an obstruction to the flow of bile into the duodenum. Treatment of these conditions lies for the most part in the domain of the physician and the haematologist, although the surgeon may be invited to remove a spleen in order to reduce haemolysis, or a gall bladder because of pigment stones.

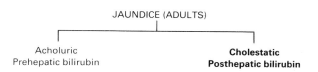

JAUNDICE (ADULTS)

Acholuric
Prehepatic bilirubin

Cholestatic
Posthepatic bilirubin

Cholestatic jaundice

Obstruction to the secretion of bile after conjugation of bilirubin has taken place in the hepatocyte can occur anywhere along the excretion pathway, in the hepatic cells themselves, in the intrahepatic bile canaliculi, the intrahepatic bile ducts, or the extrahepatic biliary passages — the left and right hepatic ducts, the common hepatic duct and the common bile duct. Whether the patient needs a surgeon or will be treated entirely medically depends (with few exceptions) on the point of obstruction being clearly outside the liver. The intrahepatic bile canaliculi and ducts are not amenable to surgical procedures for circumventing an obstruction.

This question, which in the past has sometimes been difficult to answer, is now nearly always easily solved by the use of ultrasonography. The technique accurately delineates distended extrahepatic bile ducts proximal to any extrahepatic obstruction. If distended extrahepatic bile ducts are not visible, the patient is referred to a physician: if they are visible, the case is in the province of experts using manual techniques, whether they be endoscopists, radiologists or surgeons.

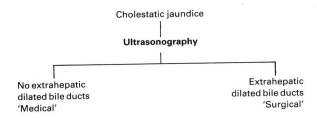

Cholestatic jaundice

Ultrasonography

No extrahepatic
dilated bile ducts
'Medical'

Extrahepatic
dilated bile ducts
'Surgical'

Urgency — evidence from tests

All patients with extrahepatic jaundice should be considered urgent because obstruction to the outflow tract damages hepatocytes. The initial investigations of the case should always include the so-called 'liver function tests', of which the most useful are the plasma concentrations of alkaline phosphatase (normal range 20–85 i.u. per litre or 3–13 King—Armstrong units per 100 ml), the transaminases (aspartate aminotransferase and alanine aminotransferase, both with normal levels of 50–100 i.u. per litre) and albumin (normal range 30–40 g/litre).

Alkaline phosphatase is excreted by the liver cells into the bile, and obstruction to the flow of bile leads to an increased rate of formation of the enzyme for reasons that are not clear, and an early and large regurgitation into the plasma. 'Surgical' jaundice therefore tends to be associated with high plasma levels from an early stage, even before the hepatocytes are damaged. However, it is only at a later stage that the effects of chronic obstruction damage the liver cells sufficiently to make them porous to the transaminases, and to interfere with their power to synthetize albumin. The urgency of the case is thus proportional to the height of the alkaline phosphatase level (roughly, the degree of obstruction) and the change in the other indices (roughly, the degree of liver cell failure).

Another useful test for the completeness of obstruction is to examine every specimen of urine for urobilinogen. If no urobilin is getting through into the intestine, then no urobilinogen is being formed in the intestine, so that there is none to be reabsorbed into the plasma and ultimately excreted via the kidney.

Urgency — clinical evidence

Palpable abdominal mass

One is not concerned in this section with a palpable liver, since any cause of cholestatic jaundice may produce sufficient turgidity in the liver to render that organ palpable. The presence of any other intra-abdominal mass, however, constitutes a strong indication for laparotomy, at least after some preliminary investigations.

If it is decided that the mass felt is the gall bladder (p. 113), Courvoisier's dictum should be remembered that in a patient with obstructive jaundice a palpable gall bladder suggests that the cause of the obstruction is not a calculus. If the gall bladder is distended, the obstruction must lie below the junction of the cystic and common bile ducts, and malignancy is more likely than calculus because a gall bladder which contains or has contained stones is likely to have become shrunken and fibrosed by inflammatory episodes and, so, incapable of becoming distended.

Any other mass in the abdomen raises the possibility of a neoplasm which has given rise to secondary deposits in lymph nodes in the porta hepatis. Once again, the suggestion of neoplasia dictates urgency.

Constitutional disturbances (See p. 125.)

Diagnosis of extrahepatic obstructive jaundice

ERCP

The ultrasound examination that has already demonstrated dilated extrahepatic biliary passages may also have suggested a possible cause, such as stones in the gall bladder — and by inference the possibility that there is one obstructing the common bile duct, or a mass in the head of the pancreas. The definitive investigation, however, is endoscopic retrograde cholangiopancreatography (ERCP). The endoscope is passed into the duodenum and the papilla of Vater identified. Any cause of obstruction at the papilla can be sampled for biopsy, or excised if small enough. If the lesion prevents cannulation of the lower end of the bile duct, a diathermy sphincterotomy is performed. Sometimes this releases an impacted stone. When cannulation of the common duct is achieved, contrast is injected into the biliary tree (Fig. 11.1) to determine if there is obstruction higher up.

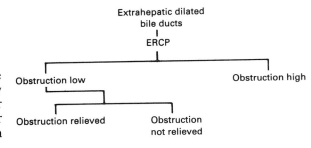

Extrahepatic dilated
bile ducts

ERCP

Obstruction low

Obstruction high

Obstruction relieved

Obstruction
not relieved

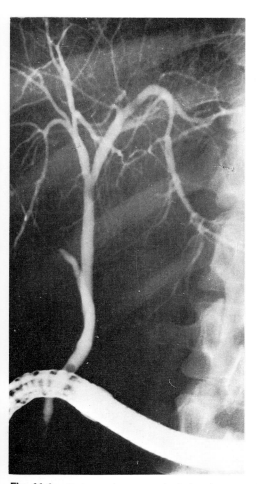

Fig. 11.1 Endoscopic retrograde cholangiopancreatogram (ERCP). Cholangiogram obtained by cannulating the lower end of the common bile duct through an endoscope passed via the mouth into the duodenum. The radio-opaque endoscope is seen lying in the curve of the antrum and first part of the duodenum. The injected contrast material in the bile duct system shows the common duct with its (normal) narrow terminal segment, the cystic duct and the hepatic ducts. The filling defect in the common duct at the upper border of the image of the endoscope is an air bubble — note its smooth rounded perimeter. (X-ray by courtesy of Dr P. B. Cotton)

The examination is not only meant to be diagnostic, but therapeutic as well. Operations on jaundiced patients carry important hazards (p. 125) so that the endoscopist's aim is to decompress the obstructed biliary tree if possible. If an obstructing stone has been removed and the endoscopist has seen a gush of bile into the duodenum, nothing further need be done. In other situations where a less definite (or no) relief of the obstruction has been achieved, an attempt is made to by-pass the region of the obstruction with an in-dwelling catheter passed up the duct and left *in situ* (via a nostril) after removal of the endoscope. With the liver decompressed and the jaundice subsiding, the urgency has been taken out of the situation and there is time to consider further management, and even perhaps to wait for liver function to improve.

Sometimes — and this usually occurs with high obstructions, i.e., those in the region of the confluence of the hepatic ducts — it is not possible to by-pass the obstruction, and then decompression is sought via a different route.

PTC

Percutaneous transhepatic cholangiography (PTC) is performed by radiologists with special experience. The patient is sedated, and the radiologist punctures the liver with a fine, slightly flexible needle and adjusts its position until bile can be aspirated into a syringe attached to the needle. In a liver without cholestasis, it is unlikely that aspiration of bile will be achieved; it is only when biliary obstruction has existed for some time that the bile ducts proximal to the obstruction dilate sufficiently to make bile aspiration a common phenomenon. If bile is aspirated, a plastic cannula is threaded along the needle and into the punctured bile duct, and the needle itself can then be withdrawn. Radiographic contrast medium can then be injected and x-rays taken to demonstrate the dilated biliary system and the exact site of the block (Fig. 11.2). Bleeding is an important possible complication of this investigation. The patient's haemostatic mechanism must be tested, and corrected if found to be abnormal (p. 125), before the puncture is performed.

Other investigations

If the nature of a mass in the head of the pancreas has not been elucidated by ERCP including pancreatography, additional information may be gained from CT-scanning and, particularly, fine-needle aspiration cytology performed via percutaneous puncture of the anterior abdominal wall under ultrasound control.

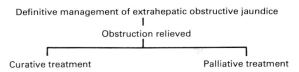

The decision whether to aim at curative or palliative treatment can be very difficult.

Carcinoma of the head of the pancreas

If a carcinoma of the head of the pancreas has presented with obstructive jaundice, experience teaches that it is unlikely that it can be cured, even by such an extensive procedure as Whipple's operation (p. 107). Some form of permanent by-pass procedure is usually indicated involving at least a choledocho- or cholecysto-jejunostomy and possibly a gastrojejunostomy (as the enlarging tumour may produce pyloric as well as bile duct obstruction).

Carcinoma of the lower end of the bile duct

These lesions, because of their unique situation, usually cause obstructive jaundice at a very early stage of their evolution, and so Whipple's operation has a reasonable chance of being curative. If careful ultrasound and CT-scanning demonstrate no evidence of lymphatic or hepatic secondaries, and this is confirmed at laparotomy, pancreatico-duodenectomy is performed. In a poor-risk patient, or one in whom metastases have been demonstrated, the lesion is by-passed.

Choledocholithiasis

Except in countries like China where primary stones form in the biliary passages in association with the liver fluke, *Clonorchis sinensis,* stones in the common bile duct have originated in the gall bladder. In younger, fit patients who have been demonstrated by ultrasound to have stones in the gall bladder, there is a strong case for cholecystectomy even if the common duct has been cleared of all stones during the ERCP. In the elderly, unfit patient the decision is much more finely balanced. Cholecystectomy in this group carries an appreciable mortality. It may be thought wiser to rely on a generous endoscopic sphincterotomy to prevent any gall bladder stones that subsequently migrate into the common bile duct from causing further bouts of obstruction.

Hepatic and common bile duct 'strictures'

At the lower end of the common bile duct, a stricture is, in the absence of previous surgery, likely to be due to a carcinoma. Endoscopic sphincterotomy will have possibly relieved the obstruction, and biopsy have confirmed the diagnosis.

Elsewhere in the biliary tree, the stricture may be a localized lesion or a more generalized disturbance of the normal anatomy with multiple strictures and irregular dilatations. Localized strictures are traumatic (especially arising from injury during a previous cholecystectomy), due to a neoplasm of the duct (cholangiocarcinoma) or to extrinsic pressure, usually from lymph nodes involved in primary (lymphoma) or secondary neoplasia.

In these higher reaches of the biliary tree, drainage will probably have been achieved from above via the percutaneous transhepatic approach. When the local oedema subsides with the relief of pressure, the radiologist will often be able to dilate the track of his catheter sufficiently to pass firmer instruments that will dilate the stricture. Using such techniques, not only can material be obtained for histological examination but a stent can be forced through the stricture to give the patient a semi-permanent route to the duodenum for his bile. Help may also be obtained by percutaneous fine-needle biopsy of masses visualized by ultrasound or CT-scanning in the region of the stricture.

Multiple irregularities may be due to primary biliary cirrhosis, the pericholangitis/sclerosing cholangitis complex and, again, cholangiocarcinoma. *Primary biliary cirrhosis* is a rare condition affecting particularly middle-aged women, associated with auto-immune disorders such as rheumatoid arthritis and Hashimoto's thyroiditis, and characterized by a positive mitochondrial antibody test. Needle biopsy of the liver provides typical histology. The disease is incurable and progressive. Chronic fibrosing inflammation of the biliary tract is often associated with chronic inflammatory bowel disease — Crohn's disease or ulcerative colitis. It may be impossible to distinguish this complex from an extensive cholangiocarcinoma.

Only *short* strictures are likely to be suitable for an attempt at cure, and the lower the stricture the easier the operation. In very high strictures there may be no possibility of a surgical by-pass. Even Longmire's operation, in which part of the left lobe of the liver is amputated and an intrahepatic bile duct, located on the cut surface, is anastomosed with a Roux-loop of small intestine, cannot drain the right half of the liver if the junction of right and left hepatic ducts is occluded. Where possible, however, the affected segment of bile duct is excised and the upper bile duct system joined to a loop of intestine. The success rate of these operations has improved since long term drainage across the anastomosis has been adopted with a tube that runs upward along the duct and across the liver to emerge through the abdominal wall. Even for short strictures due to cholangiocarcinoma, the chance of cure is not high and many surgeons elect for palliative treatment from the start.

For long strictures, only palliation with a stent is feasible.

Dangers of operations on jaundiced patients

The modern approach to the management of 'surgical' jaundice as described above obviates the necessity to perform a laparotomy on a jaundiced patient: the jaundice is relieved before any laparotomy is undertaken. Rarely, it may be necessary to operate for emergency indications before the jaundice can be relieved. Vitamin K_1 must be given intravenously to attempt to correct any tendency towards impairment of blood coagulation as a result of deficient absorption of the fat-soluble vitamin from the intestine. Broad spectrum antibiotic cover is needed if there has been any suspicion of cholangitis or septicaemia. Deeply jaundiced patients (plasma bilirubin exceeding 170 μmol/l) (10 mg/100 ml) are peculiarly susceptible to renal failure (the so-called 'hepatorenal syndrome'); there is evidence that the incidence of this complication can be reduced by increasing urine output during the operation, and for the next 24 hours, with infusions of the osmotic diuretic, mannitol.

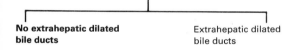

| No extrahepatic dilated bile ducts | Extrahepatic dilated bile ducts |

Diagnosis of intrahepatic obstructive jaundice

For most patients with cholestatic jaundice in whom the extrahepatic bile ducts are not dilated, there are no surgical implications. The reader is referred to medical textbooks for a discussion of the main diseases and their diagnosis and management. Two conditions already mentioned under 'surgical' jaundice may appear exclusively in this 'medical' group. Primary biliary cirrhosis usually only affects the smaller intrahepatic radicles, and so may chronic fibrosing inflammation of the biliary tree in which case the condition is called pericholangitis rather than sclerosing cholangitis. Intrahepatic cholangiocarcinoma may be clinically and radiologically indistinguishable from these conditions.

Much more important to the surgeon is a group of patients who, despite lack of extrahepatic bile duct dilatation, may have a very serious surgical significance — the group that presents with severe constitutional disturbance.

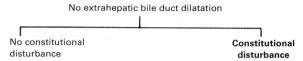

No extrahepatic bile duct dilatation

| No constitutional disturbance | **Constitutional disturbance** |

Constitutional disturbance

If jaundice is associated with a swinging fever, rigors, sweating and prostration, the urgency of the situation cannot be exaggerated. Had the ultrasound examination shown a dilated common bile duct, it would have been virtually certain that the obstructed duct had become infected, resulting in ascending cholangitis and septicaemia with or without an hepatic abscess. Immediate treatment with a mixture of antibiotics covering the widest possible spectrum would have been mandatory, but it would be necessary to bring the septic focus under control before the antibiotics could possibly prove effective. The way to do this with ERCP, etc., has already been described.

Unfortunately ascending cholangitis can occur without dilatation of the extrahepatic ducts and the primary focus need not be in the biliary apparatus itself although gall bladder and common duct stones can be responsible. From the surgical viewpoint, important sources of infection include other intra-abdominal diseases such as appendix abscess. The jaundice is not due to mechanical obstruction but to the overwhelming interference of the ascending infection with the function of the hepatocytes. This is a situation to test the most acute clinician.

In half the cases there is no obvious intra-abdominal source of the infection even though septicaemia and liver abscess are ultimately proved. While awaiting the results of blood culture, however, it is important to bear in mind other possible causes of this clinical picture and perform any tests suggested by any feature of the history or examination. *Hepatic amoebic abscess* may be accompanied by cysts and vegetative forms of the causative organism, *Entamoeba histolytica,* in the stools, and several fresh specimens should be sent for examination but negative results do not exclude the diagnosis. Sigmoidoscopy may reveal the characteristic shaggy, flask-shaped ulcers of colonic amoebiasis, but it is rare for the colon and liver to be affected simultaneously. Serological tests are available, for example a latex agglutination test and an indirect haemagglutination test.

Malaria should be spotted in blood films, infectious mononucleosis gives a positive Paul–Bunnell test and antibodies against the Epstein–Barr (EB) virus can be demonstrated, while the spirochaetes of leptospirosis or relapsing fever may be found in the blood at an early stage of the disease and antibodies to these organisms can be found at a later stage. The various forms of hepatitis A, B, and non-A, non-B can also produce this picture. Much rarer causes, at least in Britain, are yellow fever, tuberculosis and syphilis, and the appropriate serological and bacteriological tests should be undertaken.

The first batch of investigations may on their return provide evidence of one of the specific infections, and any specific remedies available can be started. Penicillin is useful for syphilis and relapsing fever, and is usually given to patients with leptospirosis (of which the common form, due to *Leptospira icterohaemorrhagiae,* is called Weil's disease and is contracted from rats in sewers and similar dark, wet places) although it is of less certain value in that condition. Treatment for tuberculosis is considered in Chapter 2.

If no specific diagnosis has been made, more blood samples are taken in the search for septicaemia, and diagnostic endeavour is turned to the possibility of liver abscess, which may be single or multiple. Ultrasound and/or CT-scanning give the diagnosis both of a liver abscess and of a subphrenic abscess, two conditions which can be clinically indistinguishable.

When a liver abscess is diagnosed, and unless there is a known focus of sepsis to which the liver abscess is clearly secondary, the possibility of an amoebic origin should be carefully considered. The symptoms and signs are on the whole less severe than with a pyogenic abscess, unless secondary infection has occurred. Diagnostic aspiration yields the typical anchovy-sauce pus, but only in the absence of secondary infection, and the organisms may be demonstrated by staining techniques. Treatment with metronidazole (Flagyl), together with repeated aspirations if necessary, is effective but open drainage is required for the abscess with secondary infection.

In a few patients the investigations reveal no specific cause and fail to substantiate a diagnosis of septicaemia. This is a serious situation with a high mortality. Usually one treats with a combination of powerful antibiotics on the assumption that the patient is septicaemic and that the failure to confirm this is technical. Should the acute illness improve, the possibility of gallstones being responsible is urgently investigated with ERCP or PTC.

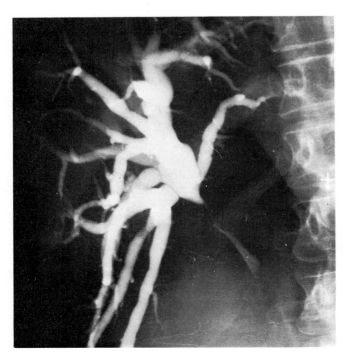

Fig. 11.2 Percutaneous transhepatic cholangiogram (PTC). A fine flexible needle has been passed through the parietes and into the dilated duct system within the liver. There is an obstruction to the common hepatic duct just below the confluence of the intrahepatic ducts. The obstruction was due to a carcinoma of the hepatic duct, and a previous attempt at surgical removal had been unsuccessful (note the wire suture near the lower margin of the picture). (x-ray by courtesy of Dr R. Dick)

Flow-chart 11.1

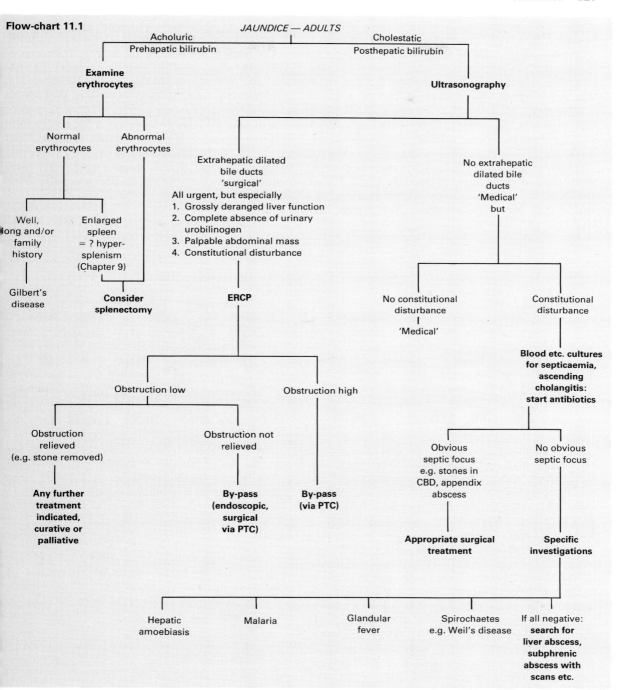

Neonatal and childhood

There are several reasons for separating jaundice in very young subjects from jaundice in adults. First, the proportion of congenital anomalies, many of which are incompatible with survival to adulthood and therefore are only seen in this age group, is high. Secondly, neonatal jaundice is such a common phenomenon and so often rapidly self-limiting that this benign type is often called physiological jaundice. Thirdly, the general surgeon is unlikely to be involved with management until the attending obstetrician or paediatrician has ruled out 'non-surgical' causes of jaundice.

Fourthly, the important biochemical findings that enable adult patients to be sorted into different management groups are nothing like so clear-cut in the neonate. For example, pure haemolytic disease can give rise to bilirubin in the urine, while some cases of complete atresia of the bile ducts yet manage to have some urobilinogen in the urine. Moreover, levels of alkaline phosphatase are much higher in infancy, and again in adolescence, than the accepted upper limits of normal in adults.

The management of an infant who is born jaundiced, or who develops jaundice within the first few days afterwards, is therefore to exclude the more obvious and common conditions that can be responsible at this time and then to await resolution during the next 2–3 weeks on the assumption that the jaundice is physiological. Provided that the level of bilirubinaemia is not too high, the infant is therefore usually about 3 weeks old before other causes of the jaundice are seriously considered and investigated.

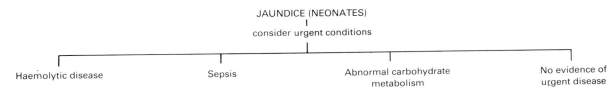

Conditions to exclude

Haemolytic disease

This is the most important category of conditions that must be excluded. The most important example is rhesus incompatibility, in which the erythrocytes of a rhesus-positive infant are attacked by antibodies that have crossed the placenta from a rhesus-negative mother. With adequate antenatal care which should include examination of the mother's serum for rhesus antibodies and, where indicated, examination of the amniotic fluid, there should be advance warning of this problem. Its incidence has recently been greatly reduced through the prophylactic injection of all rhesus-negative mothers with anti-D antibody at the time of birth. This prevents the immunization of the mother with fetal red cells carrying the D-antigen. Examination of the blood film, grouping of mother and infant, and the Coombs' test rapidly indicate the diagnosis. Occasionally, blood groups other than the rhesus factor can cause similar trouble, and it is important to recognize that the Coombs' test, especially in ABO incompatibility, may be negative.

The infant's problem may be simple anaemia, and transfusion is indicated if the haemoglobin concentration is falling rapidly. More serious, however, is the problem of deep jaundice: serum bilirubin levels that exceed 350 µmol/litre (20 mg/100 ml) are liable to damage the basal ganglia of the brain (kernicterus), and this severe and irremediable complication must be prevented by one or more exchange transfusions in which the infant is bled and simultaneously transfused.

Other types of excessive haemolysis occur, for example due to malaria or to abnormalities of the red cells, and these should be picked up on the standard haematological investigations.

Sepsis

The infant liver is very susceptible to the effects of infection anywhere, and an important site to remember in the neonate is the umbilical cord, whence infection can track directly to the liver via the umbilical vein.

Metabolic disorders

The urine of a jaundiced infant should be routinely tested for non-glucose-reducing substances. The very rare conditions of galactosaemia and hereditary fructose intolerance, due to the lack of specific enzymes, are associated with liver failure. In hypothyroidism, persistent jaundice may well point to the diagnosis; the classical features of cretinism are rare.

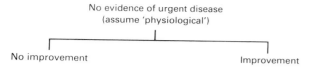

No evidence of urgent disease
(assume 'physiological')

No improvement   Improvement

Management of 'physiological' jaundice

In the usual mild case no active measures are necessary. If the bilirubinaemia reaches 85 μmol/litre (5 mg/100 ml) the level can be reduced by exposure of the infant to sunlight or, failing that, to an artificial ultraviolet lamp. Provided that the jaundice fades in 2–3 weeks, nothing further needs to be done.

Persistent jaundice

This is the group in which surgical intervention has to be considered. Many patients need a diagnostic laparotomy, although cases that can be cured by surgery are only a small proportion of the total. Possible non-surgical causes include drugs given to the mother or to the infant (vitamin K, sulphonamides, salicylates, etc.), virus hepatitis of various kinds, pyogenic infections (especially acute urinary infection), and rare conditions such as congenital syphilis and toxoplasmosis. Serological tests and examination of the urine for bacteria and cytomegalovirus are important at this stage. When the jaundice has persisted 3 months without definite diagnosis of one of the preceding conditions, histology of the liver is required. Needle biopsy may be sufficient, but there should be no undue reluctance to advise laparotomy in order to obtain an adequate specimen and to inspect the anatomy of the biliary tree, with cholangiography if indicated. The adequacy of the specimen is crucial to the definition of possible hepatic enzyme defects such as absence of glucuronyl transferase (Crigler—Najjar), or of various transport defects (Gilbert's syndrome affecting transport into the liver cells, Dubin—Johnson and Rotor syndromes affecting transport of conjugated bilirubin from the liver cells).

Corrective surgery

There are two conditions amenable to surgical treatment: choledochal cyst and extrahepatic biliary atresia.

Choledochal cyst

This is a congenital anomaly in which there is a huge cystic dilatation of the common bile duct. Cholestasis results. The cyst is readily palpable; it must be removed and the common duct repaired in whatever manner proves feasible.

Extrahepatic biliary atresia

If the atresia does not affect the main ducts at the porta hepatis and the intrahepatic ducts, it may be technically possible to drain bile from the liver by an anastomosis to a loop of jejunum. This requirement is encountered in only about 10 per cent of infants with biliary atresia, but it is impossible to be certain of the exact anatomy without doing a laparotomy. Since anaesthesia and a major operation are contraindicated in the other conditions that may cause persistent jaundice (provided that the diagnosis can be established in other ways), it is important to be able to diagnose biliary atresia with confidence. It should be remembered that the presence of urobilinogen in the urine does not exclude complete atresia. If phenobarbitone or cholestyramine given to the baby produce a fall in the level of bilirubin in the serum, it is unlikely that there is complete atresia. Another test is to inject radioactive-labelled Rose Bengal intravenously. This dye is excreted by the liver, and if less than 10 per cent of the radioactivity is recovered from the stools in the next 3 days it can be deduced that there is obstruction of the main bile duct. None of these tests is reliable, but if they are positive laparotomy should be delayed till about 4 months if the baby's condition does not deteriorate, in the hope that the obstructed bile ducts will have reached a size that will facilitate the difficult operation needed.

Flow-chart 11.2

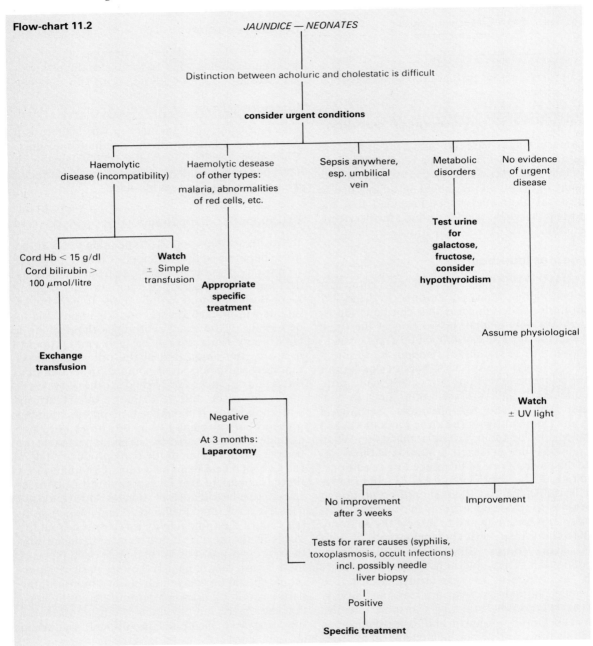

JAUNDICE — NEONATES

Distinction between acholuric and cholestatic is difficult

consider urgent conditions

Haemolytic disease (incompatibility)

Haemolytic desease of other types: malaria, abnormalities of red cells, etc.

Sepsis anywhere, esp. umbilical vein

Metabolic disorders

No evidence of urgent disease

Cord Hb < 15 g/dl
Cord bilirubin > 100 μmol/litre

Watch
± Simple transfusion

Appropriate specific treatment

Test urine for galactose, fructose, consider hypothyroidism

Exchange transfusion

Assume physiological

Negative

At 3 months:
Laparotomy

Watch
± UV light

No improvement after 3 weeks

Improvement

Tests for rarer causes (syphilis, toxoplasmosis, occult infections) incl. possibly needle liver biopsy

Positive

Specific treatment

Further reading

Cotton, P. B. (1972). Cannulation of the papilla of Vater by endoscopy and retrograde cholangiopancreatography (ERCP). *Gut* **13,** 1014–25.

Cuschieri, A. and Berci, G. (1984). *Common Bile Duct Exploration*. Boston, Dordrecht, Lancaster. Martinus Nijhoff.

Faris, I., Thomson, J. P. S., Grundy, D. J. and Le Quesne, L. P. (1975). Operative cholangiography: a reappraisal based on a review of 400 cholangiograms. *British Journal of Surgery* **62,** 966–72.

Gibson, R. N. (1985). Interventional radiology of the pancreaticobiliary tract. *Current Opinion in Gastroenterology,* **1,** 678–684.

Gregg, J. A., Carr-Locke, D. L. (1984). Endoscopic pancreatic and biliary manometry in pancreatic, biliary and papillary disease, and after endoscopic sphincterotomy and surgical sphincteroplasty. *Gut* **25,** 1247–54.

Le Quesne, L. P. (1974). Choledocholithiasis: incidence, diagnosis and operative procedures. In: *Abdominal Operations,* Vol. 1, 6th edn. Ed. by R. Maingot. New York, Appleton-Century-Crofts.

Okuda, K. et al. (1974). Non-surgical percutaneous transhepatic cholangiography — diagnostic significance of medical problems of the liver. *American Journal of Digestive Diseases* **19,** 21–36.

Sherlock, S. (1981). *Diseases of the Liver and Biliary System,* 6th ed. Oxford, Blackwell Scientific.

Chapter 12

Change in Bowel Habit; 'Piles'

These two presentations are described in the same chapter because they frequently overlap, both in the acute and the chronic forms.

Acute presentations

Changes in bowel habit presenting as acute emergencies consist of massive bleeding per rectum or massive diarrhoea. Absolute constipation resulting from large bowel obstruction is rarely acute: the symptoms gradually increase over a period of days or weeks until the obstruction is finally complete; the resulting acute-on-chronic picture is described in Chapter 26, on intestinal obstruction. The complaint of 'piles' may also present as an acute attack.

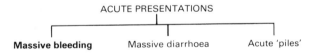

ACUTE PRESENTATIONS

Massive bleeding   Massive diarrhoea   Acute 'piles'

Massive bleeding per rectum

This is rare. The patient should be immediately admitted to hospital and a blood clotting screen performed. It is most important to consider whether the source of the bleeding could possibly be the stomach or duodenum, because although blood from that area usually takes an appreciable time to traverse the small and large intestines and therefore appears in the altered tarry black form of melaena, very rapid bleeding can appear as fresh blood. Thus gastroduodenoscopy and/or an emergency opaque meal radiological examination should be performed unless one is confident upon other grounds that the bleeding originates lower down. If the source does turn out to be the stomach or duodenum, it is very likely that an operation will

be necessary to control a haemorrhage of such proportions.

In most cases the bleeding is manifestly not very rapid, and so the unaltered blood must have arisen from the lower digestive tract. A source of bleeding is sought in the perineum and anal canal by external and digital examination, but sigmoidoscopy during the phase of acute bleeding is usually futile. Most patients settle down spontaneously with the usual conservative management for haemorrhage, and indeed blood transfusion is often unnecessary. When the bleeding has stopped, and preferably after the lapse of a day or two to ensure that the lower bowel has cleared itself of blood, investigations are commenced to seek the source of the bleeding. The usual order of performing these investigations is a sigmoidoscopy, barium enema, upper gastrointestinal endoscopy, colonoscopy. If the first three investigations demonstrate a lesion that is the likely source of the bleeding, colonoscopy is unnecessary. Sigmoidoscopy should always precede barium enema because the latter is not accurate in the rectum and lower sigmoid colon, and if the films are mistakenly reported as normal one might be tempted to forget to perform the sigmoidoscopy. In some centres there is a tendency to omit the barium enema and rely on colonoscopy.

A large variety of causative lesions may be unmasked by these investigations, although it should be noted that just because a lesion is demonstrated, it is not necessarily the cause of the bleeding. The commonest are diverticular disease of the sigmoid, carcinoma of the sigmoid or rectum, and a polyp of the large bowel; less often one finds evidence of Crohn's disease, ulcerative colitis, ischaemic colitis, familial polyposis, amoebiasis, etc. Each condition is dealt with on its merits, but certainly an episode of severe bleeding would influence the surgeon in favour of surgical management where the underlying cause is a chronic disease such as diverticular disease that may be treated conservatively or by operation.

Even in cases where colonoscopy is not necessary for diagnosis, the procedure may be valuable as a method of treatment. Small and moderate-sized (up to 3 cm) polyps can be approached through this instrument, and removed by diathermy snare. Care must be taken to include the stalk of the lesion in the excision, so that infiltration of the base with neoplastic cells can be demonstrated and, if it is present, appropriate major resection of colon undertaken.

Sometimes no causative lesion is disclosed by this programme of investigation. It is probably safe to wait and see whether the bleeding recurs. If there is another episode, the whole procedure of investigation should be repeated, and indeed extended by ERCP (p. 123) to seek lesions in the biliary and pancreatic passages. Arteriography occasionally pin-points the site of bleeding provided that the blood loss is at least 1 ml/min. The usual lesion demonstrated by this technique is angiodysplasia, particularly of the caecum. The decision about when to proceed to laparotomy is always difficult because even at laparotomy the source of bleeding remains obscure in an appreciable proportion of cases. Factors in making the decision include the number of bleeding episodes, their frequency and their severity, but in the last resort the decision depends on the judgement of the individual surgeon faced with the problem of the individual patient.

Finally, it may on rare occasions be necessary to proceed to exploratory laparotomy during an episode of severe haemorrhage, even the first, if the rate of blood loss is so large as to threaten life. The operation itself does not differ in principle from the one described (p. 277) in the management of haematemesis and melaena, but in practice it is one of the most difficult in general surgery, since the bleeding can be arising anywhere in the alimentary tract or in the outgrowths of the tract such as bile and pancreas. In general, when the blood loss is bright red rather than tarry, the lesion is likely to be distal rather than proximal. Per-operative endoscopy can be of great help.

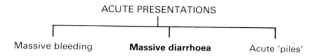

ACUTE PRESENTATIONS

Massive bleeding   **Massive diarrhoea**   Acute 'piles'

Massive diarrhoea

Massive diarrhoea threatens life by loss of fluid from the exracellular compartment. Anyone who has diarrhoea and shows signs of extracellular depletion (p. 269) or who is losing in any measured time interval of a few hours 2 litres of fluid more than he can drink, should therefore be admitted to hospital. With the exception of epidemics of cholera, this is a rare situation: most patients with acute diarrhoea present with less severe fluid loss and can be safely treated at home.

The gravest forms of massive diarrhoea occur in patients who are already in hospital, and particularly who have recently had a surgical operation. The dangerous conditions of staphylococcal enteritis, necrotizing colitis and antibiotic-associated enterocolitis are real possibilities in such patients, and the diagnosis of simple acute gastroenteritis should never be accepted in them until those alternative diagnoses have been excluded.

Management consists of replacing the fluid and electrolyte losses as in any patient with extracellular depletion (p. 315), sending blood for routine analysis and also for specific tests for typhoid, cholera and other diseases producing severe diarrhoea, and taking two separate scrapings of the rectal wall via a sigmoidoscope and sending them for bacteriological examination. The bacteriologist should set up anaerobic and aerobic cultures, but he must also examine immediately a smear from the aerobic specimen, stained with Gram's stain. In this way, a diagnosis of staphylococcal enteritis can be made without undue delay. This condition arises when staphylococci take over as the predominant organisms in the bowel, the usual flora having been destroyed by appropriate antibiotic therapy. Thus any patient who has been on antibiotic treatment, but particularly those who have undergone a course of preoperative sterilization of the bowel in preparation for colonic surgery, is at risk from this condition though its actual incidence is very small. If the diagnosis is confirmed, specific treatment with one or more agents to which staphylococci would be expected to be sensitive is immediately begun. Another organism producing antibiotic-associated enterocolitis is *Clostridium difficile*. Treatment is vancomycin by mouth (and intravenously too if the patient has a foreign body such as a heart valve in his circulation) plus metronidazole.

During the sigmoidoscopy it may well be that no view is obtained of the colonic mucosa because of obscuration by the diarrhoea fluid. If the mucosa can be seen, it will probably be reddened and friable and the pattern of mucosal blood vessels will have been lost. These changes should not be interpreted as necessarily due to ulcerative colitis, as they are more likely to be a non-specific reaction to the vast discharge of diarrhoea fluid. However, a biopsy is taken if the view is sufficiently good to make this a safe procedure: histological examination of this may in due course substantiate a diagnosis of necrotizing entercolitis. The aetiology of this condition is entirely unknown, but it is a rare complication of any abdominal operation. There is no specific treatment. In the case of *Cl. difficile* enterocolitis a tenacious 'pseudomembrane' forms on the bowel wall and is characteristic.

Another possibility which should be carefully considered if the patient has just had an abdominal operation is that the cause is a mechanical short-circuit of the alimentary tract, either iatrogenic or resulting from some complication of the operation. For example, it is not unknown for a surgeon, in performing a gastroenterostomy, to unite the stomach with a loop of distal ileum instead of with the first loop of the jejunum, and the resulting intestinal hurry can produce a devastating diarrhoea. Again it is probable that vascular damage to a loop of bowel, perhaps resulting from traction or twisting of the vascular pedicle or from dislodgement of an atheromatous plaque during the manipulations of the operation, can damage the integrity of a large area of mucosa with a similar loss of extracellular fluid into the lumen. These possibilities should be discussed with the surgeon who performed the operation. A gastroscopy might be indicated, for example.

The supportive treatment is maintained and a careful watch kept for complications — of which the most important is peritonitis — while the results of the bacteriological investigations are awaited. Several of the conditions producing massive diarrhoea may produce perforation of the bowel; for example, typhoid, vascular lesions, and necrotizing enterocolitis. If spreading abdominal pain, tenderness and guarding and an increasing haemoconcentration despite apparently adequate replacement of losses with saline, suggest peritonitis a laparotomy is essential. If possible, the affected segment of bowel is repaired, exteriorized, or resected, but the prognosis is poor (except in the case of solitary perforation of a typhoid ulcer).

In due course, positive bacteriological results may be received from the laboratory and appropriate treatment given for such conditions as typhoid. Sometimes no cause is ever found for the severe illness, but such cases usually settled spontaneously within 1 week.

For ulcerative colitis presenting acutely, see p. 148. Of increasing importance is the variety of infections of the gastrointestinal tract spread by sexual activity — the group of conditions collectively known as the 'gay bowel'.

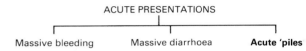

Acute 'piles'

When a layman complains to his general practitioner or to a medical officer in a casualty department, that he has a sudden and severe 'attack of piles', he means that he is experiencing an acute episode of anal pain. In the layman's vocabulary, 'piles' is a term describing anything that feels wrong in the region of the anal canal, and the doctor should beware of confusing the patient's use of the term with the common (but not exclusive) medical use as a synonym for an internal haemorrhoid. This point is expanded later (see p. 138).

The chief causes of acute anal discomfort are strangulated prolapsed internal haemorrhoids, acute anal fissure, subcutaneous perianal haematoma (thrombosed external pile) and the much less common prolapsus ani and proctalgia fugax. They are easy to distinguish from each other on the basis of the history and a simple clinical examination.

Prolapsed strangulated internal haemorrhoids

The history is usually clear-cut: a patient who has been having trouble with internal haemorrhoids, either prolapsing or bleeding or both, defaecates and feels the piles prolapse. The lumps do not return spontaneously, and he is unable to replace them within the anal canal. Gradually they become more and more painful until he can hardly walk and sitting is agony.

On inspection the diagnosis is obvious: the masses of one or more plum-coloured segments of shiny anal mucosa, weeping blood-stained mucus and partially covered on their peripheral asepct with oedematous anal skin (Fig. 12.1), are unmistakable. With the patient in the left lateral or

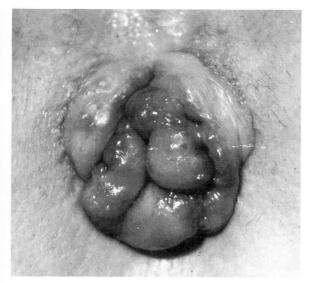

Fig. 12.1 Prolapsed strangulated internal haemorrhoids. The plum-coloured segmental protrusions of anal mucosa, with oedematous perianal skin on their outer aspect, are unmistakable. (Photograph by courtesy of Mr J. P. S. Thomson)

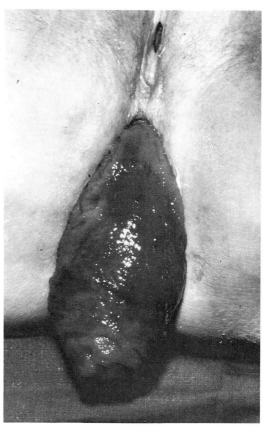

Fig. 12.2 Complete anorectal prolapse in an elderly woman. The deeply injected mucosa suggests that the prolapsed tissue is about to become gangrenous, but this complication rarely, if ever, occurs. (Photograph by courtesy of Mr J. P. S. Thomson)

knee—elbow position, the doctor may be able to replace the haemorrhoids and this gives excellent pain relief, but relapse is common. Tepid baths, compresses with astringent lotions, suppositories of astringents such as hamamelidis, are all comforting measures, but these can all be carried out in the patient's home if the home circumstances are good, and there is no need for admission to hospital. The condition subsides gradually during the next 2—3 days, and the fibrosis resulting from the inflammation may tighten the anal mucosa sufficiently to prevent the patient having further symptoms of haemorrhoids. A sigmoidoscopy should always be performed, however, when the symptoms have subsided. In selected patients, forceful digital dilatation of the anal canal can achieve rapid relief.

Prolapsus ani

The history, apart from the fact that pain is usually much less prominent, is identical with the foregoing, but in young children or in elderly patients the diagnosis on inspection may prove to be this. There are two forms: mucosal prolapse and whole-thickness prolapse. The mucosal form is really only an extreme degree of circumferential prolapse of the anal mucosa, not well demarcated into the segmental arrangement we know as haemorrhoids. In the full-thickness form (Fig. 12.2) there is an actual telescoping of the anterior anorectal wall down through the canal, and in this case a groove can be felt posteriorly between the prolapsing wall and the posterior margin of the anus. The lack of such a groove anteriorly distinguishes this condition from the much rarer intussusception presenting at the anus. Patients with full-thickness prolapse should be admitted to hospital.

After conservative management similar to that for prolapsed haemorrhoids, injection treatment may be undertaken in adults and children to try to prevent mucosal prolapse. Details of this treatment

Flow-chart 12.1.

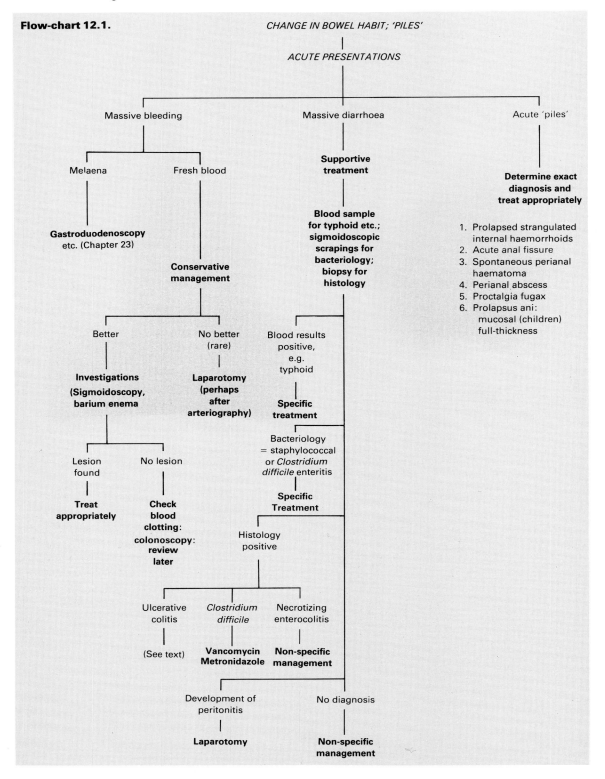

CHANGE IN BOWEL HABIT; 'PILES'

ACUTE PRESENTATIONS

Massive bleeding · Massive diarrhoea · Acute 'piles'

Massive bleeding:
- Melaena → **Gastroduodenoscopy** etc. (Chapter 23)
- Fresh blood → **Conservative management**
  - Better → **Investigations (Sigmoidoscopy, barium enema**
    - Lesion found → **Treat appropriately**
    - No lesion → **Check blood clotting: colonoscopy: review later**
  - No better (rare) → **Laparotomy (perhaps after arteriography)**

Massive diarrhoea:
- **Supportive treatment**
- **Blood sample for typhoid etc.; sigmoidoscopic scrapings for bacteriology; biopsy for histology**
  - Blood results positive, e.g. typhoid → **Specific treatment**
  - Bacteriology = staphylococcal or *Clostridium difficile* enteritis → **Specific Treatment**
  - Histology positive:
    - Ulcerative colitis → (See text)
    - *Clostridium difficile* → **Vancomycin Metronidazole**
    - Necrotizing enterocolitis → **Non-specific management**
      - Development of peritonitis → **Laparotomy**
      - No diagnosis → **Non-specific management**

Acute 'piles':
- **Determine exact diagnosis and treat appropriately**

1. Prolapsed strangulated internal haemorrhoids
2. Acute anal fissure
3. Spontaneous perianal haematoma
4. Perianal abscess
5. Proctalgia fugax
6. Prolapsus ani: mucosal (children) full-thickness

are exactly as for the injection treatment of haemorrhoids (p. 139). Whole-thickness prolapse, if it recurs, needs much more elaborate surgical procedures for its cure. Probably the commonest procedure used at the moment is an abdominal operation in which the rectum is mobilized and pulled up, and then a plastic sponge is inserted between the gut and the sacrum in order to promote adhesions.

Acute anal fissure

The history is frequently typical. During defaecation the patient strains to pass a constipated motion and then, immediately after passage of the stool, feels a sudden pain at the anal verge, often of an intense boring nature. There is frequently a speck of bright red blood on the toilet paper afterwards. The pain persists and intensifies over several minutes or an hour or so, and makes sitting uncomfortable, but later settles to a dull ache. However, it becomes worse again during the next act of defaecation.

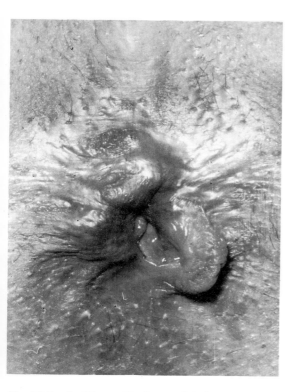

Fig. 12.3 Anal fissure. The linear split in the posterior wall of the anal canal leads down to, and is partly overshadowed by, the large skin tag ('sentinel pile'). (Photograph by courtesy of Mr J. P. S. Thomson)

On inspection the anus is tightly contracted, and any attempt to pass a finger is exquisitely painful. There is localized tenderness at one point on the anal verge — usually posteriorly in the mid-line, but in women it may sometimes be anteriorly in the mid-line.

If it is possible to pass a dilator liberally coated with an ointment containing a local anaesthetic, the intense spasm of the muscles of the anal canal rapidly subsides. If the patient cannot tolerate this, dilatation of the anal canal should be performed under general anaesthesia: this confirms the diagnosis by demonstrating the linear fissure in the wall of the lower part of the anal canal (Fig. 12.3), and also cures the condition. Anti-constipation measures should then be advised. Very occasionally, the lesion turns out to be a carcinoma of the anal canal.

Subcutaneous perianal haematoma

The history is identical with that given by a patient with an acute anal fissure, except that there is usually no bleeding and a lump may be noticed. On examination a small haematoma is found in the perianal skin. The usual explanation given for its production is the bursting of a small subcutaneous blood vessel as a result of straining at stool. If the patient presents within a day or two after the onset, severe pain can be relieved by incising into the haematoma (under local anaesthesia) and evacuating the contents. If the pain has already started to subside, the condition is best treated with local astringent applications.

Proctalgia fugax

It is rare for a patient actually to present with this condition: *fugax* means fleeting, and the patient gives a history of having experienced a sudden, and very severe pain deep in the anorectal region, often with a lancinating series of exacerbations that shoot deep into him from the buttock region, often occurring in the middle of the night, somewhat relieved by the pressure on the buttocks of sitting down on something hard, and disappearing spontaneously and fairly suddenly.

One should test to see whether moving the coccyx with the index finger in the rectum and the thumb outside reproduces the pain, and it may be worth doing serological tests for syphilis since the very rare lightning pains of tabes dorsalis may resemble proctalgia. In general, there is no treatment except reassurance, and the condition, while painful, is self-limiting and entirely harmless.

Chronic presentations

The history

The importance of a true change in bowel habit as a pointer to serious disease cannot be over-emphasized. The symptoms can be difficult to assess because some people cannot be said to have any regular bowel habit. The significance of a change in bowel habit also depends on its duration: a person who claims that he has been constipated for 10 years is unlikely to be suffering from any serious disease. Again, the range of normality is so wide: one patient may normally have three bowel actions a day, another only one every three days. Nevertheless, *any* deviation from a patient's norm, no matter how minor, must be considered significant if it is persistent and has been present less than, say, two years. (Serious disease is unlikely to have been present more than two years without some other feature of the disease becoming manifest.)

It is important that the doctor make sure that the patient and he are using terms in the same sense. *Constipation* means the passage of a hard stool, with the consequent necessity to strain. *Diarrhoea* means the passage of a liquid or semi-liquid (i.e. unformed) motion. An increase or decrease in the number of motions may be significant, even if there is no alteration in the consistency of the stool. Particularly important is a history of alternating bouts of constipation and diarrhoea, since this combination suggests a stenosing lesion of the left side of the colon. In this region of the colon, the bowel contents are solid and tend to obstruct the narrowed lumen so for some days there is little or no stool and what there is is hard; however, the scybalous masses dammed up behind the obstruction rub against and irritate the colonic walls which respond by secreting mucus in large quantities so that, when chance clears the obstructing lump of faeces from the stricture, there is a flood of mucous diarrhoea. Any other feature of the history suggestive of intestinal obstruction should also be carefully sought.

Incontinence is a complaint that always needs careful assessment. An occasional leak of flatus or a little liquid may be a sequel to anorectal operations for haemorrhoids, fissure, etc. A continuous leak of a small quantity of mucus may be discharged from a fistula. A patulous sphincter on digital examination may be part of a neurological disorder, but is probably commonest in elderly patients with anal prolapse. Here the cause is probably damage to the internal pudendal nerve by such factors as childbirth.

Dyschezia signifies that the rectum and anal canal still feel (and indeed are) loaded with faeces after defaecation. *Tenesmus*, the feeling that a solid object is stuck in the anal canal, arousing an intense desire to defaecate that cannot be satisfied, is a much more alarming symptom but both can be associated with an anorectal neoplasm.

The characteristics of anal *pain* due to acute anorectal disturbances have already been discussed (p. 134). Third-degree haemorrhoids, i.e. those that are permanently prolapsed, are uncomfortable to sit upon, while a chronic fissure is associated with pain similar to, but less intense than, that with an acute fissure. The pain of a perianal abscess builds up gradually and develops a bursting, throbbing quality: its typical site is to one or other side of the anus. The pain of a pilonidal abscess is similar, but is localized behind the anus. It is important to appreciate that malignant disease of this region does not usually produce pain. By contrast, all anal or perianal conditions may be associated with *itching*.

If the patient has noticed a *lump* at the anus, he will probably complain of 'piles' irrespective of whether the lump is a prolapsed internal haemorrhoid, a skin tag in association with an internal haemorrhoid ('external pile'), a skin tag in association with a fissure ('sentinel pile'), a subcutaneous perianal haematoma ('thrombosed external pile'), or a prolapse. The synonyms in parentheses show that surgeons are also prone to use the word 'piles' in many different senses. Occasionally, multiple perianal lumps turn out to be the typical filiform warts transmitted by sexual contact (Fig. 12.4).

Finally, the *characteristics of the stool* should be elicited. Apart from any change in the consistency, ask about colour, greasiness, mucus and — the commonest important feature — blood.

Intestinal hurry and steatorrhoea produce pale, loose motions; the complete loss of pigment resulting in a clay-coloured stool is typical of obstructive jaundice; steatorrhoea produces a greasy motion that floats on water, the passage of pure mucus implies the irritation of colonic mucosa by prolapse, by obstructed faeces of a pelvic abscess, or by the inflammation of, say, ulcerative colitis. In the last-named disease, the inflamed mucosa

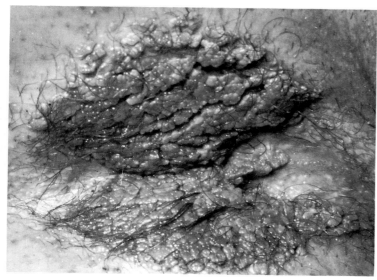

Fig. 12.4 Anal warts. These filiform lesions, transmitted by sexual contact, may be complained of by the patient as 'piles'. (Photograph by courtesy of Mr J. P. S. Thompson)

bleeds as well as weeps mucus so that the mucous discharge is pink or red. The venous engorgement of strangulated mucosa produces the much darker red or purplish mucus ('redcurrant jelly') said to be typical of intussusception but also occurring in infarcted bowel following mesenteric vascular occlusion. The black tarry stool of melaena means that there is bleeding from the upper gastrointestinal tract (i.e. in the region of oesophagus, stomach or duodenum) or that the patient is taking an oral preparation of iron. Dark blood well mixed in the stool represents bleeding coming from a site that is most likely to be the left side of the colon, and probably from a malignancy. Bright red blood lying on the surface of the stool, or noted on the toilet paper used after defaecation, suggests bleeding from a lesion of the lower rectum or anal canal; statistically this usually means a benign lesion such as internal haemorrhoids, or a fissure, or proctitis.

The examination

There are two major aspects to the examination. The first is to look for evidence of intestinal obstruction (Chapter 26), because this condition makes the situation an emergency in the sense that the patient should be admitted to hospital immediately, and because the treatment of many of the diseases being considered in this Chapter is drastically altered by the presence of intestinal obstruction. The second aspect is that the perineum, anal canal and rectum must be examined by inspection, digital exploration and proctosigmoidoscopy, and any practitioner who is not prepared to perform all these manoeuvres, especially the sigmoidoscopy, and interpret the findings should at this stage transfer the patient to a surgeon. Rectal examination and sigmoidoscopy are mandatory in any patient who complains of any of the symptoms under discussion in this Chapter, although the exact timing of the sigmoidoscopy may need to be varied in certain circumstances as mentioned in the appropriate contexts below.

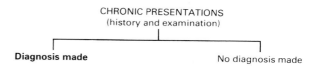

Patients with intestinal obstruction are admitted to hospital and handled as in Chapter 26. In patients without evidence of intestinal obstruction, the routine examination described either yields or fails to yield a diagnosis.

Diagnosis made

The diagnoses made fall into two groups: minor anorectal conditions and the rest. Minor anorectal conditions may be very painful, but are essentially benign. In most cases they can be treated definitively without further investigation.

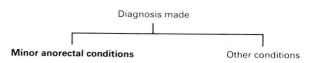

Internal haemorrhoids of the first degree (bleeding only, no prolapse) usually respond satisfactorily to injections of 5 per cent phenol in almond oil, delivered into the submucosal layer at the level of the anorectal ring. The ensuing chemical inflammation and resultant fibrosis fix the redundant anal mucosa and submucosa to the muscular wall of the canal. Third-degree haemorrhoids (permanently prolapsed) usually require an operation, probably a formal haemorrhoidectomy. Second-degree haemorrhoids, which prolapse on defaecation but later retract spontaneously, may respond to injection or banding but will occasionally need some surgical procedure, whether a haemorrhoidectomy or a forceful dilatation of the anal canal (Lord's procedure). The selection of a patient for treatment and the choice of procedure clearly depend largely on the severity of symptoms: many patients can be kept comfortable by the prevention of constipation and the regular use of astringent suppositories, as there is a natural tendency to remission of symptoms for variable periods of time.

A chronic fissure-in-ano oftens responds to regular dilatations, performed by the patient himself with a conical dilator liberally smeared with an ointment containing a local anaesthetic. It is probably the local anaesthetic that is the curative agent rather than the dilatation. In the early stages sigmoidoscopy may be intolerable because of pain, but the procedure must be carried out later when the pain has settled. If this conservative management does not work, forceful stretching of the anal sphincters or sphincterotomy to divide the internal sphincter and release the spasm or, if there is much scar tissue present, excision of the fissure as part of sphincterotomy are all good operations. Any associated sentinel skin tag is excised at the same time. Like external haemorrhoids, such skin tags promote pruritus and are better removed.

A patient with the tell-tale induration of a perianal abscess close by the anal verge should be admitted to hospital, and the abscess deroofed and drained under general anaesthesia. Sigmoidoscopy should be avoided at this stage, and apart from a digital examination to exclude a carcinoma of the rectum, no attempt should be made to explore the anal canal in search of the internal opening of a fistula although this is a likely cause for the abscess, because such manipulations in oedematous tissues may create a fistula. Should the condition recur and require drainage again (this happens in about half the patients), after a few days, when the inflammation has subsided, the patient is examined under anaesthesia; if a fistulous communication with the bowel is found, the position of this vis-à-vis the anorectal sling of muscle is carefully assessed. If the fistula is entirely superficial to the anorectal sling (*low-level fistula*), the track is laid open and allowed to heal by granulation from the depths. However, a high-level fistula, which is very rare, is a difficult condition to treat since laying it open may produce incontinence, and the case should be referred to a surgeon with particular interest in colorectal diseases. A patient presenting with an established fistula is treated along similar lines. The cause of a high fistula is commonly Crohn's disease.

A pilonidal abscess presents in the subcutaneous tissue of the natal cleft, to one or both sides of the mid-line and several centimetres posterior to the anal verge. Like any subcutaneous abscess elsewhere, it should be drained by deroofing the overlying skin and laying open any tracks found to be radiating from the main cavity. The abscess often contains hairs, hence the name pilonidal, meaning a nest of hairs. Sometimes there is a history of one or more episodes of acute inflammation in the region, subsiding following spontaneous discharge, and the patient presents with one or more openings of sinus tracks in or near the natal cleft. The treatment is similarly admission to hospital, and an operation to lay open all the tracks. There has been controversy about the treatment of pilonidal sinus in the past, and there are still protagonists of the theory that it is congenital in origin and must therefore be treated by wide excision to ensure that all the buried epithelium of the congenital pit at the basis of the lesion has been removed. Such operations are difficult and have a definite recurrence rate, and since the condition is self-limiting (it is rare over the age of 35 years) and well proven to be a foreign-body granuloma, it seems more sensible to do a limited procedure as advocated here.

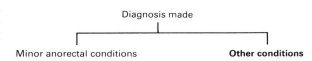

Other conditions are to be distinguished by the feature that they require further investigations, and are definitely or potentially more serious in nature. The most important of these lesions is carcinoma of the rectum. The examining finger feels a hard ulcer with everted edges, or else a polypoid

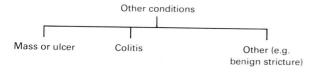

mass, in the lower rectum. The lesion is visualized through the sigmoidoscope and a biopsy taken from the region of its edge, where it adjoins normal tissue. Very occasionally the histological report is a surprise such as lymphoma, but usually the clinical diagnosis of carcinoma is confirmed. In the absence of intestinal obstruction, a barium enema examination or colonoscopy should next be performed because, of all patients presenting with a carcinoma of the large bowel, about 5 per cent have a second carcinoma elsewhere in the colon. After due preparation of the large bowel by mechanical cleansing (enemas or vigorous purgation), the growth is excised. Since it was low enough to be palpable per anum, the operation needed will probably be an abdominoperineal resection of the rectum and anal canal: experience shows that a margin of 3 cm must be obtained below the palpable growth if one is to be reasonably sure of a complete excision, and considering the low level of this tumour it is clear that the anal sphincters have to be sacrificed. An occasional exception arises when it is found that the lesion was palpable per anum because it had intussuscepted down from the upper reaches of the rectum, and an anterior resection of the rectum with restoration of continuity of the alimentary canal and preservation of the sphincter is then on the cards. Less often, the lesion is too high to be felt but is seen through the sigmoidoscope, and anterior resection is usually then feasible.

A *polyp* may also be felt, and seen via the sigmoidoscope or indeed occasionally prolapsing through the anal canal. Polyp is the name given to any pedunculated mass, without prejudice to its histological nature. Some of these polyps in the anal canal have long stalks and are manifestly benign, but any polyp greater than 2 cm in diameter must be assumed to be malignant unless proved otherwise by histological examination. The lesion is visualized via the operating sigmoidoscope and removed by diathermy snare, care being taken to include normal tissue at the base of the tumour. If there is no histological evidence of malignant invasion of the base, all is well; if there is invasion, an excision of the rectum follows — either abdominoperineal or anterior resection, depending on the level of the tumour.

Another type of neoplasm that is sometimes encountered in the rectum feels typically like a soft velvety carpet, and histologically is reported to be a villous adenoma. This is a benign tumour, but with a marked tendency to malignant change. It weeps mucus in large quantities, and may therefore be associated with mucous diarrhoea and clinical potassium deficiency. Local operations are usually adequate for this lesion; for example, they may be floated off the submucosa by an infiltration of adrenaline 1:10 000 solution and excised with a margin of mucosa. If malignant change has occurred, the radical operation appropriate to the level of the growth is performed.

Prolapse of the rectum may be noted at this stage (p. 135). Unquestionably the most important remaining group of conditions are those involving inflammation of the colorectal mucosa.

Sometimes the appearances of the inflamed mucosa are characteristic: the experienced observer can confidently diagnose amoebic colitis from the small scattered ulcers.

Ulcerative colitis cannot be distinguished from Crohn's disease, although such features as complicated perineal fistulae or previous attacks of obstruction of the small intestine suggest the diagnosis is Crohn's. In all patients, the cause of the colitis is usually ultimately determined by laboratory methods: histological examination of deep biopsy specimens of the colonic mucosa, culture of the stools and of rectal wall scrapings, special serological tests (e.g. for amoebic disease, gay bowel). Patients with acute colitis need immediate admission to hospital so that these investigations can be performed, and in practically all of them it is advisable to investigate the rest of the large bowel by barium enema though this investigation should be deferred till the acute colitis has subsided. Finally, if the histology shows non-specific inflammation only and all the other tests are negative, one should remember that the colitis might be secondary to a more proximal cause of diarrhoea such as a gastrocolic fistula, rather than the cause of the diarrhoea, and investigate accordingly.

The management of colitis is straightforward if a specific cause with a specific remedy is found. Most cases prove to be non-specific, in the group of ulcerative colitis/Crohn's disease, although ulcerative colitis when confined to the rectum is usually called granular proctitis; the management of the whole group is described later (p. 148).

Very occasionally, an anorectal stricture will be encountered that is not malignant. The histological appearances of biopsy material may show non-specific fibrosis, and such strictures may arise in elderly patients as a result of habitual overpurgation. Specific diseases that may produce strictures of this part of the bowel include lymphogranuloma venereum and schistosomiasis, and the appropriate cultures and serological tests are carried out.

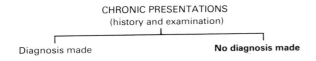

CHRONIC PRESENTATIONS
(history and examination)

Diagnosis made   **No diagnosis made**

Diagnosis not made

In general, if clinical examination and proctosigmoidoscopy have not yielded a diagnosis, one proceeds to a barium enema examination or colonoscopy. A full barium enema is a traumatic procedure, and in elderly patients (over 75 years old) who have no abdominal mass on palpation and have never passed blood per anum, experience teaches that there is only a very small return of positive results. In this group, therefore, it may be wise to defer the barium enema for 4 weeks and review the patient: if his symptoms have disappeared and no physical signs have developed, it is reasonably safe not to pursue the investigations.

It is simplest to consider first the situation that the barium enema shows no abnormality. The choice available is either to proceed to barium meal and then if necessary colonoscopy, or to review the patient in 4 weeks. The decision will depend upon the doctor's judgement of the severity and duration of the symptoms, the presence of any abnormal physical signs, and especially on the nature of the symptoms: a history of blood per anum can never be ignored unless it was bright blood that is adequately explained by a benign anorectal lesion.

If the full spectrum of investigations yields no diagnosis there is no alternative to keeping the patient under review and repeating the investigations if the symptoms have not subsided in 4 weeks.

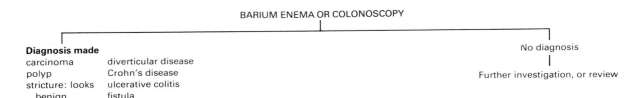

BARIUM ENEMA OR COLONOSCOPY

Diagnosis made
carcinoma   diverticular disease
polyp   Crohn's disease
stricture: looks ulcerative colitis
  benign   fistula

No diagnosis

Further investigation, or review

Finally, there is the situation that the barium enema does reveal an abnormality. There may be a filling defect, a stricture, a diverticulum, a fistula, a mucosal irregularity, or a combination of more than one of these. A filling defect greater than 2·5 cm can be assumed to be malignant, although in regions of the world where amoebiasis is common a therapeutic trial of a course of emetine is justified before operating. A lesion smaller than 2·5 cm may be a benign polyp, but the diagnosis must be proved histologically. Most strictures of the colon are due to carcinoma, and if the strictures have shoulders at their ends the diagnosis is, in practice, certain (Fig. 12.5). Very smooth, tapering strictures may have resulted from ischaemic disease of the colon and occasionally a stricture may be due to a peridiverticular abscess, or to late changes after irradiation with x-rays. Diverticula may be multiple, and they occur most commonly in the rectosigmoid region with a variable tendency to extend proximally along the left half of the colon, or solitary, in which case they are commonest in the caecal region. A fistula between the colon and the exterior, or between the colon and neighbouring abdominal organs such as the bladder, vagina or small bowel, may result from a large variety of pathological processes; the commonest is diverticular disease, followed by Crohn's disease and carcinoma. Alterations in mucosal pattern may suggest a diagnosis of Crohn's disease or ulcerative colitis.

Over and above such abnormalities, the important feature to be sought from the barium enema is evidence of impending intestinal obstruction, either in terms of the degree of narrowing of the bowel at the site of the lesion or the tendency for the bowel to dilate proximal to the lesion. A generalized dilatation of the colon in patients with ulcerative colitis is also important — this is the condition called 'toxic megacolon' which heralds perforation and therefore requires urgent laparotomy. Conversely, spasm is often an inconstant feature and its chief significance is that it may make more difficult the interpretation of the films.

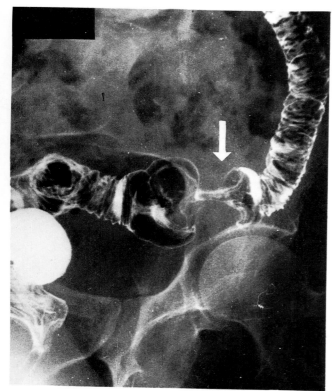

Fig. 12.5 Carcinoma of the sigmoid colon. Film from a barium enema series with air contrast. Note the stricture at the upper end of the sigmoid colon. The 'shoulders' of the stricture, particularly well marked at the proximal end (arrowed), are practically pathognomonic of malignancy.

Carcinoma of the colon

A suspicion of carcinoma indicates a laparotomy. For the question of preparation of the bowel, see Chapter 18. Fifty per cent of carcinomas of the large bowel occur in the rectum and rectosigmoid, and most of the rest occur in the left half of the colon, but there is an appreciable incidence in the caecum and a small one elsewhere in the right half of the colon. Indeed, right-sided colonic carcinoma seems to be getting commoner. Left-sided tumours are likely to present with disorders of bowel habit, including blood in the stools, while obstruction is common; right-sided tumours produce chronic iron-deficiency anaemia as a result of a slow chronic, and therefore macroscopically invisible, loss of blood in the stool.

The principle of the operation is to perform a trial dissection aimed at removing the segment of bowel containing the tumour with an adequate margin, together with as wide as possible a removal of the lymphatic glandular drainage area. If there are pathological adhesions to neighbouring structures, with or without fistulation, then such structures are excised with an adequate margin in the same block of tissue. Such a radical operation, designed to be curative, may be contraindicated if there is evidence of distant blood-borne metastases (e.g. in the liver), or if the local pathological adhesions are so extensive or involve such important structures as iliac vessels as to make wide excision unjustifiable. Nevertheless, if it is technically possible to remove the primary tumour with only a reasonable risk, this should always be done: death from distant secondaries, for instance from liver metastases, is preferable to death from the pain, bleeding and faecal discharge of an uncontrolled primary. In a palliative resection, a wide clearance of the lymphatic drainage is unnecessary.

The primary carcinoma usually does not show much tendency to spread microscopically along the bowel beyond the bounds of the macroscopically visible and palpable tumour, so from this viewpoint it is sufficient to excise a segment of bowel whose limits are at least 2·5 cm (where possible, 5 cm) beyond the naked eye limits of the tumour. However, the lymphatic channels run with the arteries, and due attention must be paid to

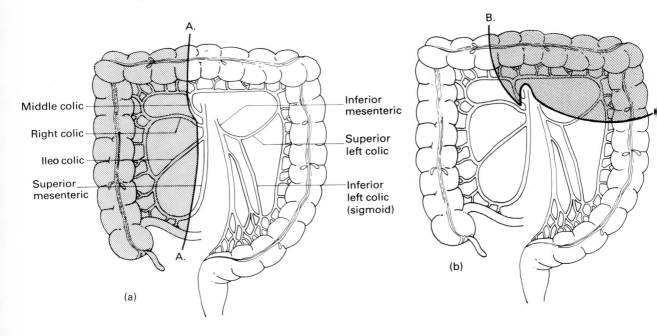

Middle colic

Right colic

Ileo colic

Superior
mesenteric

Inferior
mesenteric

Superior
left colic

Inferior
left colic
(sigmoid)

(a)

(b)

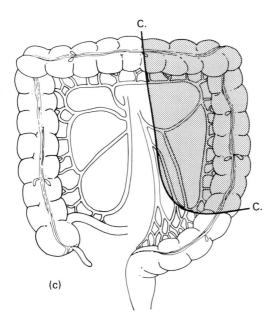

(c)

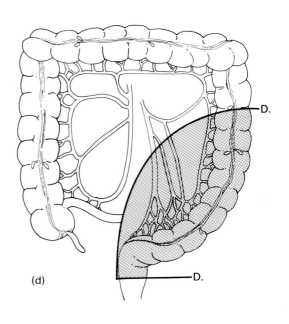

(d)

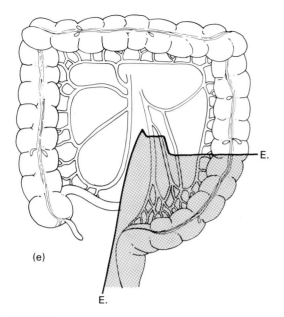

(e)

E.

Fig. 12.6 Formal resections of colon. (a) The principal arteries supplying the colon are labelled, although the exact pattern is variable. A–A indicates the limits of excision of a right hemicolectomy. The left branch of the middle colic artery is preserved. If this is not possible, the whole of the transverse colon must be excised, as in (b). (b) B–B represents the limits of excision of a transverse colectomy. The descending branch of the superior left colic artery is preserved. (c) Left hemicolectomy. (d) Anterior resection of the rectum (restorative resection). (e) Radical excision of the rectum (usually a synchronous abdominoperineal approach). Some surgeons advocate that in (c), (d) and (e) the inferior mesenteric artery should be tied and divided at its origin from the aorta.

the anatomy of the arterial supply if a wide lymphatic clearance is to be achieved yet a reasonable blood supply left to the remaining bowel. The exact details of how much bowel is resected depend upon the exact anatomy of the arteries in the individual, but Fig. 12.6 shows the average pattern of the four main operations used: abdominoperineal excision of the rectum for tumours so low that the sphincters cannot be saved; restorative resection of the rectum and the similar left hemicolectomy; transverse colectomy; and right hemicolectomy.

After abdominoperineal excision there is no alternative to an end-colostomy. After the other operations, the ideal procedure is an immediate anastomosis of the cut ends of the remaining bowel. Here the effect of intestinal obstruction becomes important. The risk of leaks at the anastomosis is greater with colon than with small bowel, probably mostly because of the greater vas-

cularity of small bowel. In obstructed patients the proximal colon may be grossly distended and its nutrition impaired: experience teaches that the incidence of leaks is unacceptable unless at least one end of the bowel is small rather than large. Thus in the presence of obstruction, immediate reconstitution is usually attempted only after right hemicolectomy; in other cases the proximal cut end is brought to the skin surface as a colostomy, while the distal is also brought to the surface if possible, or if it is too deep in the pelvis for this to be possible it is simply oversewn (Hartmann's operation). A further operation can subsequently be performed, often with difficulty, when the bowel has recovered from the effects of obstruction, to restore continuity. (See also p. 338). Factors other than obstruction, for example severe local sepsis due to perforation, may also weigh against primary anastomosis.

Non-malignant stricture

Even if the radiographic appearances suggest that the stricture is not malignant, most patients will need laparotomy, if only because of impending obstruction. If biopsy and histological examination of frozen sections confirm a non-malignant aetiology such as ischaemic or post-radiotherapy colitis, a local resection can be performed. The question of immediate anastomosis again depends upon obstruction.

Diverticula

The common problem is generalized diverticulosis maximal in the rectosigmoid region. Apart from acute complications such as local perforation (pericolic abscess), generalized perforation with peritonitis, intestinal obstruction and acute haemorrhage (discussed in Chapters 26 and 27), the usual indications for operation are fistula formation and the suspicion that a cancer of the colon is also present but is being obscured in the x-ray pictures by the spasm of the diverticular disease. In general, patients with the chronic symptoms of diverticular disease — cramping lower abdominal pain and constipation — can be kept comfortable with a high-residue diet (especially plenty of bran) plus, if necessary, antispasmodics. Occasionally, however, operation is required because of symptoms that interfere with the patient's work and enjoyment of life. The orthodox procedure is a local resection of the rectosigmoid with primary anastomosis.

Flow-chart 12.2

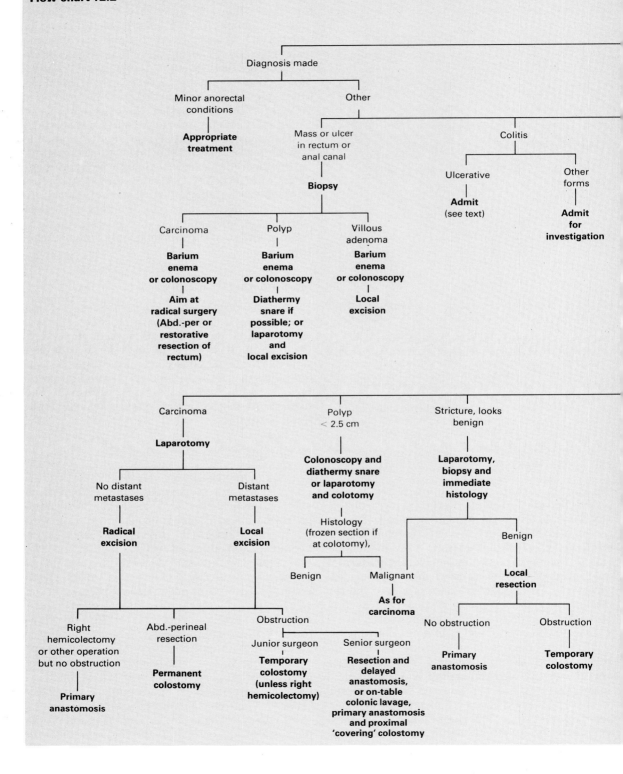

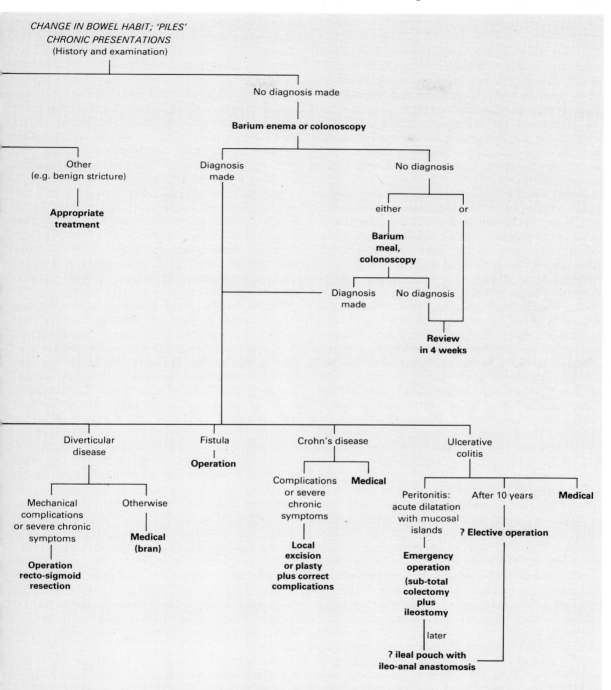

CHANGE IN BOWEL HABIT; 'PILES'
CHRONIC PRESENTATIONS
(History and examination)

Mucosal changes

The two chief conditions are Crohn's disease and ulcerative colitis. If a suspicion of either of these arises, the surgeon would be wise to enlist the aid of a physician with special interest in these conditions as their primary management is medical and the indications for and against operation can be finely balanced. It is also true that in most cases a barium meal and follow-through examination is mandatory, since the disease may not be confined to the large bowel.

In the absence of knowledge of the aetiology of these conditions, they remain descriptive labels which one hopes will help to guide management. While most patients can be confidently assigned to one or other category, there are a few with clinical features that seem to lie at a borderline between the two diseases and their management may be correspondingly difficult.

The radiological appearances of ulcerative colitis are confined to the mucosa, with loss of haustrations the most obvious feature. Crohn's disease is characterized by deep ulceration through the submucosa and into the muscles, and this corresponds radiologically to gross irregularity and thickening of the wall of the bowel, with fine spicules of the contrast medium set in the wall at right angles to the lumen. Histological material obtained via the sigmoidoscope, even when the mucosa of the region is normal radiographically and to the naked eye, may help to distinguish the two conditions.

Treatment of ulcerative colitis is now fairly standard. Mild attacks, usually of the distal colon and rectum only, can be treated on an out-patient basis with sulphasalazine, 1 g thrice daily, alone or in combination with steroid suppositories or self-administered retention enemas. In more severe attacks, usually with systemic disturbances such as fever or weight loss and abdominal pain, the patient should be admitted and systemic corticosteroids started immediately. When nausea and diarrhoea subside, sulphasalazine and retention enemas should be added. The question of urgent operation should be considered if there is a failure to respond, particularly if the temperature and pulse rate remain high, abdominal tenderness and malaise are severe, and if there is evidence of a falling body weight, and haemoglobin and plasma albumin concentration. Generalized peritonitis

due to perforation, and the combination of severe dilatation of the colon with gross irregularity of the mucosa ('mucosal islands') in a plain x-ray of the abdomen, constitute indications for immediate operation.

During remissions between acute attacks, sulphasalazine in a dose of 2 or 3 g daily has been shown to reduce the relapse rate. Finally, after about 10 years the patient with total ulcerative colitis is at risk from carcinomatous change, and elective operation is advisable unless the facilities for surveillance are excellent.

The choice of operation lies between total proctocolectomy with a permanent ileostomy and total colectomy with preservation of the lower rectum and an ileorectal anastomosis. The former procedure is standard, but in selected cases the latter may preserve reasonable defaecatory function at the risk of possible carcinoma of the retained stump of rectum.

Treatment of Crohn's disease can also be divided into emergency surgery, elective surgery and medical management. The emergency situations comprise free perforation with generalized peritonitis (a rather rare complication), bleeding, obstruction and abscess formation. Bleeding and obstruction usually settle with rest and intravenous feeding. An abscess presenting in the abdominal wall requires drainage, and a fistula from the underlying diseased bowel usually ensues. Elective operations may be advised for local complications such as fistula, abscess or chronic intestinal obstruction, or for chronic ill health (diarrhoea, blood and protein loss, malaise). The principles of such operations are to correct any local complication and to excise macroscopically diseased bowel with primary anastomosis where possible. It is known that the microscopic changes of Crohn's disease may extend very widely over areas remote from the macroscopic site, and indeed there may be areas of macroscopic disease remote from the main site, but the accent remains on conservatism because the progress of the condition can be very slow and excision, no matter how wide, is not curative.

The mainstay of treatment is medical, but treatment regimes are not as clearly defined as in ulcerative colitis. The three agents thought to have some influence on the course of the disease are sulphasalazine, corticosteroids and the immunosuppressive azathioprine.

The exceptional case

Throughout this Chapter, descriptions have been confined to the common conditions that one might expect to encounter as the basis for the various situations. Occasionally, other diseases will be found. For example, histological examination of a mass in the caecum removed by right hemi-colectomy may reveal that instead of carcinoma it is tuberculosis, sarcoidosis, lymphosarcoma, etc. The disease found may require further specific treatment. Nevertheless, the bulk of clinical practice, at least in the British Isles, will be covered by the diseases previously mentioned in this Chapter.

Further reading

Bolt, D. E. (1973). Diverticular disease of the large intestine. *Annals of the Royal College of Surgeons of England* **53**, 237–45.

Cameron, A. (1977). Left colon resection. *British Journal of Hospital Medicine* **17**, 281–9.

Goligher, J. C. (1984). *Surgery of the Anus, Rectum and Colon,* 5th edn. London, Baillière Tindall.

Gottrup, F., Diederich, P., Sorensen, K., Nielsen, S. V., Ornsholt, J. and Brandsborg, O. (1985). Prophylaxis with whole-gut irrigation and antimicrobials in colorectal surgery. A prospective, randomised double-blind clinical trial. *American Journal of Surgery* **149**, 317–22.

Lee, E. C. G. (1984). Aim of surgical treatment of Crohn's disease. *Gut* **25**, 217–22.

Lennard-Jones, J. E. (1984). Medical treatment of ulcerative colitis. *Postgraduate Medical Journal* **60**, 797–802.

McCormack, T. T., Bailey, H. R., Simms, J. M. and Johnson, A. G. (1984). Rectal varices are not piles. *British Journal of Surgery* **71**, 163.

Nicholls, J., Pescatori, M., Motson, R. W., Pezin, M. E. (1984). Restorative proctocolectomy with a three loop ileal reservoir for ulcerative colitis and familial adenomatous polyposis. *Annals of Surgery* **199**, 383–8.

Patey, D. H. P. and Scarff, R. W. (1946). Pathology of post-anal pilonidal sinus: its bearing on treatment. *Lancet* **ii**, 484–6.

Plumley, P. F. (1966). A simple regime for preparation of colon before large-bowel surgery. *British Journal of Surgery* **53**, 413–14.

Chapter 13

Lump in the Groin

There are two difficulties about this chapter: one is the difficulty in defining the groin, the other is that many lumps present in the groin and the scrotum together.

Inguinoscrotal swellings are left for discussion with true scrotal swellings in the next chapter. For our purposes, we define the groin as the region between the upper end of the symphysis pubis and the anterior superior iliac spine on each side, bounded below by the crest of the pubis and then the skin crease separating groin from thigh, and extending upwards from this base for an arbitrary 5 cm above the line of the inguinal ligament.

Difficult though it is to define the groin, it is not usually difficult in clinical practice to decide whether a lump should be categorized as being in this region. Most lumps in fact lie in the inferomedial corner of each groin, around the region of the pubic tubercle. Indeed, this point is such an important landmark that the clinician must satisfy himself that he can find it rapidly and accurately, even in a fat or uncooperative patient. The author finds the technique demonstrated in Fig. 13.1a to be the most useful. The examiner's hand is placed on the patient's ipsilateral anterior superior iliac spine, with the middle finger on the spine and the fingers straight and side by side and pointing medially and downwards at 30 degrees to the horizontal. The hand is then moved medially and downwards along the direction it is pointing until the middle finger encounters a first bony point — this is the pubic tubercle. There are alternative methods. However,

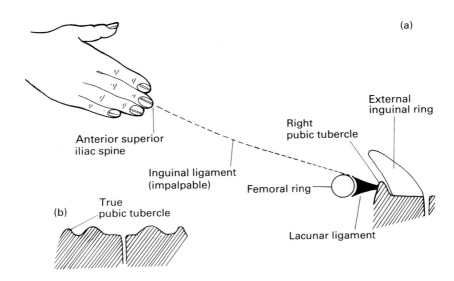

(a)

Fig. 13.1 The inguinal region. (a) To find the pubic tubercle, the examiner places his hand as shown, touching the anterior superior iliac spine with his middle finger, and then moves his hand medially and downwards at 30 degrees to the horizontal until he meets bone: this point is pubic tubercle. (b) The approach from lateral to medial rather than from the mid-line laterally prevents the examiner being misled by the bump on the superior border of the body of the pubis.

palpating outwards from the pubic symphysis along the pubic crest till one comes to the prominence of the tubercle fails if the crest is shaped as in Fig. 13.1b, a situation the author has met more than once; while following the tendon of the adductor longus muscle upwards requires the cooperation of the patient in adducting the straight lower limb against the examiner's resistance.

Lumps in the skin raise the same considerations as skin nodules anywhere else (p. 13): when they are clinically diagnosable, the specific treatment for the condition is advised; when they are not

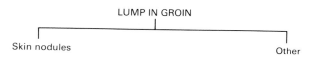

clinically diagnosable, they are biopsied if rather large, or excised and submitted for histological examination. Further treatment depends on the histological findings.

Lumps deep to the skin need separate consideration according to whether they lie, or do not lie, at one of the hernial orifices.

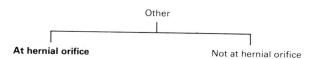

The external hernial orifices

The decision that the lump is at an external hernial orifice is crucial, so the clinician's knowledge of the positions of these orifices must be exact.

There are four recognized orifices in each groin: inguinal, femoral, Spigelian and obturator. In the author's experience, the obturator hernia is most unlikely to be clinically distinguishable from a femoral hernia. The reason for this is that the obturator hernial orifice itself is deep in the thigh, remote from the examiner's finger; the obturator hernia, by the time it comes to lie superficially in the readily palpable subcutaneous tissue, occupies more or less exactly the position of a femoral hernia. The Spigelian hernia is rare, so the common inguinal and less common femoral hernial orifices receive most attention in the following description.

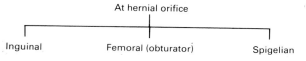

Inguinal hernial orifice

The external orifice of an inguinal hernia, i.e. the opening through which the hernia reaches the subcutaneous tissues and becomes readily palpable, is the external inguinal ring. This is an obtuse-angled triangular defect in the aponeurosis of the external oblique muscle, based on the pubic crest with its apex pointing upwards and laterally.

The pubic tubercle is the essential landmark. Since the tubercle is at the lateral end of the pubic crest, it follows that the external ring, *at the horizontal level of the pubic tubercle,* is immediately medial to the pubic tubercle. The italicized phrase in the previous sentence must be emphasized: due to the direction of slope of the apex of the ring, particularly as the fibres of the external oblique aponeurosis or muscle are split further upwards and laterally by an increasing bulk of hernia, the uppermost part of the palpable hernia may be lateral to the vertical line drawn through the pubic tubercle. Nevertheless, the hernia must lie medial to the tubercle at the horizontal level of the tubercle.

Femoral hernial orifice

The external orifice of a femoral hernia is bounded medially by the *lacunar (Gimbernat's) ligament,* anteriorly by the inguinal ligament, posteriorly by the superior pubic ramus, and laterally by the femoral vein. The lacunar ligament separates the orifice from the pubic tubercle, but the ligament is a tiny triangular structure, not wider than 5 mm, and Fig. 13.1 makes it clear that the obvious medial relationship of the orifice is therefore the pubic tubercle. Once a femoral hernia reaches the groin it may enlarge considerably in size, expanding in all directions so that various parts of the lump may have quite different relations to the pubic tubercle.

However, at the neck of the hernial sac, at the horizontal level of the pubic tubercle, the hernia lies immediately *lateral* to the tubercle.

Position of the inguinal ligament

The junior student is sometimes confused by statements such as that an inguinal hernia lies above the inguinal ligament and that this fact distinguishes it from a femoral hernia, which lies below the inguinal ligament. The facts are, of course, that an inguinal hernia lies above the medial half of the inguinal ligament, but also lies at the same level as the ligament medial to the ligament's medial end (i.e. the pubic tubercle), and indeed below that level if it extends into the scrotum; that a femoral hernia lies originally below the inguinal ligament but, as it enlarges, may well overflow the ligament to lie above it; and that in any case the inguinal ligament itself is only a geometrical landmark. One knows the position of the two ends of the ligament, since one can feel the pubic tubercle and the anterior superior iliac spine; but between these two bony points the ligament is impalpable and invisible to the external observer.

Spigelian hernial orifice

The orifice of this rare type of hernia is a defect in the aponeurosis of the oblique muscle of the anterior abdominal wall at the lateral edge of the rectus sheath, below the linea semilunaris. In this region, the aponeurosis of the lateral muscles forms the anterior layer of the rectus sheath, and there is no posterior layer. The defect is usually quite small and, if it lies in the upper part of the area, is easily distinguished from the external inguinal ring; the lower it lies, however, the more likely is confusion to arise. The implication of this statement is developed on p. 157.

Lump at a hernial orifice

If the lump lies at one of the hernial orifices, the clinician must assume that it is a hernia unless there is specific clinical evidence in favour of some other lesion.

Often, there is specific evidence in favour of the diagnosis of hernia: a cough impulse.

Cough impulse

A lump is said to have a cough impulse if it expands, visibly or palpably, when the intra-abdominal pressure is raised.

By tradition, the patient is asked to raise his intra-abdominal pressure by coughing. However, a cough produces only a momentary rise in intra-abdominal pressure, and therefore imparts only a momentary expansile thrust to any lump in the groin that has free communication with the abdominal cavity. It is better to ask the patient to contract his abdominal muscles by sustained voluntary effort: this results in a sustained expansile thrust in the lump, easier for the clinician to appreciate.

A hernia is the commonest type of lump in the groin to exhibit a cough impulse, but other lumps may do so and some hernias do not. These points receive emphasis in the following sections.

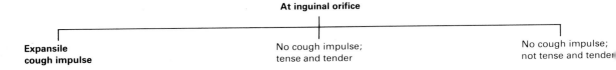

At inguinal orifice

Expansile cough impulse | No cough impulse; tense and tender | No cough impulse; not tense and tender

At inguinal orifice, with cough impulse

This is the commonest situation encountered under the general heading of a swelling in the groin. The diagnosis of inguinal hernia is made. The presence of a cough impulse in an inguinal hernia guarantees that the hernia is not strangulated.

Reducibility

An attempt is made to reduce the contents of the sac back into the abdominal cavity. One should remember the obliquity of the inguinal canal; the hernia is manipulated upwards and laterally, after first squeezing the lump without movement so that the contents of any loop of bowel that happens to be in the hernia are transferred along the bowel into its abdominal extensions, thus reducing the volume of the hernia.

Management

The *irreducible* inguinal hernia should be viewed with suspicion, as one that is likely to strangulate. Therefore, the patient should be advised that surgery is essential and his name should be put on the waiting list for urgent admission.

The *reducible* inguinal hernia can only be cured by operation, and the patient should be advised accordingly. If there is any strong contraindication to surgical treatment (e.g. severe cardiac or respiratory disease), or if the patient refuses operation, a *truss* is fitted.

Management by a truss cannot cure a hernia: the objectives are the limited ones of preventing the enlargement of the hernia and preventing strangulation. Both these objectives are achieved by keeping the hernia reduced at all times: that is why a truss is useless for an irreducible hernia. The patient must be shown how to reduce his own hernia (usually the recumbent position facilitates reduction) and apply the truss so as to keep the hernia reduced. The dangers of strangulation are explained, and he is instructed that the hernia must be reduced and the truss applied before he rises in the morning, that he must go through this routine at any time of the day should the truss slip and the hernia escape, and that apart from bathing he must not remove the truss until he is in bed at night. Even in the case of those patients who are most frightened of a surgical operation, a few weeks of life with a truss is often sufficient to convert them to accept the advantages of an operation.

Direct or indirect?

Some clinicians teach that it is possible, and important, to distinguish between the *oblique (indirect)* and the *direct inguinal hernia* on clinical grounds. The oblique sac is probably a remnant of the processus vaginalis of the fetus: it leaves the abdominal cavity at the internal inguinal ring, lateral to the inferior epigastric artery, traverses the inguinal canal within the coverings of the spermatic cord, and may be long enough to extend with the cord into the scrotum. The direct hernia leaves the abdomen via a defect in the fascia transversalis below the arch of the conjoint tendon, and medial to the inferior epigastric artery. It does not lie within the coverings of the cord and therefore does not show a great tendency to follow the cord into the scrotum.

The reason it is said to be important to distinguish between the two types is that the direct type is not likely to strangulate because the defect is a diffuse area without deeply defined edges, and that it is therefore safe to treat a direct hernia with a truss. The criteria by which it is said to be possible to make the distinction are: that an inguinoscrotal hernia must be indirect; and that a hernia which, after reduction, can be prevented from reappearing when the patient coughs by pressure over the internal inguinal ring, must be indirect.

The author does not subscribe to the view that it is possible with certainty to distinguish between these two types of hernia clinically, nor indeed to the view that it is important to do so. The diagnostic problem is twofold: a direct hernia may extend into the scrotum, although admittedly this is not a common event; and the internal ring has no immediate bony relationships, so its position and extent cannot be accurately defined from the exterior. It is usually said that the internal ring lies just above the mid-point of the inguinal ligament and is not more than two finger-tips in width. Clearly the true position of the ring might be a little more medial than the clinician realizes, in which case his pressure on the wrong spot fails to control an indirect hernia. This also happens when the internal ring is expanded medially by a large and long-standing oblique hernia. The converse error can also occur: a defect in the lateral third of the posterior wall of the canal, close to the internal ring, may be controllable by digital pressure at a point mistakenly thought to represent the internal ring itself, in which case the direct hernia will be diagnosed as indirect. In these circumstances, it is fortunate that there is little importance in making the distinction: the direct hernia carries a small but definite risk of strangulation, and operation should be advised for all inguinal hernias (in the absence of strong contraindications).

The operation

One advantage of the policy of not attempting to distinguish between direct and indirect hernias is that the surgeon approaches the operation with an open mind: he is thus less likely to miss a direct bulge in a patient with an obvious indirect sac, and less likely to miss a small congenital sac in a patient with a large direct hernia. Any indirect sac is excised at its neck, i.e. at the internal inguinal ring — the operation known as *herniotomy* — and the internal ring is narrowed to fit snugly aound the cord. Any weakness of the posterior wall is repaired with strong non-absorbable material inserted from the strong tissues of the conjoint tendon above to the strong tissues of the inguinal ligament below, and extending from the pubic tubercle medially to the internal ring laterally — the operation of *inguinal herniorrhaphy*.

In *infants* the inguinal canal runs straight backwards through the abdominal wall: the internal ring lies directly behind the external. All inguinal hernias in infants are indirect, and herniotomy alone is necessary. In young adults with an oblique sac and good musculature, herniotomy alone may be sufficient. As age increases, however, so does the likelihood that herniorrhaphy will be needed even if the main clinical swelling is due to an indirect sac.

At inguinal orifice, without cough impulse

Two situations may be distinguished: either the lump is *tense* and *tender*, or it is not.

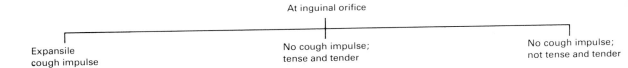

At inguinal orifice

Expansile cough impulse

No cough impulse; tense and tender

No cough impulse; not tense and tender

Tense and tender

At any hernial orifice, a tense, tender lump without a cough impulse must be diagnosed as strangulation of the appropriate hernia unless there is strong evidence to the contrary, and the inguinal orifice is no exception to this rule.

Strangulation is defined as the constriction of the vascular pedicle of a part of the body, to an extent sufficient to impede the venous drainage of the part. The essence of strangulation is that the veins, containing blood at a much lower pressure than that in the arteries, are obstructed while the arteries are still patent. In consequence, the pressure in the veins, venules and capillaries of the strangulated region rises until it exceeds the pressure applied by the strangulating agent, and the region is choked full of stagnant blood. Distended capillaries are damaged capillaries, and they leak protein-rich liquid into the interstitial space, and into the lumen of any hollow viscus that is involved. The increased pressure in the tissues produces the *tenseness* of a strangulated external hernia; the *tenderness* is produced by the accumulation of acid metabolites and pain substances as a result of stagnant anoxia and anaerobic metabolism. The moistness of the tissues predisposes towards infection, and the onset of an early, wet type of gangrene. Note the differences between strangulation and *ischaemia*, the latter being produced by an obstruction to the arterial inflow (p. 348).

The only alternative diagnoses to strangulated inguinal hernia that are at all common are inflamed lymph node and torsion of an undescended or retractile testis.

If the diagnosis of inflamed lymph nodes can be substantiated, there are urgent reasons not to operate on the patient: operation simply opens up tissue planes and invites the spread of infection and possibly even septicaemia. However, failure to operate on a patient with a strangulated inguinal hernia that contains bowel will result in peritonitis with a high morbidity and mortality rate. In modern circumstances, with antibiotics to combat the risk of spreading infection, not to operate is a greater risk than to operate. Therefore, if there is no definite clinical indication that the lump is an infected lymph node, exploration should be undertaken immediately.

A firm clinical indication of lymphadenitis is provided by pink streaks in the subcutaneous tissues, leading proximally towards the groin: they are infected lymph vessels (*lymphangitis*). A less definite pointer is provided by finding an infected, or possibly recently infected, lesion somewhere in the area from which infection would drain to the inguinal lymph nodes. The area in question is the skin and subcutaneous tissues of the external genitalia and the perineum, the anal canal, and the whole of the lower limb and the ipsilateral half of the trunk up to about the umbilical level. Depending on how strong the evidence is that the lump is inflammatory, the primary source of infection is dealt with on its merits, antibiotics prescribed and operation deferred for a reasonable length of time.

However, if substantial doubt remains or recurs with regard to the diagnosis of lymphadenitis, it must be reiterated that it is far safer to explore immediately.

Torsion of an undescended or retractile testis is suggested (but not proved) by the absence of the testis from the hemiscrotum on the affected side. This condition in any case requires exploration immediately, since the torsion produces a strangulation-like effect. Unless the testis can be untwisted within 6 hours of the onset of symptoms, it is unlikely to be found viable.

The relationship between strangulation of a hernia and intestinal obstruction requires careful comment. First, strangulation and obstruction are often spoken of as though they were synonymous. This is a serious error and results in much confusion. It is true that strangulation of a loop of bowel (usually small intestine) within an external hernia is an important cause of intestinal obstruction. However, a strangulated external hernia need not necessarily contain bowel at all; the strangulated tissue may be omentum, urinary bladder, or even (rarely) portions of a much more remote viscus such as liver or kidney. And if the hernia does contain bowel, it may not include the whole circumference of the bowel: a segment only may be caught in the hernia and strangulated, leaving the rest of the lumen unobstructed — the so-called *Richter's hernia*.

Secondly, in a patient diagnosed as having small-bowel obstruction (p. 310), the likeliest cause if he has previously undergone laparotomy is intraperitoneal adhesions; in the absence of any previous laparotomy, the likeliest cause is strangulated external hernia.

Thirdly, the search for a strangulated external hernia, in a patient with intestinal obstruction, needs to be extremely thorough and careful. The reason for this statement is that the strangulated hernia is often quite small and not painful, and

may well not have been noticed by the patient who is likely to be concentrating on his generalized abdominal symptoms of abdominal pain, nausea and vomiting.

The *principles of the operation* for a tense tender lump at the external ring may be briefly described. The lump is exposed: if it is a twisted testis, the cord is untwisted and if the testis looks viable it is fixed in that region. At a subsequent operation, when the inflammation has subsided, an attempt is made to lengthen the cord sufficiently to permit the testis to be placed in the scrotum. If the testis is not viable, it is excised.

Much more often, the lump proves to be a strangulated inguinal hernia. The sac is opened, the blood-stained exudate aspirated, and the strangulated tissues held gently but firmly by an assistant. Only then does the surgeon free the constriction at the neck of the sac. In this way, strangulated tissue is prevented from falling back into the peritoneal cavity before its viability can be assessed. Should the strangulated tissues be of minor importance (e.g. omentum), they are excised. In the case of small bowel, a period of at least 5 minutes is spent to see if viability can be confidently diagnosed: the anaesthetist is asked to ensure a high oxygenation of the patient's blood, and warm packs are applied locally to encourage vasodilatation. At the end of the period, viability is judged by the sheen of the peritoneal surface, the pinkness of the muscle of the bowel wall, the presence of peristalsis and, particularly, the presence of pulsation in the small arteries near the bowel wall. Special attention is paid to the constriction rings at each end of the loop, where the bowel entered and left the neck of the sac. Viable bowel is returned to the peritoneal cavity, non-viable bowel is resected and (in the usual circumstance that the bowel is small intestine) an immediate end-to-end anastomosis is performed. The hernia is repaired and the wound closed.

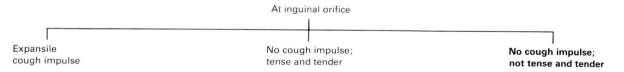

At inguinal orifice

Expansile cough impulse

No cough impulse; tense and tender

No cough impulse; not tense and tender

Not tense and tender

A few conditions that give rise to lumps in this category at the external inguinal ring can be fairly confidently diagnosed on clinical grounds. One of

these is an *encysted hydrocele of the cord*. This lump is a patent, isolated segment of a processus vaginalis that has become obliterated normally above and below the segment: it contains liquid, and is therefore a smooth, spherical or oval, transilluminable swelling which can be moved downwards by traction on the ipsilateral testis. Another is a *retractile* testis or an *undescended* testis: in either case the ipsilateral hemiscrotum is empty, but the retractile testis can be coaxed down into the scrotum by gentle pressure on the inguinal region in warm surroundings, while the undescended testis cannot be so manipulated.

The encysted hydrocele of the cord should be removed to confirm the diagnosis: the retractile testis needs no treatment, while the undescended testis should be brought down into the scrotum (if possible) by surgical operation before puberty is reached, otherwise, normal spermatogenesis is unlikely to occur. If puberty has already been passed, the same operation (orchidopexy) is advised for cosmetic reasons, but assuming that a normal testis is present on the other side the surgeon is more likely to sacrifice the testis should orchidopexy prove difficult. The undescended testis should not be left where it is because the tendency to malignant change is high.

Other lumps in this category will probably not be diagnosable on clinical grounds. The general principle of surgery that an undiagnosed lump should be excised and submitted to histological scrutiny will be followed.

At femoral orifice

```
            At femoral orifice
                   |
     ┌─────────────┴─────────────┐
Cough impulse              No cough impulse
```

At femoral orifice, with cough impulse

The obvious diagnosis is femoral hernia, but two alternative possibilities should be considered: the *saphena varix*, and the *cold abscess of the psoas sheath*.

Saphena varix

The upper end of the long saphenous vein, as it dips through the deep fascia to join the femoral vein, lies within 3 cm of the pubic tubercle (below and lateral to the tubercle). Should it become varicose and dilate, the degree of dilatation does not need to be very great before the varix overlies the femoral canal.

The diagnosis is suggested by the blue colour of the venous blood in the varix shining through the patient's skin, and confirmed by the *fluid thrill* experienced by the examiner's hand palpating the swelling when the patient coughs. This fluid thrill is a prolonged vibration, quite unlike the sharp impact in a hernial sac. Almost always, it is possible to trace a connection between the varix and varicosities of the external saphenous further down the limb, by the method of tapping (p. 197). The management is as part of the management of the varicose veins of the limb in general (p. 198).

Cold abscess of the psoas sheath

This is a rare condition nowadays, produced by a tuberculous focus somewhere in the spine, which breaks down to form a cold abscess of caseating material that tracks along the sheath of the psoas muscle to present in the groin. The patient is usually ill, there may be evidence of tuberculosis elsewhere, and the fluctuant mass may show cross-fluctuance with a similar mass above the inguinal ligament since the abscess may be large enough to present in the right iliac fossa as well.

Clearly the florid example of this condition is unlikely to be confused with a femoral hernia, but the safe rule to adopt is that the spine should be examined clinically and radiologically in any patient with an apparent femoral hernia who displays unusual clinical manifestations.

Treatment of a cold abscess of the psoas sheath follows the same principles as those used in treating a cold abscess elsewhere: drainage of the necrotic material and systemic antituberculous chemotherapy.

Femoral hernia

In the absence of any evidence to the contrary, the lump is diagnosed as a femoral hernia and treatment by operation recommended.

Treatment by a truss is not possible for a femoral hernia, even if the hernia is fully reducible. The femoral canal, through which the hernia reaches the thigh, is deep in the groin and overlain by the pubis, and its direction towards the abdominal cavity is medial rather than backward: in these circumstances it is impossible to design a satisfactory truss that will maintain reduction.

The tendency towards strangulation is much higher for a femoral than for an inguinal hernia, so the patient's name should be put on a 'soon' rather than a 'routine' waiting-list.

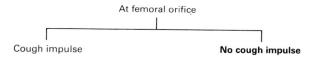

At femoral orifice

Cough impulse   **No cough impulse**

At femoral orifice, without cough impulses

Two situations may be distinguished: that the lump is tense and tender, or that it is not.

Tense and tender

Virtually the same remarks apply as in the case of a similar lump at the external ring. The possible diagnoses are strangulated femoral instead of strangulated inguinal hernia, or lymphadenitis, or torsion of an ectopic testis instead of torsion of an undescended testis. Except in undoubted cases of lymphadenitis, exploration is undertaken. The operation follows the same lines as already described, but technically a strangulated femoral hernia is a more difficult surgical exercise than a strangulated inguinal hernia. To release the constriction at the neck of the sac it is usually necessary to incise the lacunar ligament, and this ligament can usually not be seen clearly unless the approach is from above the inguinal ligament. A combined approach, i.e. from both above and below the inguinal ligament, is therefore recommended.

Not tense or tender

The usual situation is that the lump feels like a lipoma — a soft, fluctuant, lobulated subcutaneous swelling. This means that it is almost certainly a femoral hernia, because a femoral hernia frequently develops a large pad of fat in its extraperitoneal fatty layer when it reaches the thigh. The sac in such a femoral hernia is probably only a small fraction of the whole mass, at the root of the swelling. The large fat pad prevents the positive cough impulse in the sac from reaching the examiner's hand, and also prevents reduction of the hernia. Neither irreducibility nor absence of a cough impulse in themselves suggest strangulation in a femoral hernia.

Early operation is advised for a femoral hernia, as already discussed. Very occasionally, the mass turns out to be indeed a lipoma; much more usually, it is a femoral hernia, and the fat and sac are excised and the defect repaired.

Occasionally, a swelling in this category is diagnosable as something else on clinical grounds. An ectopic testis (hemiscrotum empty) is an example.

If the lump deos not seem to be a typical femoral hernia, and cannot be diagnosed, it is excised and submitted to histological examination.

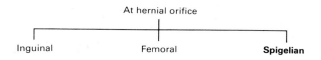

At hernial orifice

Inguinal   Femoral   **Spigelian**

At Spigelian orifice

Little need be said about this presentation. The diagnosis of hernia should be assumed and operation advised: urgently if there is evidence of strangulation, soon if there is not.

The real importance of the Spigelian hernia is when it has been misdiagnosed as an inguinal hernia. If a surgeon opens the inguinal canal and fails to find the inguinal hernia he expects, he should consider the possibility that his diagnosis before operation was faulty, and raise his skin flaps further upwards and downwards to inspect the Spigelian and femoral orifices.

Other than skin nodules

At hernial orifice   **Not at hernial orifice**

Lump not at a hernial orifice

The possible diagnoses are legion. The lump arises in the subcutaneous tissue, or deep fascia, or muscle or bone, or from artery, vein or nerve. Careful examination will probably reveal from which layer of the tissues it arises, but apart from the occasional typical lesion such as an aneurysm of the femoral artery, it is unlikely that the diagnosis will be achieved without exploration and biopsy.

Flow-chart 13.1

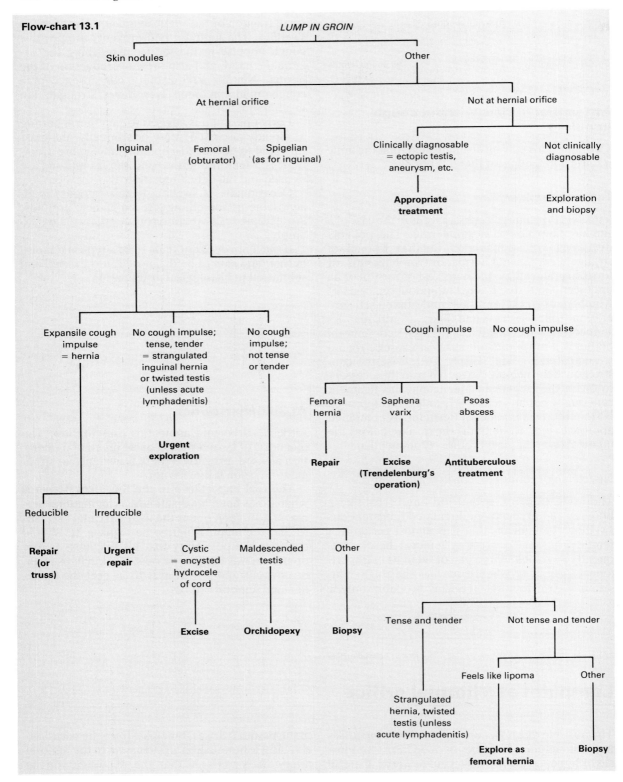

Minimal criteria for inguinal hernia

This is a common and important problem. The contents of an inguinal hernial sac may be reduced at the time that the patient is examined, yet there is a history of a lump, and maybe of discomfort or pain, in the region.

The general practitioner's role is twofold: if he thinks the story is sufficiently suggestive of a hernia, he should send him to a surgeon for a specialist opinion; even more important, should he actually find a hernia, he must describe this finding carefully so that he makes it clear to the surgeon that he has actually seen and felt a lump.

From the surgeon's viewpoint, if no lump is present when he examines the patient, then the general practitioner's description of having found a lump is invaluable: the diagnosis of hernia must be accepted, and acted upon. If the general practitioner himself has not found a lump, the problem is more difficult. The author's practice is to accept a good history of a lump (i.e. that the lump appears on standing and disappears on lying down, etc.) from a patient who seems a good witness, but not to accept a history simply of pain.

Some clinicians have taught that it is possible to detect an empty sac by invaginating the root of the scrotum into the inguinal canal and feeling a cough impulse. This manoeuvre is extremely uncomfortable for the patient, and how one can tell that an impulse on coughing is *expansile* if one cannot feel a lump is not clear to the author. Of course, the finger in the inguinal canal does feel a diffuse thrust on coughing, due to the contraction of all the muscles of the abdominal wall, just as does a finger anywhere on the abdominal wall; it is the *expansile* nature of the thrust in a *lump* which characterizes the non-strangulated external hernia.

Further reading

Davies, H. (1977). Inguinal and femoral hernias. *British Journal of Hospital Medicine* **17**, 178–86.

McEvedy, P. G. (1966). The internal approach for inguinal herniae. *Postgraduate Medical Journal* **42**, 548–50.

McVay, C. B. (1971). The normal and pathologic antomy of the transversus abdominis muscle in inguinal and femoral hernia. *Surgical Clinics of North America* **51**, 1251–61.

Ralphs, D. N. L., Brain, A. J. L., Grundy, D. J. and Hobsley, M. (1980). How accurately can direct and indirect inguinal hernias be distinguished? *British Medical Journal* **280**, 1039–40.

Chapter 14

Scrotal Swellings; The Empty Scrotum

The first decision to make is whether the lump is in the *skin* of the scrotum. If it is, it may be easily diagnosable by its clinical features. The sebaceous cyst is a common lesion in scrotal skin, and is frequently multiple. If a diagnosis can be made clinically, the appropriate treatment (if any is necessary) is carried out; otherwise the lump is excised and submitted to histological scrutiny.

Logically, the lump may be in the *subcutaneous fat* or *dartos muscle*: such lesions are rare, and will normally need to be excised and examined histologically.

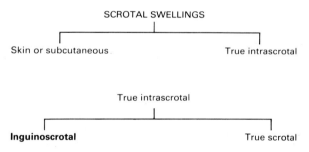

Deeper than that, the lump may be called a true *intrascrotal swelling*. A major subdivision now needs to be made. Many lumps palpable in the scrotum are also palpable in the groin: the question is, does the lump arise within the scrotum and has it, by virtue of simple enlargement, encroached upon the territory of the groin? or does the lump emerge from the abdomen via the inguinal canal and, by virtue of its size, encroach upon the territory of the scrotum? The first type of lesion may be called a *true scrotal* swelling, the second type an *inguinoscrotal*. If the lump is obviously confined to the scrotum there is no problem. In other cases, the distinction is made by trying to get the fingers of one's two hands to meet above the swelling in the groin: if they do, the lump is scrotal; if not, it is inguinoscrotal. In making this observation, it will be found easiest to have the patient standing up.

Inguinoscrotal swellings

Two situations may be distinguished, according to whether or not the mass has a cough impulse (see p. 152).

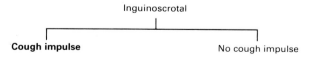

Cough impulse present

The presence of an expansile cough impulse means that the mass consists basically of a persistent processus vaginalis communicating with the peri-

toneal cavity. However, a persistent processus vaginalis is not in itself palpable, but becomes so only because it is distended with intra-abdominal contents (i.e. an *inguinal hernia*) or with liquid. In the latter case, the whole processus has usually remained patent right down to the tunica vaginalis enveloping the testis, and the inguinoscrotal swelling then extends so completely into the scrotum as to make the testis impalpable. The condition is then often called a *congenital hydrocele*. Inguinal hernia and congenital hydrocele are distinguished by the fact that the former does not, the latter does, transilluminate when a torch is applied to one aspect of the swelling through the superficial tissues. Both conditions require surgical exploration, excision of the processus, and the reduction and repair of any inguinal hernia, so the fact that both conditions may coexist is less of a clinical problem than it might be.

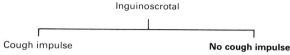

Cough impulse absent

Occasionally, the testis is not palpable and the mass is transilluminable. These findings mean that the swelling is a very large hydrocele of the tunica vaginalis, communicating with that part of the processus which lies in the inguinal canal; but that the top end of the processus has become obliterated and does not communicate with the peritoneal cav-

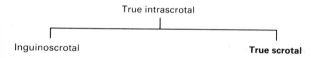

True scrotal swellings

Here the question of a cough impulse no longer arises, and the important subdivision is based upon whether or not the testis is palpable. It is not always easy to answer this question, especially if the scrotal swelling is very large: the clinician should bear in mind the characteristic size and shape of the testis, and its sensibility to pressure which produces pain not only locally but also referred to the central or upper part of the abdomen. He should also remember that while the testis usually lies in front of the epididymis and cord, the relative relations of these structures is occasionally reversed.

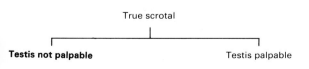

Testis not palpable

A further subdivision is made according to whether the swelling is transilluminable or not.

ity. In other words, this condition is not fundamentally different from a simple hydrocele, and its treatment is identical. It is sometimes called an *infantile hydrocele*.

Usually, the testis is palpable. If the mass is transilluminable, it is an encysted hydrocele of the cord which extends downwards far enough into the scrotum, and upwards far enough into the inguinal canal, to be called inguinoscrotal, but not far enough upwards to communicate with the peritoneal cavity. If the mass is not transilluminable, and if it is tense and tender, then a strangulated inguinal hernia should be diagnosed and immediate treatment undertaken (p. 154). If the mass is not transilluminable, but is not tense and tender, it is unlikely that an exact diagnosis will be reached on purely clinical grounds unless other characteristic features are present. Usually, surgical exploration will be necessary to establish the diagnosis and remove the swelling.

Transilluminable

This is the common situation, and diagnostic of a *hydrocele*, sometimes called a *vaginal hydrocele*.

The important point about the management of a hydrocele is that, whatever else is ultimately done, the hydrocele must be aspirated immediately through a needle and syringe so that the underlying testis can be palpated. While most hydroceles are primary (i.e. occur for no known reason), a minority are produced by an associated disease of the testis, either inflammatory or neoplastic. If the testis feels normal, the hydrocele may be accepted as primary; if it feels abnormal, the situation becomes one of a testicular mass (q.v., p. 163). Another point which should be emphasized is that the fluid from a primary hydrocele (and, for that matter, from most secondary hydroceles) is usually clear and straw-coloured; should atypical liquid be obtained, it should be sent to the laboratory for bacteriological and cytological examination.

A primary hydrocele sometimes does not reaccumulate after the first tapping. Should it do so, however, the choice of management lies between repetitive tapping to keep the patient comfortable, and surgical operation. The choice usually depends on the patient's decision, but occasionally operation is contraindicated by some serious medical problem. If operation is undertaken, the tunica may be plicated (Lord's operation) or excised from the front up to the region of the cord and epididymis posteriorly, and the free margin oversewn to achieve haemostasis; or else the tunica may be cut open and turned inside out and then resutured (Jaboulay's operation).

Not transilluminable

This is a much more difficult problem. One possibility is that the testis is obscured by the accumulation of some material in the tunica vaginalis that does not transilluminate. A *haematoma* of the tunica, also called a haematocele, will produce this combination of physical signs, and if there is an appropriate history of trauma it is reasonable to wait a week or two to see whether the condition resolves spontaneously. Occasionally, the bleeding may be spontaneous — i.e. due to trauma so slight that the patient does not remember the incident — or to an abnormal tendency to bleed. If such an abnormal tendency to bleed can be demonstrated by the appropriate investigations, it is again reasonable to wait two weeks; but in the absence of a coagulopathy, the situation shoud be assessed as *not* due to a haematoma.

If the testis is not obscured by blood clot in the tunica vaginalis, the alternative possibility is that the palpable mass is the testis which has been altered in size and shape by some disease process so as not to be recognizable as testis: normal testicular sensation has similarly been destroyed. This makes the situation comparable with that of a definite mass palpable in the testis, and is described on p. 163.

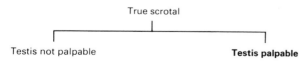

Testis palpable

Again a basic subdivision of this situation is possible: this time, according to whether or not the situation presents with the symptoms and signs of acute inflammation.

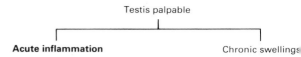

Acute inflammation

The basic picture is that the distinction between testis and epididymis is blurred, and the whole mass of testis and epididymis together is acutely tender and painful while the overlying skin of the scrotum may be reddened and warm.

Every effort must be made to distinguish between two important possible aetiologies, since the management of these two conditions is quite different — acute non-specific epididymo-orchitis and torsion of the testis.

A definite discrimination cannot always be achieved, but the following points may be made.

Acute epididymo-orchitis is favoured by a history of recent acute urinary infection; by evidence based on history, examination and urinalysis of a concurrent acute urinary infection; by a history suggestive of chronic retention of urine or of some other factor known to predispose to infection of the urinary tract such as urethral instrumentation; and by systemic symptoms and signs of infection such as headache, pyrexia and rigors. Note that a *gradual onset* of symptoms should not in itself be considered to point towards an infective aetiology.

Torsion of the testis is favoured by a rapid onset, by a history of mild trauma just before the onset, and by the patient being aged less than 25 years, especially between 12 and 16 years; also by finding that the affected testis lies high in the scrotum, and particularly if it can be discerned that its long axis is horizontal rather than vertical. The possibility of twisting seems to be associated with a high investment of the tunica vagninalis, extending up along the lower end of the cord. It is not an uncommon condition, affecting 1 in 160 males by the age of 25 years.

In the many patients in whom the diagnosis is not clear-cut, a decision has to be made whether to explore as a case of torsion, or whether to treat with chemotherapy or antibiotics as a case of urinary tract infection. The younger the patient, and the more recent the onset of the symptoms, the readier is the author to operate. Urinary tract infection in the male is much commoner in older men than in childhood and pubescence, the pain of torsion is more likely to become rapidly intense so that a really short history is much more commonly encountered in this condition, and finally if torsion has been present in severe degree for longer than 8 hours, it is most unlikely anyway that the testis will still be viable when untwisted. One should tend towards operating rather than not.

Whether or not the affected testis has been explored, if there is certainty or a reasonable suspicion that torsion might have been present, it is wise to explore the other side of the scrotum and fix the opposite testis by performing Jaboulay's operation on the tunica, turning it inside-out. Experience teaches that if a testis twists on one side the accident is likely to occur on the other side also; and of course while loss of one testis is a cosmetic embarrassment, loss of both is a human tragedy.

If no twist of the cord is found at exploration, the wound is closed and there is no indication later to explore the other side. If a twist is found, it is undone and the testis watched at least 5 minutes to see whether it seems viable. If it does, it is replaced and fixed in the scrotum; if it is obviously gangrenous, it is excised. The opposite testis should be explored and fixed at the same operation.

Torsion of the testis is a condition with serious implications. Even if the twisted testis is saved, over 80 per cent of patients subsequently show depression of sperm counts, and the depression correlates well with the duration of torsion. It seems possible that a damaged testis excites autoantibodies to spermatozoa and that these antibodies attack the opposite testis.

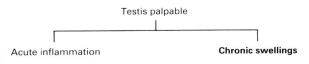

Chronic swellings

The diagnosis of chronic swellings depends on two factors: their precise anatomical location, whether in testis, epididymis or cord; and whether they are cystic, transilluminable lesions or solid ones.

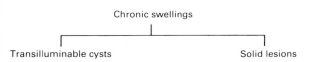

Transilluminable cysts occur at the upper pole of the testis, where they are called *cysts of the appendix testis* or *of the hydatid of Morgagni*, or in the epididymis or cord — epididymal cysts or cysts of the cord. All these cysts are thought to arise from the persistence of embryonic vestigial structures. They should all be removed by a surgical operation, as they nearly always recur after aspiration and can grow uncomfortably large. At operation, some of these cysts contain cloudy liquid and microscopical examination indicates the presence of sperms: those cysts are referred to as *spermatoceles,* but they are not diagnosable as such clinically (unless aspirated), and they have no special clinical significance.

A *solid mass* in the *cord* or *epididymis* requires exploration and excision biopsy except possibly in the instance of *tuberculous epididymitis.* The physical signs produced by the latter are so characteristic (irregularly enlarged, hard epididymis, thickened, beaded cord) that if there is any definite evidence of tuberculosis such as positive culture from sputum or urine, it is reasonable to accept the diagnosis as proven. Treatment is by antituberculous chemotherapy, and only if the lesion shows signs of beginning to break down to form a cold abscess is the scrotum explored and the affected tissue excised. However, should for any reason the diagnosis be in doubt, it is safer to explore and excise the thickened area for histological and bacteriological examination.

Solid lesions in epididymis or cord, other than tuberculous epididymitis, cannot usually be diagnosed even when exposed at operation; however, should the tumour look yellow it is likely to be an interstitial cell tumour, usually benign. These solid lesions should be removed with a reasonable margin.

A *solid mass* in the *testis* should always be considered to be neoplastic until proved otherwise. A large number of diseases can be entertained as a differential diagnosis, but despite full investigations one usually has to end up exploring the mass on the working diagnosis of neoplasia.

Possible diagnoses are tuberculoma, syphilitic gumma, and foreign-body granuloma produced by extravasation of spermatic material into the interstitial tissues of the testis in consequence of minor trauma. Unless the clinical evidence in favour of one of the first two is very strong, and there is an almost immediate response to the appropriate chemotherapy, exploration is carried out. An inguinal incision is used, and the cord and scrotal contents are mobilized from above, care being taken to keep in a surgical plane remote from the testis and its mass. In practice, exploration becomes synonymous with removal because naked-eye appearances are rarely characteristic of non-neoplastic

Flow-chart 14.1.   *SCROTAL SWELLINGS*

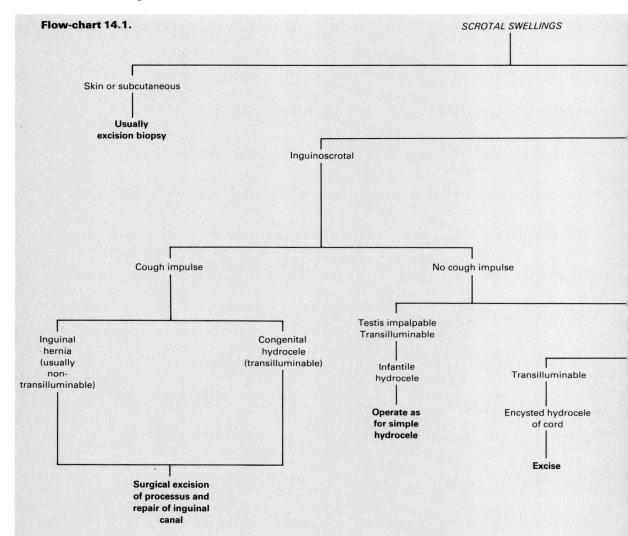

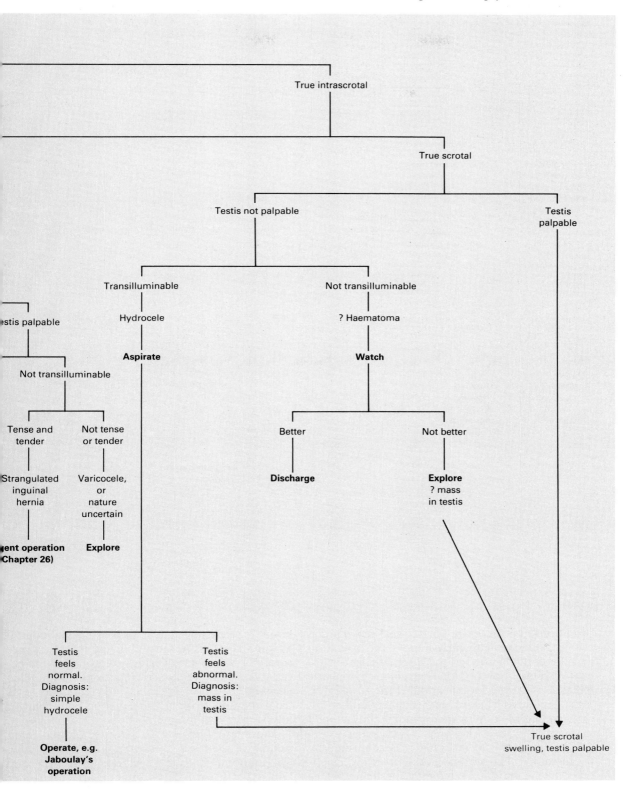

True intrascrotal

True scrotal

Testis not palpable

Testis palpable

Transilluminable

Not transilluminable

Hydrocele

? Haematoma

Aspirate

Watch

estis palpable

Not transilluminable

Better

Not better

Tense and tender

Not tense or tender

Discharge

Explore ? mass in testis

Strangulated inguinal hernia

Varicocele, or nature uncertain

gent operation Chapter 26)

Explore

Testis feels normal. Diagnosis: simple hydrocele

Testis feels abnormal. Diagnosis: mass in testis

Operate, e.g. Jaboulay's operation

True scrotal swelling, testis palpable

Flow-chart 14.1 (continued).

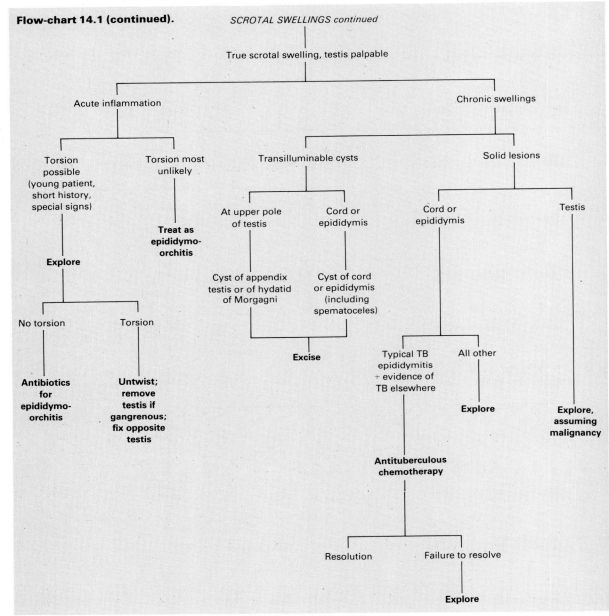

SCROTAL SWELLINGS continued

conditions; it is therefore advised that the inguinal canal be opened at an early stage of the operation and the cord clamped at the internal ring to prevent dissemination of blood-borne and lymphatic metastases during mobilization of the testis. The testis, epididymis, cord and their coverings are then excised right up to and including the clamped segment.

If the diagnosis of malignancy is confirmed by the histological appearances, radiotherapy is delivered to the para-aortic lymph nodes in an exten-sive field stretching high up the posterior abdominal wall. The reason for mobilizing the testis very carefully within its coverings is to obviate the necessity to irradiate the scrotum for possible spilled deposits, because screening the remaining testis from the effects of such irradiation is difficult or impossible.

There are basically two forms of malignant tumour of the testis: the *seminoma* and *teratoma*. The teratoma tends to affect a younger age group (20–40 years), while the seminoma affects an older

Flow-chart 14.2.

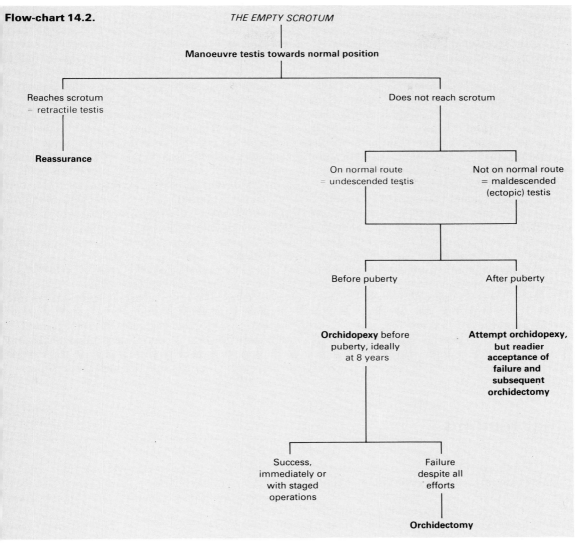

THE EMPTY SCROTUM

Manoeuvre testis towards normal position

Reaches scrotum = retractile testis

Reassurance

Does not reach scrotum

On normal route = undescended testis

Not on normal route = maldescended (ectopic) testis

Before puberty

After puberty

Orchidopexy before puberty, ideally at 8 years

Attempt orchidopexy, but readier acceptance of failure and subsequent orchidectomy

Success, immediately or with staged operations

Failure despite all efforts

Orchidectomy

(30–50 years). Both are biologically very malignant tumours, with distant spread being an early feature; however, a combination of surgery and radiotherapy as described, plus cytotoxic drugs is nowadays resulting in a much improved cure rate. The 5-year survival for all patients with a semi-noma now averages 95 per cent with combination therapy; the corresponding figure for the even more malignant teratoma is 60 per cent. Even blood-borne metastases in the lungs may respond dramatically to chemotherapy plus local irradiation.

The empty scrotum

Comments on this topic are made elsewhere also (p. 155).

If the testis does not lie in the scrotum, it may be *retractile, undescended,* or *ectopic* (maldescended).

The *retractile* testis occurs only before puberty: the powerful contraction of the cremaster muscle pulls the testis up into the inguinal canal, but in a warm room the patient clinician can, by gentle pressure on the inguinal canal, coax the testis downwards to occupy its normal position in the scrotum. No treatment is needed for this condition except reassurance for the parents: the testis settles in the scrotum at puberty.

The *undescended* testis is either not palpable at all (i.e. the testis is intra-abdominal), or can be felt at the external ring on its normal route towards the testis; but while it may be possible to manipulate such a testis for some distance towards the scrotum, it is not possible to get it into its normal intrascrotal position. Management depends upon whether the condition is unilateral or bilateral, and on whether the patient is pre- or postpubertal.

The aim of management is to get one, or preferably both, testes into the normal scrotal position before puberty, since otherwise the patient may be azoospermic. The production of spermatozoa is very sensitive to temperature, and only the relatively cool environment of the scrotum permits spermatogenesis. Moreover, the longer after puberty that a testis remains above the scrotum, the less likely is spermatogenesis to occur when the testis is placed in the correct position.

If one testis is in the normal position, the other side is explored before puberty (ideally at the age of about 8 years), and if possible the cord is mobilized sufficiently to enable the testis to reach, and be fixed in, the scrotum (orchidopexy). If puberty has already been reached, the same procedure is attempted for mainly cosmetic reasons. If orchidopexy is not possible, the testis should be removed because such organs show a high tendency to neoplasia.

If both testes are undescended, efforts are made — probably at different times — on both sides, and again definitely before puberty, to bring down each testis. If enough length of cord cannot be immediately obtained, staged operations achieving a lesser degree of lengthening at each step can be tried. Sometimes, especially with bilateral abdominal testes, it is finally necessary to sacrifice both organs and to produce or maintain the patient's secondary sexual functions with exogenous androgens.

The *ectopic* testis may lie anywhere in the inguinal, suprapubic and femoral regions. A common situation is above the inguinal ligament, in the so-called superficial inguinal pouch superficial to the external oblique muscle. Its management is identical with that of the undescended testis, but orchidopexy is usually easier because the cord is usually quite long enough to reach the scrotum.

Further reading

Blandy, J. P. (1966). The surgical management of testicular tumours. *British Journal of Hospital Medicine* **1**, 133–8.

Browse, N. L. (1978). The external genitalia. In: *An Introduction to the Symptoms and Signs of Surgical Disease*, pp. 300–22. London, Edward Arnold.

Dayan, A. (1966). The pathology of testicular tumours. *British Journal of Hospital Medicine* **1**, 126–30.

Thomas, W. E. G., Cooper, M. J., Crane, G. A., Lee, G. and Williamson, R. C. N. (1984). Testicular exocrine malfunction after torsion. *Lancet*, 1357–9.

Whittaker, R. H. (1975). Orchidopexy and orchidectomy. *British Journal of Hospital Medicine* **14**, 282–94.

Williamson, R. C. N. (1976). Torsion of the testis and allied conditions. *British Journal of Surgery* **63**, 465–76.

Chapter 15

Dysuria; Retention; Anuria

Introduction and definitions

There is much misunderstanding of the terms 'dysuria', 'retention, and 'anuria', and much looseness in their use. *Dysuria* in particular means different things to different doctors. Further cause for confusion is that the terms *dysuria* and *retention* are not mutually exclusive, while in practice *anuria* may readily be mistaken for retention.

The safe way to use the word *dysuria* is in the sense of its literal translation from its Greek stem, a disturbance of the act of micturition. *Retention* means that after an act of micturition, or an attempt at an act of micturition, there is still a significant amount of urine in the bladder. A patient with retention may or may not have dys-

uria: some patients with retention think they are passing urine normally, and are unaware that they are failing to empty the bladder, although most patients do have some obvious disturbance of micturition. *Anuria* means that the kidneys are not forming urine, so that once the bladder has been emptied it remains empty. However, during the period that the patient is only passing a few drops of urine at a time as he squeezes the bladder empty, the situation may be misinterpreted as retention.

Patients with dysuria/retention present with one of several typical clinical pictures that modify subsequent management.

Symptom patterns

Bladder outflow tract obstruction

The patient complains of frequency of micturition, and of various difficulties in connection with the act. The frequency is manifested by passing urine at shorter intervals than the normal four hours during the day, and by nocturia (i.e. the patient is woken from sleep during the night by having to pass urine). First and foremost of the difficulties with micturition is difficulty in starting the stream. Characteristically, the patient finds that he has to wait several seconds in a relaxed attitude before the flow will start, and this hesitancy is only aggravated if he strains; occasionally, however, a patient does find that he needs to strain. Once the flow starts, it is a thin stream with poor projection, and he has to strain more than normal to keep it going. When

the flow ceases, the cut-off is not sharp: dribbling continues for several seconds. The patient may be aware that his bladder still contains appreciable quantities of urine, and a few minutes later he may find it possible to pass more (*pis en deux*). In such a subject, if the call to micturition is voluntarily denied he may experience urgency, with painful suprapubic spasms, and even incontinence.

Most, if not all, of these symptoms can be mimicked by an overactive detrusor muscle. The root cause of such an instability remains unknown, but unlike the common cause of bladder–neck obstruction — benign hypertrophy of the prostate — it probably starts in childhood and certainly becomes clinically important at a much younger age. Again unlike prostatic obstruction, both sexes are affected though men more than women. Frequency is due to the impingement on the consciousness of the sharp contractions of the detrusor as soon as the volume in the bladder increases to perhaps 100 ml (instead of the usual 300–600 ml), and the apparently poor flow is related to the small volume in the bladder.

Acute urinary infection

The patient is often aware that his urine has an offensive smell and a turbid appearance. He complains of severe frequency, possibly having to urinate as frequently as every 15 minutes; of suprapubic pain partially relieved by micturition; and of a burning or stinging sensation in the urethra as the urine flows along it. These are the symptoms of cystourethritis; if the patient has pain in one or both loins, he may have pyelitis as well. Urinary infection is a common complication of an obstructed bladder, and patients with the latter condition should be asked whether they have had bouts of severe exacerbations of their symptoms in the past.

Strangury

This word means a severe pain at the root of the penis, sometimes with radiation along the urethra, associated with an urge to urinate but not relieved by the act. It is produced by irritant lesions at the base of the bladder or in the prostatic urethra; for example, calculi or carcinoma.

Haematuria

The complaint of having passed blood in the urine must always be taken seriously, to the extent that the patient should be referred to hospital even if the blood only appeared in one sample of urine. It is true that haematuria can occasionally be mimicked by the passage of red dyes in the urine, for example derived from beetroot eaten in excess, or from various purgatives such as phenolphthalein, or other drugs. In the author's experience, it is safer to ignore a history of the ingestion of such materials.

One should carefully inquire about the timing of the blood-staining relative to the act of micturition. If the whole sample of urine is uniformly blood-stained, it is likely that the source of the bleeding is in the upper urinary tract — kidneys and ureters — so that there has been time for mixing in the bladder. If the blood is not evenly mixed throughout the specimen, the earlier it appears in the sample the lower in the urinary tract is the bleeding lesion likely to be. A neoplasm of the urethra may discolour the first third of the stream only, while a similar lesion in the bladder may bleed only when it comes into contact with the opposite wall of the contracting bladder, and therefore only discolour the final third of the stream. It is vital to establish whether the haematuria is painful or painless (see p. 171).

Pneumaturia

A complaint of gas bubbles in the urine should also be taken seriously, since it may imply a fistulous connection between the bladder and the large bowel. In a proportion of cases, this diagnosis will not be substantiated, and the likely cause was a urinary infection with gas-forming micro-organisms or frothing of the urine after it was passed, as a result of lowered surface tension due to proteinuria.

```
                    DYSURIA/RETENTION
                           |
        ┌──────────────────┴──────────────────┐
Without trauma                        Following trauma
```

Management of atraumatic dysuria/retention

The patient who has been involved in trauma and may have urological complications presents an entirely separate situation which is discussed in the next section. The management of the case without a history of trauma is described here.

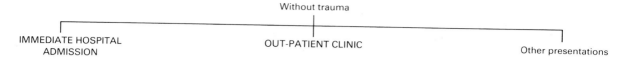

The general practitioner's role

Certain cases require immediate referral to a hospital casualty department with a view to immediate admission. They include patients with painless haematuria at the time of the consultation, or with strangury, or with complete or near-complete inability to pass urine either in conjunction with a palpable bladder (complete retention) or if the bladder is not palpable (i.e. one must assume anuria is present).

Other patients require referral in due course to the out–patient clinic of a hospital since they will need a thorough urological investigation, including cystoscopy. This category includes patients with a history of possible haematuria, with symptoms of outflow tract obstruction in combination with a palpable bladder (incomplete retention), or with a history of recurrent urinary infections for which the practitioner can find no explanation, or of pneumaturia.

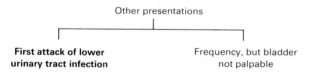

This leaves a residue of patients for the practitioner to consider more closely. The commonest problem is probably the patient with lower urinary tract infection in whom there is no relevant abnormality to be found with respect to history or physical signs. In a first attack, a mid-stream specimen of urine should be sent to the laboratory for culture and sensitivities of any organisms grown, and examination of the deposit; meanwhile the patient is started on a course of a suitable chemotherapeutic agent such as a highly soluble sulphonamide or ampicillin. The exact agent can be altered in the light of the bacteriological report in due course, and if the patient has not responded well. When the attack subsides, the question of investigation for an underlying serious cause arises. All children, all male patients and all patients in whom haematuria had occurred, should be investigated even after only one attack. In women, cystitis without a serious underlying cause is quite common, so that apart

from testing the urine for sugar the investigation of women aged 15–50 can reasonably be deferred till a second attack.

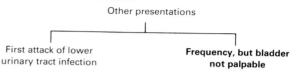

The other common problem for the practitioner is the patient complaining of frequency of micturition but whose bladder is not palpable. The commonest cause of frequency in the elderly male is outflow tract obstruction, but even in him there are many other causes, ranging from habit and insomnia through excessive intake of fluids or diuretics to diabetes mellitus or insipidus or chronic nephritis. From our viewpoint, the practitioner must pick out from this group those whose history is suggestive of bladder neck or urethral obstruction or of a hyperactive detrusor muscle (irritable bladder) and refer them to a surgeon or urologist.

Management in hospital

Every patient under investigation for dysuria/retention symptoms needs an estimation of blood urea, an intravenous pyelogram (IVP) and/or ultrasound, and examination of a mid-stream specimen of urine (MSU), but there is some variation in the order and much in the urgency of these investigations according to the type of problem presented, and of course other investigations are also required in certain patients, particularly the estimation of the flow–rate of micturition so as to decide whether outlet obstruction is present.

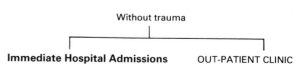

Emergency admissions

These comprise the patients with present painless haematuria, with strangury, and with complete retention.

IMMEDIATE HOSPITAL ADMISSION

Painless haematuria   Strangury   Complete or near-complete
                                                                                     inability to pass urine

Painless haematuria is nearly always the result of a neoplasm. In some patients the bleeding may be so profuse as to be alarming, but even with mild haematuria, immediate admission is indicated since the bleeding may suddenly increase in rate and anyway urgent investigation is required. Another reason is that in patients who have bled previously, and in whom full investigation has failed to reveal a source, there is at least a chance of determining by immediate cystoscopy the site of the lesion by seeing blood issuing from the appropriate ureteric orifice. This information can be crucial: a small renal haemangioma can be very difficult to diagnose, even by such sophisticated investigations as renal arteriography, and yet recurrent bleeding from such a lesion can be profuse enough to threaten life. It must be admitted, however, that such a case occurs rarely, and that cystoscopy during bleeding usually shows the surgeon only a bladder full of blood and throws no light on the source.

The usual trio of routine investigations, MSU, IVP and blood urea, is performed, and the intravenous pyelogram may demonstrate the lesion. Ultrasound is, more and more, displaying its value in the demonstration of space-occupying lesions of the urinary tract. If, as is likely, the appearances suggest a transitional-cell carcinoma of the lining of the urinary tract, then irrespective of the site of the lesion it is essential that the whole lower urinary tract be examined by cystourethroscopy. Carcinoma of the uroepithelium is frequently multifocal. Occasionally, some other lesion will be demonstrated — a renal carcinoma (Fig. 15.1a) that has eroded through the epithelium lining a calyx or the pelvis of the kidney, renal tuberculosis, calculous disease which for some reason has now given rise to pain, and so on. If no lesion is demonstrated, the surgeon

proceeds to cystourethroscopy. If the x-ray appearances are suggestive of a lesion somewhere in the upper tract, then the ipsilateral ureter is catheterized via the cystoscope with an acorn—ended catheter, and radiographic contrast solution injected up the ureter to give a retrograde ureterogram and pyelogram, and these films may resolve the doubt. Endoscopic techniques are now also available for direct inspection of the ureter, and are gradually supplanting the radiographic technique. Finally, if all these investigations are negative, it is worth making sure that there is no abnormality of the bleeding or clotting time.

If all these first-line investigations prove negative, the second-line must include urine cytology for malignant cells (despite the normal cystoscopy), examination of early morning specimens of urine for acid-fast bacilli (despite the normal IVP) and, in appropriate cases, examination of the urine for Schistosoma ova, and the sickle cell test. If these also prove negative, the surgeon has the choice of keeping the patient under review or subjecting him to the more powerful, but significantly more dangerous, investigation of renal arteriography (Fig. 15.1b). The decision will depend on such factors as the number of attacks of haematuria, the age of the patient (is he in the cancer age range?), his social history (is there tuberculosis in his family? does he work in a factory making chemicals such as aniline dyes that are known to have a carcinogenic effect on uroepithelium?), and so on. Should even renal arteriography prove negative, there is no alternative to keeping the patient under surveillance, and it is in this sort of case that if the patient bleeds again a cystoscopy while he is bleeding may prove invaluable.

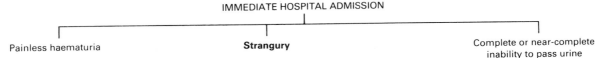

IMMEDIATE HOSPITAL ADMISSION

Painless haematuria   **Strangury**   Complete or near-complete
                                                                                     inability to pass urine

Strangury may occasionally be produced by a severe urinary infection, and if this seems a possibility it is wise to defer cystoscopy at least for a few hours until chemotherapy and antibiotics

have begun to get the infection under control. Urethral instrumentation during an acute urinary infection has a high incidence of the complications of pyelitis and septicaemia. In most cases,

(a)

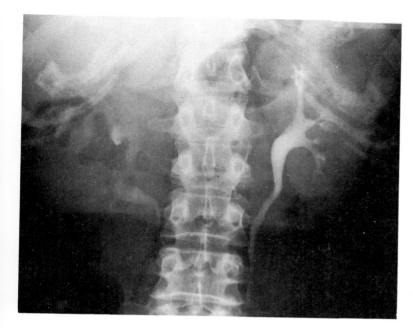

(b)

Fig. 15.1 Carcinoma of the kidney. (a) The deformity of the calyces of the right kidney, particularly the upper and middle calyces, shows that there is a lesion in the upper pole of the right kidney, possibly a carcinoma. (b) The renal arteriogram, the right artery has been selectively catheterized, and the blush of abnormal blood vessels at the upper pole confirms the diagnosis of carcinoma of the kidney.

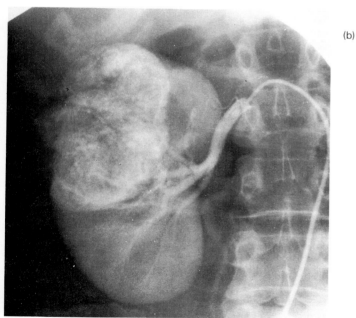

however, a patient with strangury should have a cystoscope passed immediately. This investigation usually produces a diagnosis of carcinoma of the bladder neck, which on histological examination may be of bladder or prostatic origin, or of a calculus impacted at the bladder neck. Bladder stones can usually be removed endoscopically, if necessary after crushing with a lithotrite also passed endoscopically, but occasionally the bladder has to be opened by the suprapubic route to remove a very large stone. For ultrasonic techniques of lithotrity, see p. 343.

| Painless haematuria | Strangury | **Complete or near-complete inability to pass urine** |

Complete (or near-complete) retention is an indication to attempt to pass a urethral catheter into the bladder. If this manoeuvre fails, there is probably an obstruction in the urethra although a very large prostate can be difficult to negotiate. If the prostate is very large, suprapubic catheterization (stab) is safer than repeated attempts at urethral catheterization, and this may be considered the best management even if a urethral stricture is suspected. In cases where the prostate is small, however, some urologists would make a further attempt to negotiate the urethra under anaesthesia. The cause of the obstruction in practice is always a stricture, consequent upon trauma or gonococcal urethritis in the past. The simplest technique is to pass a series of filiform bougies: the first few impact at the lower end of the stricture, but by their presence they ultimately guide the next one through the stricture. One can then fit a bougie of rather larger diameter to the end of the bougie that has been successfully passed, and the new one then be passed into the bladder in the wake of the original one that curls up in the bladder. The process is repeated till a reasonable dilatation has been achieved, whereupon an ordinary catheter can be passed to decompress the bladder. Occasionally this 'faggot' method with filiform bougies is not successful. The experienced urologist may have better success with attempts at bouginage under direct vision through a urethroscope, but general surgeons without special experience of the use of this instrument will have to drain the bladder by the suprapubic route: once the local engorgement and oedema provoked by retention have subsided, it usually becomes easy to pass a urethral catheter.

After a urethral stricture has been dilatated and the bladder decompressed, further management may be by repeated dilatations as often as necessary to maintain an adequate channel, or by urethroplasty, an operation in which the scarred urethral tissues are excised and a new tube constructed, usually by inlaying skin taken from the shaft of the penis.

The other situation that arises when an attempt is made to pass a urethral catheter is that the catheter does pass into the bladder and urine flows to the exterior. Thus the cause of the retention was obstruction at the prostate rather than in the urethra: the catheterization has been diagnostic as well as therapeutic. Most patients who have suffered complete retention require some form of operation involving the widening of the bladder neck, but in a few relatively young men (under the age of 55) who have not had much dysuria before the acute episode (acute retention) it is reasonable to maintain catheter drainage for 24–48 hours to let oedema subside and then remove the catheter in the hope that spontaneous micturition is now possible. The vast majority require surgery, either with or without a preliminary trial of catheter drainage: the exact form of operation used depends primarily on the size of the prostate gland (p. 175), and the timing depends upon whether the picture is truly acute or if the patient has had a chronic disturbance of micturition for some time before the acute episode (acute-on-chronic retention), with consequent damage of the kidneys. Suspicion of this latter possibility is aroused by such features as a long history of dysuria, a bladder that is very large (up to the region of the umbilicus) but feels fairly soft and non-tender, and a raised blood urea. It is renal function that matters, however, and since an intravenous pyelogram is necessary to help with the estimation of the size of the prostate, a simple rapid assessment of renal function is provided by noting how soon the kidneys excrete contrast at a sufficient concentration to show the pelvis and calyces. In general, if the kidneys are seen in the 5-minute film there is no contraindication to operating on the next available operating list; however, if the kidneys are damaged (i.e. if the blood urea is markedly raised), a period of several days of catheter drainage should be permitted before subjecting the patient to operation.

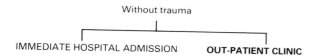

Without trauma

```
         ┌──────────────────────────┴──────────────┐
IMMEDIATE HOSPITAL ADMISSION              OUT-PATIENT CLINIC
```

Out—patient referrals

The routine management of these problems is to request the usual triad of urinary investigations — examination of the urine, blood urea estimation and intravenous pyelography — and then reassess.

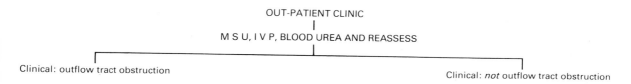

```
                         OUT-PATIENT CLINIC
                                 │
                 M S U, I V P, BLOOD UREA AND REASSESS
       ┌─────────────────────────┴──────────────────────────┐
Clinical: outflow tract obstruction          Clinical: *not* outflow tract obstruction
```

The vast bulk of these problems consists of middle-aged or elderly males with prostatic bladder neck obstruction or younger patients with an irritable bladder. The diagnosis is simple if there is a significant degree of retention, as shown by residual contrast material in the bladder in the after-micturition film of the pyelogram, and if the patient cannot achieve a urinary flow-rate above 10 ml/min (normal 18–25 ml/min). This is the picture of bladder neck obstruction, and an operation to enlarge the bladder neck is indicated. Some patients have frequency, urgency, etc., without retention and with a flow–rate in or approaching the normal range; they probably have a hyperactive detrusor and it is in this group that micturating, video—cystography with simultaneous pressure/flow studies can be of help. The basic defect of bladder neck obstruction is that when the detrusor muscle contracts in order to initiate micturition, it fails to pull apart the internal urinary meatus. In consequence, the detrusor at first responds with more vigorous contractions. Later the muscle tires, and emptying can be achieved only by voluntary contraction of the muscles of the abdominal wall. In the final stages, the bladder cannot be emptied completely. In the early stage of detrusor hypertrophy there often seems to be a coexistent irritability of the detrusor muscle, which goes into spasms of contraction that are the cause of urgency and frequency. This state of affairs is usually remedied by a suitable operation on the prostate and bladder neck, even in the absence of retention. However, should the video-cystography with pressure/flow studies not support the diagnosis of

bladder neck obstruction, but does indicate detrusor instability, the cure is not to be found in a surgical operation. Various drugs have been tried to reduce bladder irritability but so far with not much success: this is an unsolved problem. In the absence of detrusor instability the cause for the patient's symptoms must be sought elsewhere (see below).

The balance between the strengths of the detrusor and the internal sphincter can be affected by a number of neurological disorders such as tabes dorsalis, multiple sclerosis, Parkinson's disease and lesions of the cauda equina. Apart from the very rare occasions in which a reversible neurological defect has been corrected, the management of the imbalance is usually an operation on the bladder neck.

The essence of the operation for bladder neck obstruction seems to be to excise a wedge of the posterior lip of the internal urinary meatus, and it makes little difference how this is achieved. By and large, transurethral resection in the hands of a specialist urologist is the best operation and most urologists are prepared to do this procedure with prostates up to 100 g in size. If the prostate feels normal per rectum (smooth and of a firm consistency like that of the thenar eminence of the hand, with well preserved sulci between the lateral margins and the walls of the rectum, and a well marked median groove), it should be readily enucleable. The retropubic approach is best, because the tendency for a persistent urinary fistula after this operation is less than after the bladder has been opened. However, the retropubic approach is difficult unless the prostate is markedly enlarged (over 60 g), and for smaller prostates transurethral resection is preferable. On the other hand, if the prostate feels hard and irregular (in which case it is usually small also), it would be most unwise to attempt to enucleate it because it may be malignant and the operation of choice is an endoscopic resection of the prostate and bladder neck. Hard prostates are the seat of either carcinoma or chronic inflammation, and no effort should be spared to establish a diagnosis of carcinoma before the definitive operation, since treatment with oestrogens may improve the symptoms sufficiently to obviate the operation. If, in the absence of previous manipulative disturbance of the prostate by, for example, catheterization or even rectal examination, the serum acid phosphatase concentration is higher than 6 i.u./litre, it is likely that there is a carcinoma of the prostate which has spread beyond its capsule. Radiological evidence of osteoblastic metastases in the neighbouring pelvic bones is also highly suggestive. However, there is no substitute for a histological diagnosis, and an attempt should be made to get one in every case by needle biopsy via the perineal or transrectal routes.

There is also a perineal approach to a total prostatectomy for carcinoma of the prostate, but this is not often used these days.

Details of the operations cannot be given here. For the management of the patient after prostatectomy, see p. 228.

There remain for consideration those patients who have non-obstructive and non-irritable bladder urinary symptoms (i.e. urinary infection or pneumaturia) or who have symptoms which might have been due to obstruction but that diagnosis has been excluded by the preliminary investigations. A cystoscopy is mandatory, but if this does not yield the diagnosis, further investigations will be necessary. One cannot here detail all the various possibilities, but they may be grouped under the headings of congenital anomalies, abnormalities of propulsion in the urinary tract, calculous disease, inflammations and infections, and neoplasms. The first three will probably have been dignosed already by the pyelogram, although further radiographic examinations may be needed to define the exact anatomy of the defect, while the second and third categories are considered to some extent in Chapter 28. The category of infective diseases may require special bacteriological techniques, such as the examination of three consecutive early-morning specimens of urine for the Mycobacteria of tuberculosis or the examination of freshly voided urine for the ova of schistosomiasis. The treatment of infective diseases falls into two parts: the eradication of the causative organisms by the appropriate drugs, and the correction of the obstructive effects of healing by fibrosis. Neoplasia is treated primarily, where feasible, by excision, but especially in the bladder there is a place for a combination with radiotherapy or chemotherapy.

Management of post-traumatic dysuria/retention

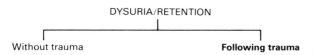

The possibility that the urinary tract has been damaged must be carefully assessed in any patient who has suffered trauma to the trunk. Management depends on whether there is damage to the spinal cord and on whether there is any reason to suspect that the lower urinary tract has been damaged (i.e. the bladder and urethra).

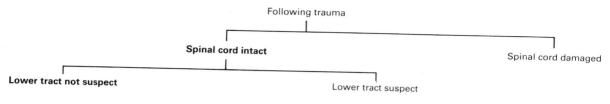

Lower urinary tract not suspect

If the patient is conscious, he is asked to void; if unconscious, a catheter is passed. If a normal-looking specimen of urine is obtained, and in particular if it is free from blood, it can reasonably be assumed that the upper urinary tract is intact. However, if there is frank blood in the specimen, damage to a kidney (or, rarely, a ureter) must be assumed to be present. In this case an intravenous pyelogram is performed in order to check not only the side and exact site and nature of the injury but also to determine whether the undamaged kidney on the opposite side is working normally.

In general, damage to the kidneys or ureters is treated conservatively unless one of the following indications for operation arises: shock due to massive bleeding, continued bleeding as shown by an increasing bulge in the affected loin, peritonitis due to rupture of the affected organ into the peritoneal cavity, and (later) infective complications such as perinephric abscess and septicaemia. What can be done at operation depends upon the exact details of the injury: if possible, the kidney is repaired, but if it is seriously disorganized and the opposite kidney is known to be functioning well, it may be necessary to perform a nephrectomy — a vital reason for getting an IVP done first!

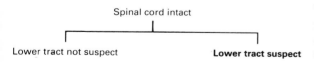

Lower urinary tract suspect

Reasonable grounds for suspicion include that the area injured was lower abdomen, perineum, external genitalia, or a fracture of the pelvis with displacement. If the patient gives a history of already having passed urine without difficulty, and the specimen passed is available and can be seen to be free of blood, and moreover if none of the specific indications of injury to the lower urinary tract mentioned below is present, it can be accepted that the tract is intact. In all other cases, the procedure detailed in the next paragraph is followed. The specific indications mentioned previously are: blood oozing from the external urethral meatus, generalized or lower abdominal peritonitis, bruising and swelling of the shaft of the penis, or induration of the lower abdominal wall extending downwards on to the upper 3−4 cm of the thigh due to extravasation of urine.

The patient is asked not to attempt to pass urine. Do not attempt to pass a urethral catheter. Attempts at urethral catheterization may aggravate the damage and convert a partial into a complete tear; therefore suprapubic catheterization should be instituted to allow the perineal tissues to heal with minimal fibrosis and hence with the best chance of avoiding subsequent stricture formation. Of course, if a complete tear is present an open operation to repair the torn tissues is ultimately inevitable.

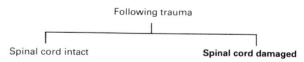

The bladder after spinal damage

The exact pattern of the disturbance of bladder function depends upon the completeness as well as upon the site of injury to the spinal cord. Full details cannot be given, but in the early stages complete retention is usual. The bladder must not be allowed to distend or there will be delay in the transition to the next stage, the automatic bladder. Bladder drainage is therefore performed, usually with a suprapubic catheter inserted using a stab technique. After a variable number of days or weeks, the bladder discharges itself when stimulated by local sensations such as stroking the medial side of the thigh, and catheters can be discarded.

Flow-chart 15.1   *DYSURIA/RETENTION*

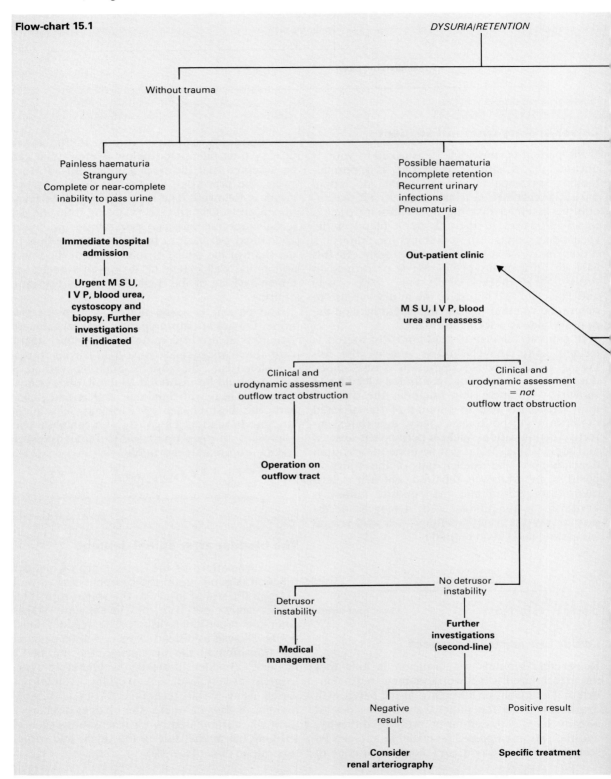

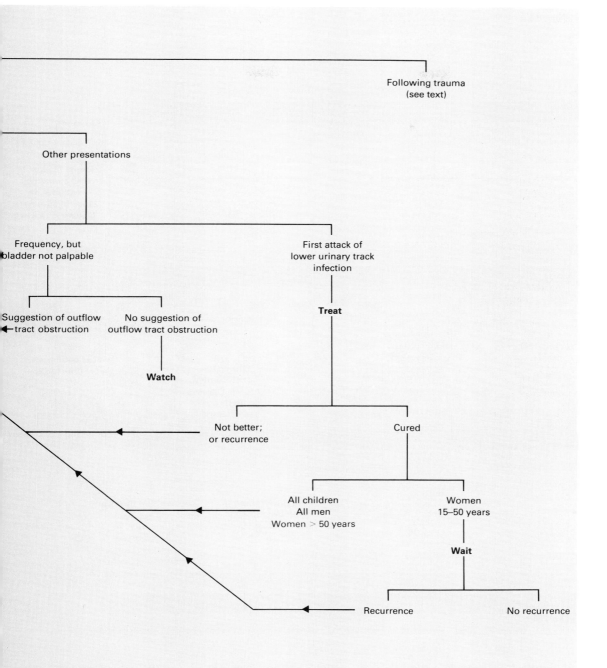

Following trauma
(see text)

Other presentations

Frequency, but
bladder not palpable

First attack of
lower urinary track
infection

Treat

Suggestion of outflow
tract obstruction

No suggestion of
outflow tract obstruction

Watch

Not better;
or recurrence

Cured

All children
All men
Women > 50 years

Women
15–50 years

Wait

Recurrence

No recurrence

Flow-chart 15.2

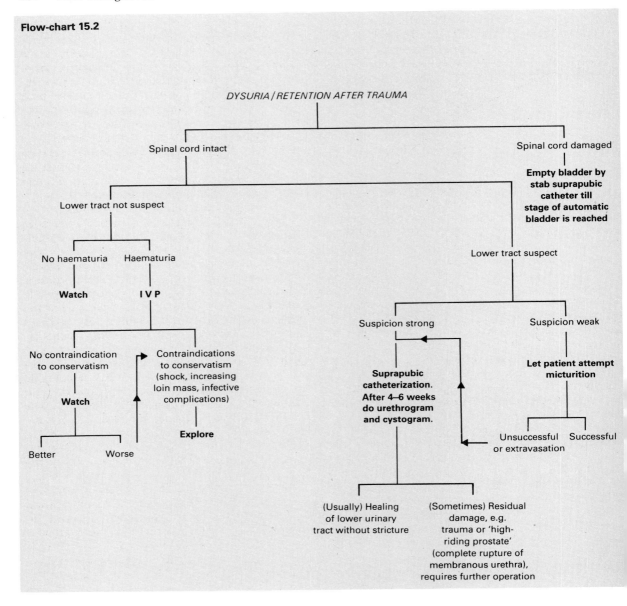

Anuria

The diagnosis of anuria is established by catheterizing the intact bladder some time after the last act of micturition and finding it empty.

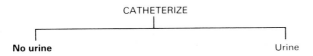

There are three groups of cases: pre-renal, renal and postrenal. The prerenal group is due to inadequate perfusion of the kidneys with arterial blood as part of the picture of shock. The renal group comprises all those conditions in which disease of the kidneys themselves results in a destruction of excretory function. The postrenal group results from obstruction of the outflow of urine from the kidney. While these are convenient categories, there is considerable overlap: long-continued renal hypoperfusion or ureteric obstruction each result in secondary renal damage which after a time becomes irreversible.

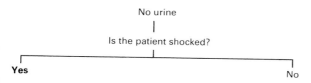

In a shocked patient it is usually wise to pass a urethral catheter so that the urine output can be monitored continuously. If anuria has already developed, the most important therapeutic measure is to restore the circulation in general, and therefore the circulation to the kidneys, to normal. In the case of the commonest form of shock — oligaemic — this will entail replenishing the circulation with an adequate volume of a fluid similar in nature to the fluid lost (p. 222). Some clinicians believe that renal damage (the so-called 'tubular necrosis') which might perpetuate the period of anuria is more likely to be prevented if a diuretic such as frusemide (Lasix) is given, but the author is unconvinced. For the special case of the patient who has obstructive jaundice, see p. 125.

Difficulties in diagnosis do sometimes arise in this group: the causative period of hypotension may have been brief or even unnoticed, or there may be oliguria (a urine output of less than 500 ml in 24 hours) rather than complete anuria, and there may be some other factor which might explain the oliguria. These conditions frequently arise in the early postoperative period, when a low urine output may be due to the postoperative metabolic response, to renal damage due to hypotension at some time during the operation, or to a combination of both causes. Helpful guides are: the specific gravity of the urine which should be high (greater than 1020) if the important factor is the postoperative response, but fixed at 1010 if the main cause is renal damage; and the rate of rise of the blood urea. If the latter exceeds 8 mmol/litre (50 mg/100 ml) in 24 hours, it is likely that the kidneys have been damaged.

In patients who are not shocked, there will in the majority be clinical evidence of the nature of the disease that has produced the anuria: acute nephritis, a long history of chronic nephritis or of bilateral ascending pyelonephritis, a carcinoma of the cervix that has spread to involve both ureters, and so on. If there is no guide to the cause, the surgeon's primary duty is to ensure that the case is not of the obstructive type: it is a tragedy if a patient is allowed to die from anuria due to bilateral ureteric obstruction from some readily correctable cause such as calculi. Careful renal ultrasound is the standard first investigation to exclude obstruction in renal failure.

Only if this investigation is inconclusive does the surgeon proceed to the much less safe alternatives of pyelography with a high dose of contrast which may show normal calyces and ureters in late films; or cystoscopy and bilateral ureteric catheterization, followed by a retrograde pyelogram if indicated, to establish the patency of the ureters and to determine whether any lesion is kinking or constricting the ureters from without.

If an obstructive cause is found, further management falls into three categories. First, the disease causing the obstruction may be irremediable and itself likely to cause an early death: in these circumstances the clinician might deem it wise not to attempt any further treatment. Secondly, the obstruction might be remediable but the patient too ill to undergo a complicated operation to correct it at that time: some form of decompression of one, or preferably both, kidneys is therefore performed in an effort to preserve renal function while the patient recovers from the effects of the anuria. The standard route for emergency decompression is percutaneous nephrostomy. Under ultrasound or x−ray control, a needle is passed through skin and abdominal wall into the distended renal pelvis and a catheter passed over the needle which is then withdrawn. This technique sounds heroic, but in fact it is easy and safe and available everywhere. Thirdly, the patient is fit enough to undergo the definitive operation immediately — the removal of the ureteric calculi, the release of the ureter from the constricting effect of retroperitoneal fibrosis, and so on.

In patients with primary renal damage, the surgeon's role is limited to renal biopsy (but see below).

Finally, no matter what has caused the renal failure, the surgeon's help may be requested in keeping the patient alive. If the renal disease is likely to be temporary, all that is necessary is to

Flow-chart 15.3

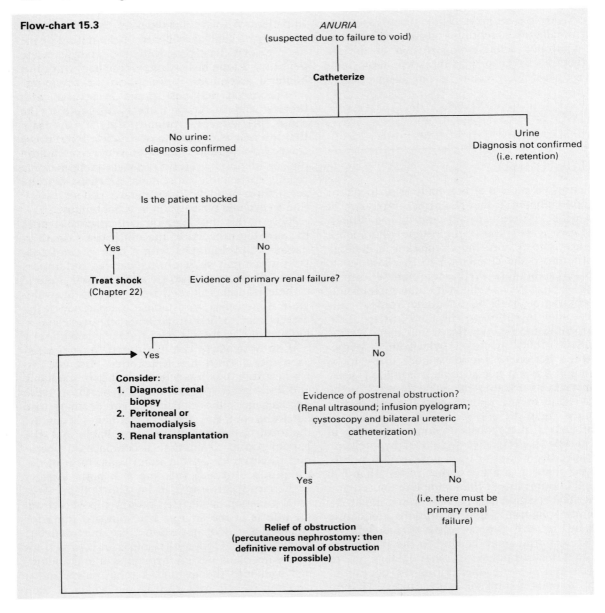

ANURIA
(suspected due to failure to void)

Catheterize

No urine:
diagnosis confirmed

Urine
Diagnosis not confirmed
(i.e. retention)

Is the patient shocked

Yes

No

Treat shock
(Chapter 22)

Evidence of primary renal failure?

Yes

No

Consider:
1. **Diagnostic renal biopsy**
2. **Peritoneal or haemodialysis**
3. **Renal transplantation**

Evidence of postrenal obstruction?
(Renal ultrasound; infusion pyelogram;
cystoscopy and bilateral ureteric
catheterization)

Yes

No

(i.e. there must be
primary renal
failure)

Relief of obstruction
(percutaneous nephrostomy: then
definitive removal of obstruction
if possible)

perform the execretory functions of the kidney by some artificial technique. The possibilities are peritoneal dialysis and renal haemodialysis. In the former, a cannula is passed through the anterior abdominal wall into the peritoneal cavity, as in paracentesis, and a balanced salt solution run into the peritoneum: urea and the other toxic metabolites that the kidneys usually excrete diffuse into the solution which, after a period to allow for equilibration, is then aspirated. In renal haemodialysis, an artery and vein are cannulated and connected to an apparatus in which the blood is circulated through tubing separated from a bathing solution by a semi-permeable membrane. The blood is cleansed of its toxic metabolites by the process of diffusion through the semi-permeable membrane. The 'artificial kidney' can be kept in the patient's own home, and connecting the patient's circulation to the machine is facilitated by the construction of an internal shunt between a convenient artery such as the radial at the wrist, and a neighbouring vein. Patients can be kept alive in theory indefinitely by a few hours of haemodialysis every few days. However, if the renal damage is irreversible, the only hope for a normal life-span lies in renal transplantation.

The technical problems of the transplantation operation itself have long been solved, but the reaction of immunity of the host against the foreign tissues of the donor still presents formidable difficulties. The best results are obtained with kidneys taken from a living volunteer donor who is closely related to the recipient, but there are grave ethical problems in this situation. The alternative solution is to use a kidney taken from a cadaver immediately after death. The problems here are again partly ethical: the kidneys deteriorate so rapidly after death that in practice the only useful source of such organs is a patient with severe brain damage who has been kept 'alive' by artificial ventilation, and who has 'died' as a result of that ventilation having been stopped. There is also the problem that the donor is not related, but methods of typing the histocompatibility antigens of donor and recipient are now advancing and giving real help in choosing a suitable donor kidney for an individual recipient. Finally, there is the problem of keeping the kidney alive while the final preparations are made for the transplantation operation: there are many preservation techniques available, but none that can be called excellent.

Once the transplantation has been carried out rejection can sometimes be suppressed by corticosteroids, x−rays, or chemical agents such as azathioprine (Imuran).

Further reading

Blandy, J. P. (1976). Lecture Notes on Urology. Oxford, Blackwell.

Blandy, J. P. (1980) Urethral stricture. *Postgraduate Medical Journal* **56**, 383–418.

Clark, P. (1985). *Operations in Urology*. Edinburgh, Churchill Livingstone.

Hindmarsh, J.R. (1984). Urological investigations. *Surgery* (Oxford) **1**,1 175−81.

Shuttleworth, K. E. D., Lloyd−Davies, R. W. and Greene, R. (1974). *Benign Enlargement of the Prostate*. London, Heinemann Medical.

Slade, N. (1976). Injuries to the kidney. In: *Urology*. Ed. Blandy, J.P. Oxford: Blackwell, 599−615.

Webb, D. R., McNicholas, T.A., Whitfield, H.N. and Wickham, J.E.A. (1985). Extracorporeal shockwave lithotripsy, endourology and open surgery: the management and follow−up of 200 patients with urinary calculi. *Annals of the Royal College of Surgeons of England* **67**, 337–340.

Whitfield, H.N. (1985) Urinary calculi. *Surgery* (Oxford) **1**, 474−7.

Williams, D. I. and Chisholm, G.D. (1976). *Scientific Foundations of Urology*, Vol 1, London, Heinemann Medical

Yeates, W. K. (1972). Disorders of bladder function. *Annals of the Royal College of Surgeons of England* **50**, 335−53.

Chapter 16

Chronic Ischaemia of the Lower Limb

Ischaemia is a reduction in arterial blood supply to a certain volume of tissue, sufficient to produce signs and/or symptoms. A flow at rest may become inadequate during exercise. Chronic ischaemia in the lower limb presents with four quite separate clinical patterns, but more than one of these may coexist in some patients and in others there is a tendency to progress from milder to severer patterns.

Clinical patterns

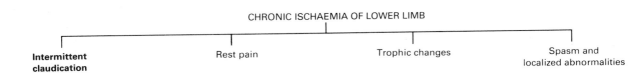

CHRONIC ISCHAEMIA OF LOWER LIMB

Intermittent claudication   Rest pain   Trophic changes   Spasm and localized abnormalities

Intermittent claudication

Claudication means limping. Intermittent claudication implies discomfort in the limb, which is not present all the time but commences after a reproducible severity of exercise of the limb and is relieved by standing still.

The type of discomfort produced is very variable from patient to patient. Limping itself is quite unusual: the use of the term 'claudication' derives from the fact that the syndrome, and its relationship to ischaemia, was first worked out in a horse which was seen to start limping every time it had walked a certain distance. In the human, the commonest symptom is pain, which is often described as being tight, or cramping, or bursting. Other symptoms include a sensation of cold, or of pins-and-needles, or numbness, or burning. The site of the pain is most often the calf, but shin, instep and thigh may be involved. Pain in the buttock may be particularly confusing, as it may be mistaken for sciatica unless great care is taken in eliciting the history.

The fact that the symptoms start each time after the same amount of exercise is one of the most characteristic features. The patient may describe how he walks each morning from his front door to a certain street-corner, and there has to stop and rest because of the discomfort. Walking uphill, or running for a bus, probably brings on the symptoms after a much shorter distance. It is important to determine the current claudication distance, and record it in the notes in such terms as '400 metres on the level at normal pace, 180 metres uphill'. It may also be crucial to the management of the case to note whether the claudication distance is static, or whether it is diminishing or increasing over the previous weeks or months.

The final characteristic of intermittent claudication is that it is relieved by standing still. The speed of relief is important: the acute symptoms should disappear within 1 minute, leaving at most only a bruised or heavy feeling. It is also important that *standing* still is enough to relieve the symptoms because this feature distinguishes intermittent claudication from the similar, but much rarer, venous claudication. The latter syndrome is due to a partial obstruction of the main venous drainage from a limb, usually in the common or external iliac vein, and consists of a severe bursting pain in the whole limb after a characteristic amount of exercise, but it is not relieved rapidly by standing still: the venous return must be further assisted by gravity, so the subject finds he has to sit or lie and elevate the limb.

In patients with intermittent claudication there may be no physical signs, or some of the stigmata referred to in the third pattern of presentation, trophic changes, may be present. Finally, on physical examination there may be direct evidence of the site, and occasionally of the nature, of the functional block reducing arterial inflow (p. 187).

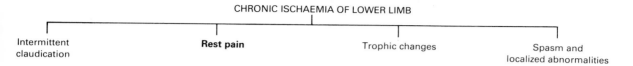

CHRONIC ISCHAEMIA OF LOWER LIMB

| Intermittent claudication | **Rest pain** | Trophic changes | Spasm and localized abnormalities |

Rest pain

Like intermittent claudication, the syndrome of rest pain, when fully developed, is diagnostic of arterial insufficiency. The commonest site is the foot, where the pain starts in the toes and works back to the heel. In severe cases pain may extend upwards to the thigh. The pain is intense, and most distressing since it is so difficult for the patient to find any relief. The various factors of exercise that bring on the pain of intermittent claudication also intensify rest pain, but one feature which is surprising at first sight is that the pain is particularly liable to come on when the patient is lying still in bed at night. The explanation of this anomaly is that the limb becomes heated under the bedclothes and tissue metabolism — and therefore the demand for oxygen — increases, while the blood pressure drops due to peripheral vasodilatation. In this situation the patient often finds some relief in throwing off the bedclothes and sitting up in bed with his legs hanging down over the side. In the most advanced cases, pain is present all the time without respite and the patient becomes morose and irritable, or even suicidal.

While this clinical picture is practically unmistakable and some stigmata of trophic origin are always present in the established case, it should be remembered that the pain of nerve or nerve-root irritation is similarly deeply felt and similarly intractable. The distinction lies in such features as the distribution of the pain and of alterations of skin sensation (stocking distribution in arterial insufficiency compared with the characteristic distribution of nerve or nerve-root), and the presence or absence of abnormalities of motor or reflex function (p. 186).

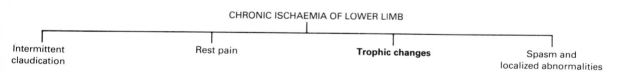

CHRONIC ISCHAEMIA OF LOWER LIMB

| Intermittent claudication | Rest pain | **Trophic changes** | Spasm and localized abnormalities |

Trophic changes

Inadequate arterial blood supply to the skin and subcutaneous tissues produces a wide spectrum of abnormalities culminating in ulceration and gangrene. An ulcer is a break in the surface lining of an organism, whether skin or mucosa, whose healing is delayed by some local pathological factor, while gangrene is death of tissue on a macroscopic scale. The lesser degrees of abnormality produced by ischaemia are typical and readily ascribable to that cause, but ulceration and gangrene are the end result of many disease processes other than ischaemia, so that their role as evidence of ischaemia must not be accepted uncritically.

In assessing trophic changes short of ulceration and gangrene, it is important to look for asymmetry between one leg and the other although it is not impossible for ischaemia to affect both legs symmetrically. The affected skin is pale and, in the more severe cases, shiny due to oedema. Hair is lost, while nails are brittle, ridged or otherwise deformed, and lose their lustre. The skin is cold to the touch, and its capillary circulation poor as demonstrated by pressing at one spot, then releasing the pressure and watching for the blanched area to be gradually recolorized as the capillaries dilate. A feature of the advanced case, where gangrene is imminent, is that marked changes in the colour of the limb occur with changes in posture. When the limb is passively elevated to an angle of 45 degrees, the skin of the leg below the knee dramatically blanches; when the limb is allowed next to hang down over the side of the bed, a dusky cyanosis appears.

An ulcer in an ischaemic limb is initiated by trauma, and the nature of the trauma can usually be elicited by a careful history. Apart from an accidental blow, which can naturally occur at any site, simple pressure over an area such as the ankle malleoli where the bone is close to the skin surface may be responsible. Such pressure commonly arises in a patient bed—bound for any reason, and the nursing care of pressure points is particularly important in the ischaemic limb. In an individual with an ischaemic lower limb, an ulcer at a pressure point or at a site of recent trauma may reasonably be assumed to be ischaemic in nature, although logically there are other possibilities (Chapter 17).

Gangrene in chronically ischaemic tissue is nearly always of the dry variety: the affected area becomes dark red, then purple and finally black, while the skin becomes increasingly wrinkled and shrivelled. The appearances at the margin of the gangrenous area depend upon the level of the blood supply there. If there is sufficient perfusion to support an acute inflammatory response, a clear—cut zone of inflammation demarcates the dead from the living tissue and the dead tissue ultimately sloughs off to leave a wound that heals. If perfusion is inadequate, the zone of inflammation is weak and indistinct, and the area of gangrene spreads.

If for some reason (such as congestive cardiac failure) the tissues are oedematous, or if infection supervenes, the gangrene is of the moist variety which is much more dangerous since it spreads rapidly and more commonly produces septicaemia. Mummification alone requires no urgent local treatment, but wet gangrene does.

Gangrene may spread from the margin of a traumatic ulcer, or, in a limb of which the blood supply falls below the critical overall level, it starts in the most poorly perfused tissues, i.e. the tips of the toes. Dry gangrene in an appropriate site in an ischaemic limb must be at least partly due to ischaemia, but other contributory factors must be carefully considered, especially if the gangrene is moist or unusually painless (p. 193).

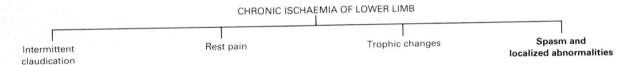

the hands. The pallor results from spasm of the digital arteries, the cyanosis from the stagnant pooling of blood in capillaries whose walls have dilated in consequence of a loss of tone induced by temporary ischaemic damage, and the final erythema from arteriolar dilatation stimulated by the anoxia via local reflexes when the spasm of contraction abates.

Spastic and localized abnormalities of arteries

There is a small group of patients that presents with skin colour changes indicative of arterial insufficiency, but in a spasmodic or intermittent pattern. An attack consists of one or both feet becoming suddenly white, and the patient experiences a sensation of cold and numbness. The colour next changes to deep purple, and finally to bright red, and in these later stages pain and tingling are prominent. The attacks are commonly provoked by exposure to cold, and the onset of the second and third phases and the ultimate return to normal can be accelerated by warming the limbs, for example by immersing them in warm water. This combination of symptoms and signs is called Raynaud's syndrome, and it in fact occurs more commonly in

In another small group of patients, the skin colour changes are permanent rather than spasmodic, but localized rather than in the diffuse distribution seen in the majority. Where the area affected is at an extremity (toes, in the present context, but also fingers, nose), the condition is called acrocyanosis, while localization to the skin of the calf is called Bazin's disease and a history that the lesion has been produced by exposure to cold defines a chilblain.

Identification of cause

In the majority of patients, the cause of chronic-ischaemia of the lower limb is occlusive arterial disease, but arterial and arteriovenous aneurysms account for a few cases and arteriospasm for a few more. The mechanism producing ischaemia in patients with aneurysms is that thrombus forms on the wall of the lesion and then fragments break off and are swept distally to occlude narrower arteries distal to the aneurysm. The crucial subdivision of arterial occlusive disease is into large and small vessel disease. The most important associated cause of damage to tissues from arterial insufficiency is a disturbance of sensory innervation. The exact nature of the association is unknown, but presumably it relates at least partly to the interference with protective reflexes that are designed to cause withdrawal of the limb from noxious stimuli such as heat, cold and pressure. The commonest condition which affects sensory innervation is diabetes mellitus, and it must also be remembered that occlusive arterial disease is more common in patients with diabetes.

The peripheral pulses

The peripheral pulses, by their presence or absence, and when present by the findings on auscultation, give most valuable information. If neither groin pulse can be felt, this means a blockage of the aortic bifurcation or of both iliac arteries. If one groin pulse cannot be felt, this indicates an obstruction somewhere between the aortic bifurcation and the beginning of the femoral artery. If both groin pulses can be felt, but the popliteal artery behind the knee, on one or both sides, does not pulsate, this locates the obstruction to the femoral artery in the thigh. (In practice, this is much the commonest situation that is encountered.) If the groin and knee pulses are absent, so will be the foot pulses. Occasionally it happens that all pulses to knee (popliteal) level are palpable, but the foot is pulseless. This indicates a block in the small vessels, which in practice suggests diabetes or collagen disease. The most extreme case of all is the patient whose symptoms are those of deficient blood supply to his muscles, but whose pulses can all be felt (see next section).

Obstructions of the main arterial system above the level of the knee raise the possibility of surgical intervention. Surgical techniques to overcome arterial obstruction below the knee can be performed but the results are poor in patients with atherosclerosis.

There are two special clinical features which may help to localize the block: in men, impotence is a common complication of a block at the aortic bifurcation, while in either sex a history of intermittent claudication in the buttock means that the internal iliac artery of the same side is blocked.

It is worth auscultating the groins. Sometimes a patient with a clear history of intermittent claudication has a femoral pulse that is strong enough to be acceptable as within normal limits, but a bruit heard with a stethoscope held over the vessel at the groin shows that there is some irregularity of the arterial tree proximal to the groin, even though it has not been sufficient to obliterate the femoral pulse. Pedal arterial blood pressure can also be simply measured in the outpatient clinic using a Doppler technique, and a low ankle/brachial systolic pressure ratio confirms ischaemia.

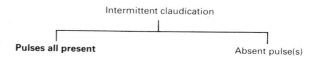

History of intermittent caludication but all pulses present

This is a challenging situation for the diagnostician. Most of these problem cases can be elucidated by re-examining the pulses after the patient has exercised: the increased blood flow through the leg muscles diverts blood from the peripheral arteries to demonstrate a deficiency in blood supply that had not been noticeable at rest. This is an important group surgically, because the cause of the relative reduction in blood supply is usually a localized block in an abdominal artery, aorta or iliacs, and such lesions usually give good results with reconstructive surgery.

In a few patients, the peripheral pulses are still present after exercise. If possible, this finding should be confirmed with the Doppler technique. There are three possible explanations: intermittent claudication of the cauda equina, McArdle's syndrome, or (in the absence of evidence of any other disease) functional overlay. Intermittent claudication of the cauda equina is sciatic pain (sometimes in association with neurological signs) produced by interference with the blood supply to the cauda equina by narrowing of the spinal canal, with or without protrusion of an intervertebral disc. A neurological opinion and careful x-rays of the lumbosacral spine clinch the diagnosis, and management is the province of the neurologist or the neuro-

surgeon. McArdle's syndrome is true ischaemic pain produced by the accumulation of pain factors, due not to an inadequate arterial supply but to the congenital lack of an enzyme (phosphorylase) vital to the efficient aerobic metabolism of the Krebs' cycle. The diagnosis is suggested by the youth of the patient and confirmed by special histochemical staining techniques of material obtained by muscle biopsy.

Management of large vessel disease

The working definition of large vessel disease is that potentially it is capable of being corrected by a surgical operation, i.e. there is a block above the level of the knee, and the popliteal pulse is absent or weak. Further management depends upon the pattern of presentation of the peripheral ischaemia in the individual patient, but in all patients one looks for evidence of contributory factors affecting sensation, such as diabetes mellitus (p. 193). Note that diabetes itself accelerates the vascular disease.

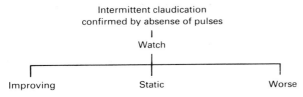

Intermittent claudication

This condition does not necessarily demand an attack upon the block. In many patients the symptoms are mild, and the important questions to ask are: do they interfere with his work? do they interfere with his leisure activities? how reasonably can one expect the patient to be prepared to modify his patterns of work and leisure? In any case it is justifiable to wait a few weeks or months, even if the answers to these questions suggest that surgery is indicated. One-third of patients with intermittent claudication get worse during such a period of observation, one-third improve, and in the remainder the condition remains static. If the symptoms are improving, or in any case do not interfere radically with the patient's capacity for work or enjoyment of life, conservative management is adopted (see below). However, if there is a case

for a surgical approach, further investigations must be undertaken to explore feasibility (p. 189).

Rest pain

This is a graver situation: not only does the pain tend to increase in severity and duration so as to become intolerable, but the integrity of at least a major portion of the limb is threatened. Rest pain should be considered synonymous with incipient gangrene. While immediate conservative measures are important in an effort to delay the onset of gangrene, further investigations to explore the feasibility of surgery are mandatory.

Trophic changes

The milder varieties, such as loss of hair and deformities of the nails, may coexist with a mild presentation such as intermittent claudication, and do not significantly influence the management of the claudication. Colour changes with passive elevation and depression of the foot, however, should be treated as evidence of incipient gangrene and, like actual ulceration and gangrene, demand further investigations, as an emergency, to explore the possibility of corrective surgery.

Arteriospastic changes

These should be thought of as a separate entity because, although they may proceed in a few cases to a situation where the spasm becomes fixed because the digital vessels are permanently occluded, it is rare to find large vessel disease in a case of arteriospasm.

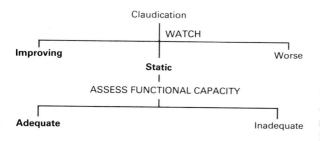

Claudication
WATCH

Improving   Worse

Static

ASSESS FUNCTIONAL CAPACITY

Adequate   Inadequate

Conservative management

Intermittent claudication

First, and this is most important, the patient is advised to give up all forms of tobacco, which has a deleterious effect upon peripheral arterial disease. Next the patient is encouraged to alter his work and leisure patterns to reduce the strain of exercise on the affected limb. The danger of minor trauma is emphasized: paring the toe-nails is particularly dangerous, and should be entrusted to a chiropodist. The limb should be kept socially clean by frequent washing, to discourage infection of any small abrasion, and drying with a soft towel should be followed by powdering of the feet and toes to reduce friction against stock-

Rest pain and trophic changes

URGENT CONSERVATIVE MEASURES

ings and shoes. The subjective sensation that the limb is cold worries many patients, and they must be warned that the ischaemic limb is particularly prone to injury by burning: hot-water bottles in bed and sitting too near a fire or radiator are highly dangerous. Athlete's foot and similar skin problems must be treated early and efficiently to avoid secondary infection. Exercise should not be completely avoided. The instruction is given to take plenty of exercise to just beyond the threshold of pain production, in the hope that the anoxic stimulus encourages the development of a collateral circulation. Anaemia, and any other factor interfering with nutrition, is corrected.

Rest pain and gangrene

When the patient complains of pain at rest, and particularly if the severe trophic changes of ulceration and gangrene are present, the advice given for intermittent claudication is modified by the fact that the patient should be admitted to hospital for bed-rest, urgently in the patient with rest pain only, immediately if ulceration or gangrene is present. The nursing care of the limb at risk is of crucial importance, and much ingenuity may be needed to ensure that there is no untoward pressure anywhere upon ischaemic tissues. As far as possible, the ischaemic tissues are exposed and kept cool, if necessary with the aid of a fan. The bed is given a slight foot-down tilt.

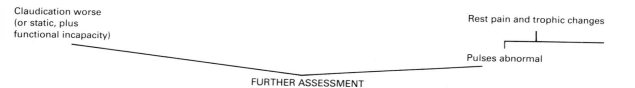

Claudication worse
(or static, plus
functional incapacity)

Rest pain and trophic changes

Pulses abnormal

FURTHER ASSESSMENT

Further investigation

If reconstructive surgery needs to be considered, the first step is a very thorough assessment to determine whether the patient is a reasonable risk. Patients with occlusive arterial disease affecting the lower limbs are only too likely to be affected by similar changes in the arteries elsewhere, especially the cerebral and the coronary vessels. There is no point in relieving a patient's intermittent claudication if he is then able to walk a little further and develop angina! A full

neurological and cardiological assessment is mandatory, with ECG and chest x-rays, and further arteriographic studies of the cerebral and coronary circulations if necessary.

 If the subject passes this assessment, Doppler ultrasound measurements of arterial pressure at various levels in the limb (in comparison with brachial pressures) are performed. Some imaging technique to show the vessels of the lower limb is undertaken. Information is sought on the site and length of any block, the patency of the

Image1: FURTHER ASSESSMENT branching to OPERATION INDICATED and LEAVE ± AMPUTATION WHEN NECESSARY.

Image2: FURTHER ASSESSMENT → OPERATION / LEAVE ± AMPUTATION WHEN NECESSARY; OPERATION branches to Unsuccessful / Successful.

vessels below the block – the 'run–off' – and the presence or absence of atherosclerosis in the arteries other than at the site of the block. Because of this last goal, it is usual to aim at a picture of the aorta and the arteries of both lower limbs, even if the symptoms and signs seem to be unilateral.

The standard technique is trans-femoral aortography. Under general anaesthesia a catheter is inserted percutaneously from the thigh to reach the aorta a short distance above the bifurcation, and a rapid injection of a large volume of radio-opaque solution made. Films are taken in rapid succession to show the bifurcation with the iliac vessels, the femoral vessels in the groin and thigh, and the region of lower thigh and upper leg. Recently a non-invasive technique using ultrasound in two planes — the so-called mobile artery and vein imaging system — has been developed and it may ultimately supplant arteriography.

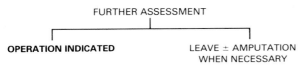

FURTHER ASSESSMENT

OPERATION INDICATED   LEAVE ± AMPUTATION
                             WHEN NECESSARY

Reconstructive surgery

The occluded segment of vessel may be excised and replaced, or it may be bypassed by some form of graft or prosthesis, or else the lumen may be restored by the reboring procedure known as disobliterative endarterectomy. In the abdomen (i.e. in the aorta and iliac arteries) disobliteration of short occluded segments may be successful, but for the more usual longer obstructions the popular procedure is excision and replacement with a prosthesis made of a knitted synthetic material such as Dacron. Below the inguinal ligament, the surgeon should discuss with the radiologist any patient with a short occlusion. There is now available a technique called balloon angioplasty, in which the radiologist (under X-ray control) percutaneously passes a catheter into the artery so that the balloon lies at the strictured site, and then distends the balloon in order to dilate the stricture. The procedure is surprisingly safe, and in selected patients can even be repeated. Should this technique fail, or be considered inappropriate (and it is important to remember that it can make matters worse), the most successful operation has been found to be a femoropopliteal bypass, using a reversed length of long saphenous vein taken from the same limb.

At the end of the operation, the patency of the new channel is checked by electromagnetic flow-meter or direct (puncture) pressure studies.

For a few days after operation there is a tendency for the limb to look red and swollen. These changes probably reflect the distensibility and leakiness of capillaries that have been damaged by a long period of chronic anoxia and are now exposed to the full force of the re-opened circulation. Ultimately, the capillaries recover their tone and these changes disappear.

After a successful operation, rest pain disappears and intermittent claudication usually improves. The relief of claudication, however, is not as certain as the relief of rest pain, and this is one reason for regarding claudication as only a relative indication for attempting reconstructive surgery. See later for the effects on ulceration and gangrene.

No matter how successful the operation, the patient's prognosis is not very good. For the prostheses, it would appear that 5 years later one-third of the patients are doing well, one-third have developed occlusion again in the same limb, many with loss of the limb, and one-third have succumbed to the effects of atherosclerosis elsewhere. For vein grafts, the results are better, with patency rates at 5 years of 80 per cent.

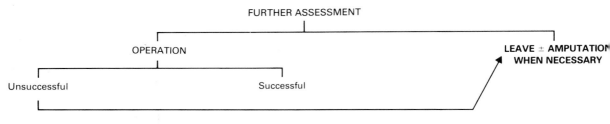

FURTHER ASSESSMENT

OPERATION   LEAVE ± AMPUTATION
                                                       WHEN NECESSARY

Unsuccessful   Successful

Ablative surgery

Where ischaemia has produced gross death of tissue with ulceration and/or gangrene, the patient is probably in severe pain, he is incapacitated in that he probably cannot walk, and he is at risk from the severe complications of infection such as septicaemia. For all these reasons it is urgent to achieve healing as quickly as possible. Healing can only be achieved by excising all dead and dying tissue through a region of the limb that is sufficiently well vascularized to support the healing of the remaining tissues by first intention. On the other hand, one naturally wishes to preserve as much as possible of the patient's limb and its function.

The timing of the operation is just as important as the details of exactly what is excised. Observation for a few hours when the patient first presents categorizes the ischaemic changes as stable (static) or unstable (advancing). If the area of gangrene is advancing, and particularly if there is any suggestion of infective complications, the situation is a surgical emergency and the sooner amputation is performed the better. If the area of gangrene is not advancing, the proximal zone of inflammation is well localized, and the patient's general condition is good, one has time to consider whether reconstructive surgery is feasible. Remember, however, that a patient's general condition rapidly deteriorates when he has rest pain, and that the condition of his coronary arteries may be crucial. The particular potential of reconstructive surgery is in the case where gangrene is limited to the distal extremity of the limb but the doubtful perfusion of areas well proximal suggests that healing of the amputation wound will not occur unless it is set at a very high level. In such a patient, a successful reconstruction of, say, a block in the femoral artery may enable a purely local amputation such as that of a single digit to heal successfully whereas without reconstruction it might have been necessary to amputate above the knee.

The advice that part of his limb needs to be amputated is always unwelcome to a patient, since he feels that the operation is destroying part of his being. The correct approach by the surgeon, to enlist the patient's full co-operation, is therefore crucial. It must be pointed out that the operation is one phase in a *constructive* process aimed at achieving healing and the restoration of function, if necessary with the aid of an artificial limb, and that the tissue being removed by the operation has already been killed by the disease, even if the process of killing is not yet complete.

Theoretically, an amputation may be performed at any level in the limb but in practice most amputations are done at certain sites of election. In patients with large vessel disease, it is unlikely that an amputation as peripheral as the ankle or foot will be successful (except after reconstructive surgery as mentioned above), and so the peripheral amputations are described with the management of small vessel disease (p. 195). The three common proximal amputations are the below-knee, the through-knee, and the above-knee (or mid-thigh).

Below-knee amputation

The function of the knee joint is maintained. To facilitate the fitting of an artificial limb, the stump must be at least 8 cm, and preferably 13 cm long, measured downwards from the tibial tuberosity. There is no advantage in constructing a longer stump, and a considerable disadvantage in that the blood supply at the periphery is very likely to be less good. If the blood supply of the limb is judged to be inadequate for a below-knee amputation, either a through-knee or an above–knee amputation should be performed.

Through-knee amputation

Bending at the knee is lost. On the other hand, the large bulk of the femoral condyles, usually re-inforced by the surgeon's incorporating the patella and its tendon in the long anterior flap, produces a very stable, directly weight-bearing stump. It should be remembered that it is very difficult to walk with two stiff knees, and so in bilateral cases a through-knee amputation should not be performed on both sides.

Above-knee (mid-thigh) amputation

Ideally the femur should be divided 25 cm below the greater tuberosity. As the length of the stump is decreased, so is the mechanical work of leverage required to manipulate a long and heavy artificial limb greatly increased. However, an artificial knee joint can be incorporated in the prosthesis, and the gain in agility, particularly in the younger, stronger patient, compensates for some loss of stability as compared with the through-knee amputation.

Selection of amputation site

No hard and fast rules can be laid down, but skin flaps constructed from pale, shiny skin are unlikely to remain viable, an operation at a level at which the patient experiences rest pain is unlikely to heal, and impalpability of the popliteal pulse is a relative contraindication to a below-knee amputation. Doppler pressure measurements can be useful, and so can transcutaneous measurements of tissue oxygen tension.

Preparation for amputation

The patient is warned about phantom limb — i.e. that after the operation he will still seem to be aware of the portion of the limb that has been ablated. It should be emphasized that phantom limb is a normal phenomenon after amputation, and that it is common for the phantom to be painful for a short time but that the pain disappears in a few days or a week or two. Since the adoption of this policy, persistent painful phantom has become less common.

Thought must also be given to the question of antibiotic cover if the amputation has to be performed as an emergency without time to get infection in the gangrenous area under control. In any case, prophylactic antibiotics to prevent clostridial infection are always used for above-knee amputations.

Where time permits, it is a good idea to have the patient visited by someone who has undergone a similar amputation and is well adjusted to his disability. In a few cases, it may even be possible to arrange a preoperative visit to the local limb-fitting centre.

The operation

The surgeon aims to produce a conical stump which will fit snugly into the cup of an artificial limb, and to try to cover cut edges of bone with muscle and fascia so as to avoid pressure necrosis of the overlying skin from within. Haemostasis must be meticulous, and suction drainage is of particular value. If the operation is an emergency procedure in the presence of heavy infection, it may be considered wise not to sew the skin flaps together, but just to let them fall together. This technique ensures that no tension develops in the subcutaneous space, and this considerably reduces the likelihood of infection.

After amputation

Any of the usual complications of any surgical operation may arise, but peculiar to amputations is the problem of joint contractures. The affected limb is nursed fairly still for a few days, and it is most important that flexion contractures at hip or knee are not permitted to develop. Such contractures result in an effective shortening of the limb, and may make the subsequent use of an artificial limb difficult or impossible. Frequent changes of the patient's position, including the use of the prone position, and some arrangement to ensure that the limb lies flat along the bed (i.e. with the knee extended), together with avoidance of the semi-recumbent posture that encourages flexion at the hip, are all helpful measures. After a few days, gentle exercises are started and bandaging of the stump commenced with more pressure distally than proximally so as to encourage oedema fluid out of the stump. When the stitches have been removed, the patient is taught to walk with crutches (if there was no time to do this before operation) and he is sent to the limb-fitting centre where he is measured for a temporary artificial limb known as a pylon ('peg-leg'). The date of his discharge from the hospital ward depends upon home circumstances, availability of home helps and physiotherapy services, etc. When he receives his pylon, he is taught to walk with this and gradually discards his crutches. Finally, when the process of shrinkage of the tissues of the stump is complete, he is measured and ultimately fitted with his definitive artificial limb. The process of rehabilitation is not complete until the amputee has returned to his usual job, or has been retrained for a new job that is within his new more limited capabilities, and is a reasonably independent member of society again.

Management with pulses present

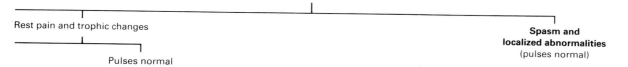

Rest pain and trophic changes

Pulses normal

Spasm and localized abnormalities (pulses normal)

Arteriospastic disease

The best treatment for Raynaud's disease is that the patient should move to a warm climate, but in the usual event that this advice is impracticable the operation of lumbar sympathectomy should be considered.

This operation consists of removal of the second, third and fourth lumbar sympathetic ganglia, together with the lumbar sympathetic chain between these ganglia. The result is that the skin of the ipsilateral lower limb becomes dry, warm and red, due to the destruction of sympathetic tone to the sweat glands and cutaneous blood vessels. It should be noted that the arterial tone in the deeper, muscular vessels is not decreased, and this explains why sympathectomy does not usually improve intermittent claudication.

The operation of lumbar sympathectomy is certain in its immediate effect, but unfortunately the effect tends to be only temporary. Ultimately the sympathetic tone reasserts itself through mechanisms not well understood. Since there is a natural tendency for Raynaud's disease to become less severe as the patient grows older, it is advisable to defer operation for as long as possible.

In men, and in all older patients, one should assume that the symptoms are Raynaud's phenomenon rather than Raynaud's disease, i.e. that there is some underlying condition such as a collagenosis which should be sought and treated. It is usually advisable to ask a physician to see the patient.

Lumbar sympathectomy is unlikely to be necessary for the minor spastic diseases such as chilblain or Bazin's disease, but it may be a useful measure in the cold, withered and weak limb one sometimes sees after anterior poliomyelitis.

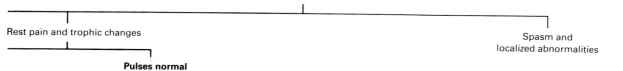

Rest pain and trophic changes

Pulses normal (small vessel disease)

Spasm and localized abnormalities

Small vessel disease

If there is no evidence of arteriospasm, and the peripheral pulses are present, then the obstruction to the arterial supply must lie in the small arteries or arterioles. If a possible cause for obstruction in the small vessels has been found proximally, for example an aneurysm which may be a source of multiple small emboli, then dealing with that cause may result in an arrest or improvement in the distal disease.

In the absence of any such cause, no curative measures are available. Any underlying disease such as diabetes mellitus or tabes dorsalis must be treated appropriately. Sympathectomy may be tried for intermittent claudication, but it is unlikely to be successful. Strenuous efforts must be made to persuade the patient to stop smoking. Areas of ulceration and gangrene on the feet are much more likely to respond to conservative surgery than in patients with large vessel disease.

Of particular interest and importance is the management of trophic ulcers These lesions occur in patients with impairment of sensation in the feet due to diabetic neuropathy or to the spinal cord changes of a disease such as tabes dorsalis. In such denervated feet there is a special danger from repeated minor trauma of which the patient is not aware. The skin over the pressure

Flow-chart 16.1

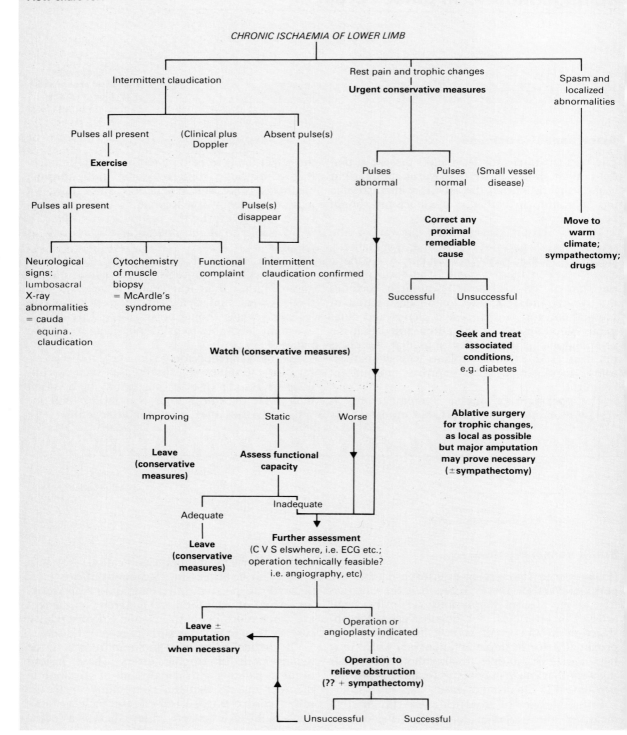

CHRONIC ISCHAEMIA OF LOWER LIMB

Intermittent claudication

Rest pain and trophic changes
Urgent conservative measures

Spasm and localized abnormalities

Pulses all present   (Clinical plus Doppler)   Absent pulse(s)

Exercise

Pulses abnormal   Pulses normal   (Small vessel disease)

Pulses all present   Pulse(s) disappear

Correct any proximal remediable cause

Move to warm climate; sympathectomy; drugs

Neurological signs: lumbosacral X-ray abnormalities = cauda equina, claudication

Cytochemistry of muscle biopsy = McArdle's syndrome

Functional complaint

Intermittent claudication confirmed

Successful   Unsuccessful

Seek and treat associated conditions, e.g. diabetes

Watch (conservative measures)

Ablative surgery for trophic changes, as local as possible but major amputation may prove necessary (±sympathectomy)

Improving   Static   Worse

Leave (conservative measures)

Assess functional capacity

Adequate   Inadequate

Leave (conservative measures)

Further assessment (C V S elswhere, i.e. ECG etc.; operation technically feasible? i.e. angiography, etc)

Leave ± amputation when necessary

Operation or angioplasty indicated

Operation to relieve obstruction (?? + sympathectomy)

Unsuccessful   Successful

areas on the sole becomes particularly thick and prone to flaking (hyperkeratosis). A minor abrasion may become infected, and track deep and silently over a wide surrounding area without this being obvious through the thickened overlying skin. The typical appearance is of a small, circular ulcer set in the centre of a large surrounding zone of keratosis. Drainage must be complete to be effective, and the whole abscess cavity must be deroofed. The extent of spread is accurately determined by probing, and the overlying skin cut away.

In all patients with such lesions, the leg should be x-rayed to determine whether the infection has spread to the underlying bones or joints. There is no prospect of healing unless all infected osseous material is excised. The sort of operation often required is amputation of a digit, or of a digit with the corresponding metatarsal or the distal half of the metatarsal (the 'ray' amputation). After such a procedure, any attempt to sew up the wound would certainly fail and so the wound should be left widely open, and constructed in such a way as to facilitate drainage when the patient is lying on his back in bed. More than one ray may be amputated in this way, or all five toes, or a transmetatarsal amputation may be done; provided drainage is adequate, healing though slow is remarkably sure. The difference from the corresponding situation in large vessel disease, where local operations are fraught with disaster, is obvious. In this context it is important to remember that a diabetic may have atherosclerosis and his pulses may be absent, and in that case his peripheral ulceration must be treated radically rather than conservatively: the important factor is the presence or absence of foot pulses rather than the presence or absence of diabetes.

After healing has been achieved, the care of the feet is most important if the situation is not to relapse. All the measures described previously (p. 189) are instituted. In addition, hyperkeratotic areas are kept pared down, and special footwear is provided, designed to distribute the pressure of weight bearing as evenly as possible over the remaining sole. It is surprising how well these patients are able to walk after local amputations, even after important weight-bearing structures such as the head of the first metatarsal have been removed.

Further reading

Blau, J.N. and Logue, V. (1961). Intermittent claudication of the cauda equina. *Lancet* i, 1081–6.

Campbell, W.B., Jeans, W.D., Cole, S.E.A. and Baird, R.N. (1983). Percutaneous transluminal angioplasty for lower limb ischaemia. *British Journal of Surgery* 70, 736–9.

Cutajar, C.L., Marston, A. and Newcombe, J.F. (1973). Value of cuff occlusion pressures in assessment of peripheral vascular disease. *British Medical Journal* 2, 392–5.

Delbridge, L., Ctercteko, G., Fowler, C., Reeve, T.S. and Le Quesne, L.P. (1985). The aetiology of diabetic neuropathic ulceration of the foot. *British Journal of Surgery* 72, 1–6.

Faris, J. (1975). Small and large vessel disease in the development of foot lesions in diabetes. *Diabetologia* 11, 249–53.

Gardham, J.R.C. (1976). The ischaemic leg. *British Journal of Hospital Medicine* 16, 43–52.

Lewis, J.D., Papathanaiou, C., Yao, S.T. and Eastcott, H.H.G. (1972). Simultaneous flow and pressure measurements in intermittent claudication. *British Journal of Surgery* 59, 418–22.

Ratliff, D.A., Clyne, C.A.C., Chant, A.D.B. and Webster, H.J.J. (1984). Prediction of amputation wound healing: the role of transcutaneous PO_2 assessment. *British Journal of Surgery* 71, 219–22.

Taylor, G.W. (1973). Chronic arterial occlusion. In: *Peripheral Vascular Surgery*, pp. 211–34. Ed. by M. Birnstingl. London, Heinemann Medical.

Varicose Veins; Ulcers

Varicose veins

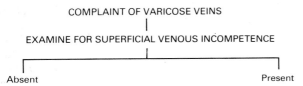

COMPLAINT OF VARICOSE VEINS

EXAMINE FOR SUPERFICIAL VENOUS INCOMPETENCE

Absent   Present

The doctor must beware of accepting a patient's diagnosis of varicose veins. On the one hand, patients often attribute a sensation of heaviness in the lower limbs towards the end of a long day of standing at work to the presence of varicose veins, or they may mistake for varicose veins the dilatations of tiny blood vessels in the skin that are correctly known as telangiectases.

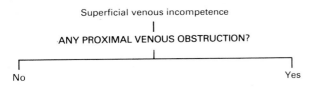

Superficial venous incompetence

ANY PROXIMAL VENOUS OBSTRUCTION?

No   Yes

On the other hand, the patient may indeed have varicose veins, but these may be secondary to a much more serious lesion that has produced them by obstructing the venous return, or the patient's symptoms may in fact be nothing to do with his varicose veins. Telangiectases require no treatment other than reassurance, while if the gravitational oedema and soreness of the lower limbs is due to acute foot strain or congestive cardiac failure or any other predisposing cause, the advice of the appropriate specialist should be sought. Similarly, while it may be unrealistic to advise that everyone with varicose veins should undergo a digital examination of the rectum to exclude a pelvic neoplasm, there is clearly little point in anything but conservative measures in the management of varicose veins in a pregnant

woman, whose veins will almost certainly return to normal a few weeks after the delivery.

Definition

Varicose veins are often defined as dilated tortuous veins, but not all varicose veins are tortuous and dilatation can be produced in any vein by obstructing the return of blood from the vein. The important distinction between a varicose and a normal vein is that the former remains full under circumstances in which the latter is empty, and this is because the valves designed to keep the normal vein empty are not working properly in the varicose vein. This may be because there is something wrong with the valves, or something wrong with the vein so that its wall has become lax and distended thereby rendering the valves useless. In either case, a varicose vein is a vein with incompetent valves.

In practice, veins with incompetent valves occur only in the lower limb, and while incompetence may occur in the valves of veins deep to the deep fascia as well as in superficial veins, it is only the superficial veins that are easily recognizable by sight and touch. In the clinical sense, therefore, varicose veins are veins of the superficial venous system in the lower limbs, with incompetent valves.

Assessment

The anatomy of the varicose veins must be established: are they of the long or of the short saphenous system, or of both? Where are the incompetent valves?

The first question is not always as easy to answer as it may appear. It is true that the long saphenous vein lies on the medial aspect of the thigh and leg and immediately anterior to the medial malleolus at the ankle, whereas the short saphenous vein enters the deep system in the mid-axial line of the limb behind the knee, and lies on the lateral aspect of the calf and behind the lateral malleolus at the ankle. Nevertheless, tributaries leading into one or the other of these systems may, in patients with varicose veins, wander over wide territories of the subcutaneous area of the limb and below the knee there may be a real difficulty in deciding whether any given tributary is a part of the long saphenous or of the short saphenous system. A technique that is useful even in a fat patient in whom the veins may be difficult to see is to map out a vein by tapping at one spot with the forefinger of one hand and picking up the vibration transmitted along its channel to a point several centimetres distant with the forefinger of the other hand, left lying lightly against the vein. In the absence of competent valves, the propagation of the impulse is excellent and it is usually a simple matter to follow the vein along its course until it definitely enters the long or the short saphenous system.

The second question is of crucial importance in treatment. In the normal way the blood in the superficial veins is sucked into the deep venous system by the so-called perforating veins that run through defects in the deep fascia. These perforating veins have valves that normally permit blood to pass only in the direction superficial-to-deep. Incompetence of the valve in a perforating vein leads to accumulation of blood in the superficial system over the area normally drained by that perforating vein. The suction force is provided by the muscle-pump effect of the muscles of the calf, which, as they contract and bulge laterally under the restraining envelope of deep fascia, squeeze the perforators and the deep veins to push blood back towards the heart in the direction permitted by the valves in the deep venous system. Thus the cure of varicose veins depends upon destroying the reflux of blood from the deep to the superficial venous system along incompetent perforators.

The highest perforating vein is the long saphenous vein itself as it dips through the cribriform fascia at the fossa ovalis, 4 cm below and lateral to the pubic tubercle, to enter the femoral vein. In many patients with varicosities of the long saphenous system, it is this uppermost valve only that is incompetent. One test for incompetence at this valve is to place the fingers of one hand lightly on the long saphenous vein in the upper part of the thigh, and ask the patient to cough. If the valve is incompetent, the forced rise in intra-abdominal pressure produced by coughing is transmitted retrogradely down the venous system to produce a palpable thrill in the wall of the saphenous vein.

Trendelenburg's test is better. The patient lies down, the examiner elevates the patient's leg passively to 45 degrees and empties the long saphenous system by the external pressure of his hand. The examiner then obliterates the upper end of the long saphenous vein by firm pressure with several fingers at a point 4 cm below and lateral to the pubic tubercle. While this pressure is maintained, the patient stands. At this stage, provided there are no incompetent perforators lower down the limb, the long saphenous system remains empty. Should there be any filling of the veins, a note should be made as to whether this filling is confined to the region below the knee or if the whole length seems to be affected. If there is no filling over a period of 15 seconds or so, the examiner's fingers are then removed suddenly, whereupon there is a rapid and dramatic filling of the venous system through its connection with the femoral vein if the uppermost valve in the saphenous vein is indeed incompetent. An appropriate modification of this test can be used to demonstrate incompetence at the junction of the short saphenous vein with the deep system.

It is usually easy to decide about incompetence of a valve at the upper end of each vein, and also to decide whether or not there are any perforators lower than the uppermost valve that are incompetent. The problem arises when one tries to define the exact position of incompetent perforators. The obvious technique to try is a modification of Trendelenburg's test in which pressure is applied at successively lower points along the course of a varicose main vein, but the results are often difficult to interpret. The Doppler technique can be used to assess the direction of flow at specific sites, and this can be most helpful. Some surgeons claim to be able to feel the windows in the deep fascia through which the perforating veins run, while infrared photography has been used in an attempt to show up the 'hot spots' of the warm blood in the dilated incompetent perforators. The delineation of the venous system by phlebography can be useful, but this is hardly a technique that can be used in the routine case of varicose veins because it is time consuming and requires the services of a skilled radiologist.

Finally, remember that the assessment is not complete until the question has been asked, could these varicose veins be secondary to some intra-abdominal lesion that is obstructing the venous return?

Management

Varicose veins do not by their presence constitute an indication for treatment, because complications such as superficial thrombophlebitis are quite rare. On the other hand, if such complications have occurred in the past, or if the patient complains of symptoms such as tiredness and aching, etc., that can justifiably be attributed to the veins and for which no other cause can be found, then treatment should be given. It should be remembered that obstruction of the deep veins can cause such symptoms. If the patient has no symptoms but objects to the unsightliness of the veins, then the fact that dangerous sequelae such as deep venous thrombosis have been shown to be commoner in patients with varicose veins should lead one to accede to the patient's request for treatment.

There are two forms of treatment: operation and injection. The principle of both forms of treatment is identical — the destruction of the incompetent perforators between the deep and the superficial venous systems. The operator divides between ligatures the long saphenous vein at its upper end, where it joins the femoral vein, and similarly divides all local tributaries of the long saphenous vein. If clinical examination had shown no incompetent perforators further down the leg, theoretically nothing further is needed. In practice, however, one is always worried about possible incompetent perforators and so an attack is made on the rest of the long saphenous vein at the same operation. One popular technique is to pass a long, flexible, metal rod upwards along the lumen of the vein from a phlebotomy at the knee. The lower end of the rod or stripper has a conical head, which can be tied securely to the lower cut end of the femoral vein at the knee. The upper end of the rod is then pulled proximally, thereby turning the long saphenous vein inside out and stripping it upwards out of the subcutaneous region of the leg. This technique has the advantage of removing the bulk of the varicosities immediately, and it also destroys the connections with any incompetent perforating veins. If the stripper will not pass, a not uncommon contingency in long-standing cases with very tortuous veins, a number of small incisions are made along the course of the long saphenous vein and segments of it are excised. It is helpful to have mapped on the leg the site of suspected perforators, so that these areas of the venous system in particular can be excised. Similar small incisions can be used to excise segments of varicose veins below the knee. Stripping should not be taken lower than the knee because of the risk that the procedure will damage the saphenous nerves.

Injection therapy consists of injecting a sclerosant substance into a varicose vein to promote a chemical thrombophlebitis which, on healing by fibrosis, obliterates the vein. With the advent of stripping techniques, injection therapy went out of fashion for several years. Recently it has been popularized again by Feegan, who has made it much more effective by paying attention to various points of detail, such as that the segment of vein being injected is isolated from the rest of the venous system by pressure at appropriate points so that the effect of the sclerosant is applied maximally at its target area. This precaution also reduces the risk that sclerosant will enter the deep veins and damage their valves. Obviously the effect of the injections will be greatest if the site of perforators has been accurately deduced. Injection therapy avoids the necessity for the patient to have a surgical operation, a procedure which is usually done as an inpatient and which is usually followed by a stay in hospital of between 1 and 3 days, and the end results are probably just as good as those obtained by operation, but the treatment may need to be repeated as recurrence is common.

Ulcers

An ulcer is a macroscopic break in the integrity of skin or mucous membrane.

In forming an assessment of an ulcer, it will be found useful to start by making as accurate a description as possible of the ulcer. Apart from the obvious features of site, size and shape, an ulcer has an edge, a floor and a base, and the condition of the neighbouring lymphatic glands requires to be reported.

The edge of an ulcer is often its most character-

Flow-chart 17.1

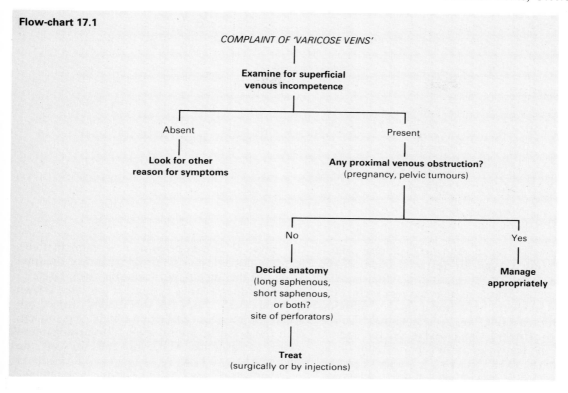

COMPLAINT OF 'VARICOSE VEINS'

Examine for superficial
venous incompetence

Absent

Look for other
reason for symptoms

Present

Any proximal venous obstruction?
(pregnancy, pelvic tumours)

No

Decide anatomy
(long saphenous,
short saphenous,
or both?
site of perforators)

Treat
(surgically or by injections)

Yes

Manage
appropriately

istic feature. In a simple traumatic, non-specific infected ulcer, the edges are terraced as new epithelium grows in from the surroundings. The edge of a tuberculous ulcer is undermined, that of a basal cell carcinoma (rodent ulcer, p. 14) is rolled, while that of a squamous cell carcinoma is everted. By contrast with these, a peptic ulcer of stomach or duodenum has vertical 'punched-out' edges.

The floor of an ulcer consists of the tissues exposed by the deficiency in the integument. The nature of these tissues is important because it decides whether a skin graft is likely to be successful; split-skin grafts do not take well on bone, for example. In order to see the structures in the floor of the ulcer it is often necessary to remove a slough of dead tissue lying superficial to the floor. This slough may itself be of diagnostic value; for example, the wash-leather appearance of the slough in a gummatous ulcer, a lesion of tertiary syphilis.

Where there is a clear history of trauma, the diagnosis of a traumatic ulcer will not be in doubt. The factor of superadded infection will probably be obvious from the appearance and smell of the discharge from the ulcer, and can be assessed more accurately by the appropriate

bacteriological investigations. There are three kinds of common ulcer which are so typical that they are usually treated without getting histological confirmation of their nature. Two of these are described elsewhere: the ischaemic ulcer (p. 185), and the perforating ulcer (p. 195). The third of these is the gravitational ulcer, which is described below. If an ulcer does not fall into any of the categories mentioned in this paragraph, there should be no question of treating it until histological examination of a biopsy of the edge of the ulcer has revealed the underlying cause.

Gravitational ulcer

The characteristic feature of a gravitational ulcer is its site: on the medial or lateral aspect of the leg anywhere from the malleolus below and extending upwards about half-way up the leg on the medial aspect, one-third of the way on the lateral aspect. In severe cases, an ulcer on the medial aspect may merge with one on the lateral aspect to become circumferential.

Infection is always present, and the floor of the ulcer is slough. In cases where there is an attempt at healing, the new epithelium grows in

Flow-chart 17.2

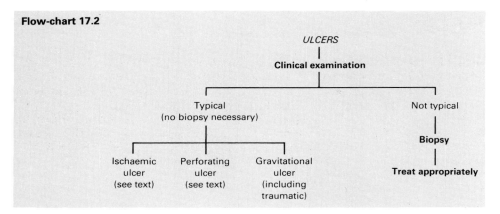

from the edges as a thin, transparent bluish zone covering a typically terraced edge. If the ulcer has been of long-standing, the base is tough, fibrous, avascular scar tissue which is unstable and likely to break down again with minor trauma after healing has been achieved. This is particularly true of those ulcers on the medial aspect of the leg whose base is periosteum of the tibia.

The cause of a gravitational ulcer is unknown, but the erect posture and weight bearing play some part. All gravitational ulcers can be made to heal by putting the patient to bed, with the leg slightly elevated, for a sufficient period (several weeks in a severe case). Severe venous stasis, such as follows widespread deep venous thrombosis in the limb followed by recanalization with incompetent valves, is often complicated by such ulcers. Ulcers and varicose veins may coexist, and it is tempting to argue, by analogy with the correlation with incompetence of the deep veins, that the back-pressure resulting from the incompetent valves in the superficial venous system can also produce the ulcers. Indeed, this view has been so widely held that the ulcers are often referred to as 'venous' or 'varicose' ulcers. However, both conditions are common, and are therefore likely to be encountered together by coincidence, and ordinary operations on the superficial varicosities do not have great success in curing ulcers. These facts, plus the peculiar distribution of gravitational ulcers, have led to the generally accepted theory that the cause is localized venous stasis produced by incompetence in

the valves of certain *perforators* − veins that collect blood from the superficial tissues of the lower half of the leg and perforate the deep fascia to enter the deep venous system. It has been shown that the perforators on the medial aspect are greater in number, and extend higher up the leg, than those on the lateral aspect, an arrangement which corresponds well with the sites of the ulcers.

Treatment is based on this theory. If it is important that the patient remain ambulant, the local venous hypertension is counteracted by pressure produced by elastic bandages or stockings, particularly the type of stocking said to produce a graded compression, applied over a dressing. If the ulcer proves refractory to such management, or shows a tendency to break down again rapidly after healing has been achieved, then one or both of two operative approaches may be necessary. Through a posterior vertical incision through the skin and deep fascia, the perforating veins can be demonstrated and divided between ligatures. Alternatively, the ulcer and its base of unstable tissue may be excised and the defect grafted. Ideally one would like to use a full-thickness skin graft for maximal resistance to recurrent ulceration, but the region is relatively avascular and so split-skin grafts are used. However, by the technique of serial application of several layers of split-skin after the abrasion of the previous layer, a reasonable thickness can be achieved. Pinch grafts — whole thickness skin in the middle, partial thickness at the periphery — are also helpful.

Further reading

Burnand, K., O'Donnell, T., Thomas, M. L. and Browse, N. L. (1976). Relation between post-phlebitic changes in the deep veins and results of surgical treatment of venous ulcers, *Lancet* **i**, 936−8.

Clyne, C. A. C., Ramsden, W. H., Chant, A. D. B. and Webster, J. H. H. (1985). Oxygen tension on the skin of the gaiter area of limbs with venous disease, *British Journal of Surgery*, **72**, 644−7.

Dodd, H. and Cockett, F. B. (1976). *The Pathology and Survery of the Veins of the Lower Limb*, 2nd ed. Edinburgh, London and New York, Churchill Livingstone.

Negus, D. (1985). Prevention and treatment of venous ulceration. *Annals of The Royal College of Surgeons of England*, **67**, 144–8.

Chapter 18

Preparation for Operation

This Chapter concentrates upon the problem posed to the medical student or resident doctor by the routine admission to a surgical ward of a patient who is to be prepared for an elective surgical operation. Some modifications that may be required if there is an urgent indication for operation will be mentioned where appropriate, and others are discussed in Chapters 3, 11 and 12.

The real difficulty and challenge of this situation is that the majority of patients admitted for an operation are fit in every way except for the particular localized lesion which necessitates operation, and so the clinician's task consists mainly of the repetitive, and therefore boring, procedure of eliciting a negative history and performing a negative physical examination. There is a natural tendency to try to save time by cutting corners, and this is the road to disaster.

One way to ensure that no relevant question or physical test is left out is to make a list of everything that should be done and check each item. In some institutions this technique has been adopted, even to the extent of collecting the information in a form suitable for feeding into a computer to facilitate keeping records, doing research, and even using computer programmes to reach a most probable diagnosis. An alternative system is to consider the problem under the four headings of general fitness, concurrent disease, anaesthesia, and specific items related to the particular operation and the individual patient.

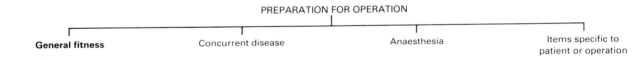

General fitness

This subject is best considered in terms of systems.

Cardiovascular

Evidence of fitness includes: lack of a past history of cardiovascular disease; lack of inappropriate dyspnoea, or of chest pain particularly on effort, and of palpitations and swelling of the ankles; a normal blood pressure, and a normal pulse rate and rhythm; and normal heart sounds on auscultation. The only special investigation usually performed as a routine to confirm cardiological fitness is the chest x-ray, which should show a heart of normal size and shape.

Respiratory

Evidence of fitness includes: lack of a past history of chronic respiratory disease such as chronic bronchitis, or of recent (within the past 2 months) acute respiratory disease; absence of dyspnoea, cyanosis, cough, stridor, wheeze, coryza and sore throat; and normal findings on physical examination of the chest. Despite all evidence of fitness, a history of smoking more than five cigarettes a day should be viewed with suspicion. To confirm respiratory fitness, a chest x-ray is performed: this should show well expanded lungs with no evidence of collapse or consolidation, and no abnormal shadows in the lung fields or mediastinum.

Digestive

The patient fit with respect to the gastrointestinal system has no history of digestive disease, and in particular has had no abdominal operation; there is no present history of digestive symptoms, abdominal pain or a change in bowel habit, and there are no abnormal physical signs on examination of the mouth, supraclavicular region (for lymph nodes), fingers (for clubbing), abdomen and rectum and anal canal. It is emphasized that every adult patient admitted to a surgical ward should have a digital examination of the rectum. In many centres, if these criteria for normality of the gastrointestinal tract are met no special investigations are done, but there is a case for doing simple liver function tests as a routine. See also urine testing in the next paragraph.

Urogenital

Evidence of normality includes absence of nocturia, a frequency of micturition during the day not greater than six times, no dysuria (Chapter 15), a good appetite, a normal sleep rhythm, and absence of pain in the loin, flank or groin. Sexual function should be inquired about if it seems possible that it might be relevant, and women should be asked about their menstrual history and whether they are taking a contraceptive pill. Premenstrual pain or irregularities in timing of the menstrual cycle that have been going on for several months can be accepted as within normal limits in the sense that they do not require postponement of the elective procedure, but it may be wise to obtain a gynaecologist's opinion in case he wishes to do some minor diagnostic procedure under the same general anaesthetic.

On examination, the tissues are normally hydrated, the kidneys may be palpable but are not tender (p. 109), the bladder is not palpable if the patient has recently passed water, and the external genitalia are normal. During the rectal examination the prostate is assessed: its size does not matter if the patient has no complaints with regard to micturition and if there is no evidence of retention, but it is important that the gland should be of the normal consistency, firm and smooth, with a median furrow.

The usual screen of special investigations is provided by a blood urea in the normal range and normal results on testing the urine — absence of albuminuria, colour in the normal range without blood. The other test on urine performed as a routine is for glucose (see the section on metabolism), and should be negative.

Blood and reticuloendothiel

These two systems should be thought about together as there is considerable overlap.

The normal patient has no history of a bleeding tendency and no complaints suggestive of anaemia such as fatigue, dyspnoea, pallor. There is no history of allergic disease or collagenoses.

On examination, there is no pallor of skin or mucous membranes, neither spleen nor liver is palpable, and no abnormal lymph nodes can be felt. The last aspect requires judgement and experience: the occasional small soft lymph node in any region can be considered to be within normal limits (the groins commonly contain several large easily palpable nodes without any serious pathological cause) and the territory draining any region containing a node judged to be pathologically affected is carefully examined for minor trauma or infection that could account for the findings.

The screening investigations are a haemoglobin estimation and examination of a blood film to make sure that there is no obvious abnormality of the erythrocytes or leucocytes, an erythrocyte count and the calculation of mean corpuscular volume and mean corpuscular haemoglobin concentration, and a total leucocyte count. The haemoglobin concentration and the haematocrit are equally valuable as baseline measurements in the assessment of changes in the body fluids giving rise to haemoconcentration (p. 315). Although not always routinely done, the author believes it is advisable that every patient admitted to a surgical ward should have his blood grouped and serum saved in case crossmatching of blood for transfusion should become necessary. All patients of Negro or Mediterranean or Arab origin should also have their blood examined for sickle cell disease or trait.

Metabolic

Metabolic disorder is unlikely to be present if the patient says that in general he feels fit, if he looks normal in terms of facies, skin, configuration, and secondary sexual characteristics, if he does not appear to be unduly tense, agitated or lethargic, if his blood pressure is within normal limits, and if his urine contains no glucose and the plasma electrolyte concentrations are normal.

Neurological

If there are no symptoms of neurological disorder, reliance is usually placed on an abbreviated examination of the nervous system. The exact details of this vary with the clinician, but it might reasonably include rough testing of the second to twelfth cranial nerves, the eliciting of normal limb reflexes and plantar responses, and the demonstration that power in the limbs is within normal limits.

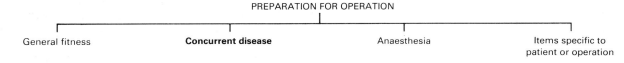

PREPARATION FOR OPERATION

General fitness   **Concurrent disease**   Anaesthesia   Items specific to patient or operation

Concurrent disease

Cardiovascular

Four common patterns of cardiovascular disease require consideration.

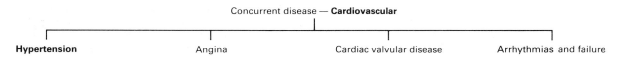

Concurrent disease — **Cardiovascular**

Hypertension   Angina   Cardiac valvular disease   Arrhythmias and failure

Hypertension

The important surgical implications depend upon the age of the patient: is he in the age group in which it is common to meet so-called essential hypertension, i.e. over about 50 years? or is he younger, and should one therefore consider the possibility that the hypertension is secondary to some condition which is potentially remediable, sometimes by surgery?

The younger the hypertensive patient, the more likely is it that one will find a primary cause. Unless the condition for which the patient has been admitted is urgent, it is wise to try to find the cause of the hypertension first in the hope that it may be possible to correct this, thereby improving the prognosis of anaesthesia and surgery.

Coarctation of the aorta usually presents in children and young adults, although it may draw attention to itself by its complications or associated cardiac abnormalities in infancy or occasionally be missed until the patient has arrived at middle age. The lesion is a narrowing of the arch of the aorta, usually quite localized, and at a site just distal to the point at which the ductus arteriosus enters the descending aorta, but sometimes it extends over a long segment of the aorta and sometimes it is at a different site.

The effect of the narowing is to produce hypertension in the upper half of the individual, while in the lower half the blood pressure is normal or only slightly raised. In consequence, the patient's physique is better developed in his upper half than in the lower, and these individuals tend to have strong arms and a deep, muscular chest, with an arm-span greater than their height. The most characteristic finding is that the femoral pulses are impalpable, or weak and delayed compared with the radial. The blood pressure lower in the thighs than in the arms can be measured with a sphygmomanometer, but a special cuff must be used. If the coarctation is sited more proximally than usual (i.e. between the innominate and left subclavian arteries), the left radial pulse may be weaker than the right. Large anastomotic channels develop between the high pressure territory and the low, and these particularly arise from the intercostal arteries and may produce a hum on auscultation over the back of the chest. These vessels also erode the bone in the region of the necks of the ribs, producing characteristic appearances in a chest x-ray.

Coarctation is normally an indication for correction by a surgical operation, and if this diagnosis is made clinically a cardiologist and cardiac surgeon should be consulted. The diagnosis is confirmed by angiocardiography. In this investigation, a cannula is introduced into the left ventricle via a brachial artery and a large, rapid injection of radiographic contrast material given. X-ray films are taken of the contrast being ejected from the ventricle and along the arch of the aorta. The technique is not only valuable in demonstrating the exact position of the narrowing and its length, but also for giving warning of associated anomalies such as aneurysms, persistent patency of the ductus arteriosus, and other congenital cardiac lesions such as defective heart valves.

The operation in experienced hands carries a low mortality, but is more dangerous at the extremes of youth and age. The large anastomotic vessels in the chest wall test the surgeon's technical skills when he is opening the chest. If the lesion is of the uncomplicated short-segment type, it is usually found possible to mobilize the upper and lower ends left after the narow segment has been excised and to sew them together to restore the aortic continuity. With long-segment lesions or cases with local anatomical complications, the gap is bridged with a Dacron prosthesis. After the operation, the usual care after a thoracotomy is needed (p. 226).

Hypertension secondary to adrenal disease includes Cushing's syndrome, Conn's syndrome, and phaeochromocytoma. These are considered later, under metabolic diseases, p. 212.

Hypertension secondary to renal disease is usually not amenable to surgical correction, since the pathological process usually involves both kidneys. Indeed, it is often difficult to be sure whether the chronic nephritis, resulting in a scarred, contracted kidney that concentrates poorly, is a consequence of exposure to hypertension or whether the renal disease has, via renal ischaemia and the renin mechanism, produced the hypertension. Very occasionally, however, unilateral renal disease may occur in association with hypertension, and the possibility that the hypertension may be relieved by appropriate treatment for the renal lesion then requires consideration.

All younger patients with hypertension should have an ultrasound or intravenous pyelogram. Should this show a unilateral lesion such as a cyst or tumour, this is treated on its merits and very

occasionally a permanent reduction in blood pressure results. If the investigation is normal, but one kidney is smaller than its fellow by at least 1 cm, then the hypothesis that the patient has renovascular hypotension must be further explored. A good screening test is renography, in which an intravenous injection is given of a radioactive-labelled compound such as sodium iodohippurate (Hippuran) that is rapidly excreted by a normal kidney, and external counting is carried out by twin instruments centred over each loin. A slower rise of radioactivity in one loin suggests an impairment of blood supply to that kidney compared with the other side. In these circumstances it is reasonable to subject the patient to renal arteriography. This investigation is carried out as for an aortogram, the contrast being injected via a catheter inserted by percutaneous puncture of the femoral artery at the groin, its tip being inserted into the origin of each renal artery in turn. The renal arteriogram may show a small kidney with vessels of normal pattern (albeit smaller than those on the other side), or a localized lesion of the arterial supply (e.g. a stricture of the main renal artery or of a major branch). Even in the presence of such abnormalities, it is wise to obtain confirmatory evidence that the abnormal arterial supply demonstrated is producing sufficient renal ischaemia to warrant the assumption that it is responsible for the hypertension. In special centres where such sophisticated techniques are available, the right and left renal veins are selectively catheterized with a catheter threaded up from the long saphenous vein at the groin, and samples of the blood in the two renal veins separately analysed for plasma renin concentration. If the venous blood from the suspect kidney has a plasma renin concentration higher than one and one-half times that from the normal kidney, the diagnosis of renovascular hypertension can be accepted.

The treatment of renovascular hypertension depends on the anatomy of the renal arterial supply. If the arteries are normal but small, the only possibility is nephrectomy. If there is a renal artery stenosis, and if the anatomy of the malformation permits, an attempt at reconstruction is made by one of the techniques of arterial surgery described elsewhere (p. 351) of bypass, excision and reanastomosis, or disobliteration. Should this procedure fail, it may be necessary to proceed to nephrectomy, but it must be borne in mind that the opposite ('normal') kidney may already have suffered irreversible and indeed progressive damage from the effects of the hypertension.

No matter what the cause of the hypertension, the extent to which the blood pressure is reduced by a successful operation depends upon the severity of the hypertension before the operation. It would appear that only a proportion of the hypertension is remediable; the rest fixed. This means that there is some urgency in the problem posed by hypertension in the young patient.

Whether the hypertension is primary or secondary, it should be remembered that high blood pressure is an important factor in surgical reckoning. The patient may be taking hypotensive drugs, and the anaesthetist needs to

consider the effects of these upon his anaesthetic techniques. The high blood pressure may make bleeding more troublesome during the operation, and hypotensive techniques are more dangerous than in the normotensive patient. Any reduction in cardiac output is less well tolerated, and the incidence of cerebral vascular accidents and coronary occlusions during and shortly after operation is greater. Reactionary haemorrhage (p. 279) is more common, too, unless the surgeon takes particular care not to complete the closure of the wound until the patient's blood pressure has recovered from the fall that usually occurs during a general anaesthetic, and has attained something like its preoperative level.

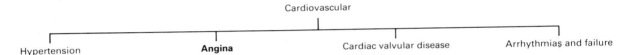

Angina

Clearly angina, or other evidence of myocardial insufficiency, is a very important factor in the preoperative assessment of the surgical patient. Usually this aspect of the patient's illness will already have come to light, and decisions about fitness for surgery and anaesthetic will already have been taken. However, sometimes the situation will only have been brought to light by the careful history of the vigilant resident. In this case he should add to the routine examination and chest x-ray an electrocardiogram (ECG)

and a lateral chest x-ray, and the opinion of a cardiologist or of a general physician should be sought. The opinion of the physician is important from the viewpoint of treatment of the angina immediately and in the long term, but remember that it is the anaesthetist who has to give the anaesthetic, and whose decision about the advisability of a non-urgent operation is therefore the definitive one. It may be that coronary artery by-pass surgery will need to be performed before the patient is deemed fit for the intended procedure.

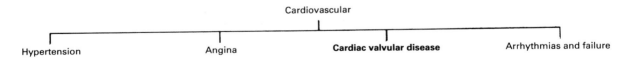

Cardiac valvular disease

Some auscultatory abnormality such as an extra heart sound or a murmur may suggest that the otherwise symptomless patient has congenital or acquired disease of one or more heart valves. In this circumstance also, an ECG is requested and a physician's opinion obtained. Assuming that the latter confirms there is an abnormality, the fact that the lesion is well compensated means that there is unlikely to be any necessity to postpone the operation. An exception to this statement is aortic stenosis, a lesion peculiarly prone

to limit cardiac output and coronary perfusion, which should therefore usually be dealt with before non-urgent surgery elsewhere. Before embarking upon any surgical operation on any patient with valvular disease, it must be remembered that deformed valves are specially prone to be attacked by circulatory micro-organisms with resultant subacute bacterial endocarditis; it has been usual to prescribe a prophylactic course of antibiotics starting just before, and continuing for about 3 days after, the operation to deal with any micro-organisms that may gain access to the circulation via the wound. This is still the routine procedure with dental operations such as tooth extractions, where the nature of the infecting organisms can be forecast with some confidence. With other operations, the newer approach (not everywhere accepted) is to have a low threshold for requesting cultures of the blood after the operation. The difficulty of routine prophylaxis for general surgery is that one does not know what organism to cover. If broad cover is given and the patient then gets a fever, it is usually impossible to prove endocarditis.

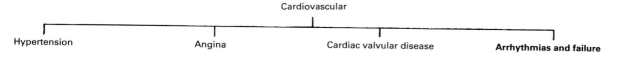

Cardiovascular

| Hypertension | Angina | Cardiac valvular disease | **Arrhythmias and failure** |

The embarrassed heart

Obvious signs that the heart is working under a strain are arrhythmias and congestive (right-sided) or left-sided cardiac failure. Specialist advice is essential. Ideally, any such disturbance should be corrected before subjecting the patient to anaesthesia and surgery, but where the indication of the operation is itself urgent there has to be a nice balancing of the risks and dangers of operating against those of not operating. In this situation, the final decision has to be the surgeon's as to how long can be spent on improving the patient's cardiac status, but he needs close co-operation from the physician and the anaesthetist.

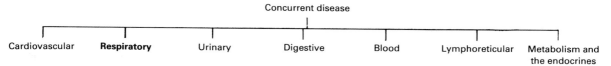

Concurrent disease

| Cardiovascular | **Respiratory** | Urinary | Digestive | Blood | Lymphoreticular | Metabolism and the endocrines |

Respiratory

The most important situation is chronic bronchitis or recent acute bronchitis, but the management of a patient with an abnormal shadow in the routine chest x-ray must also be considered.

Chronic bronchitis

This condition is said to be present if the patient complains of chronic productive cough for at least 3 months of the year, for at least 2 years. The production of an abnormally large quantity of sputum is the key to this problem, because for many reasons a patient who has just undergone general anaesthesia and a surgical operation finds particular difficulty in clearing sputum from his bronchi, and this is the root cause for a good deal of postoperative morbidity and even occasional mortality (p. 224). The preoperative management should include measures to reduce sputum production, an assessment of the patient's effectiveness in coughing, training to increase the power of coughing, and a consideration of the infective element.

The disease is rare in the non-smoker, and undoubtedly the most effective measure for reducing the production of sputum is stopping smoking. This course should be advised in the out-patient clinic, when arrangements for admission are being discussed. Particularly if the patient feels unable to accept this advice, he should be admitted 5—7 days before surgery to give time for preparation. On admission, tests of pulmonary mechanical function are performed, usually the forced vital capacity (FVC) and the forced expiratory volume in 1 second (FEV_1). The patient is asked to breathe out as rapidly as possible into a spirometer at the end of the deepest possible inspiration, and the volume expired (the FVC) is compared with the normal value to be expected for a subject of that stature. One can read off the spirometer tracing the volume of gas expired in the first second, and in a normal subject this FEV_1 should be at least 70 per cent of the FVC. A reduction in FVC signifies a *restrictive* defect, while a reduction in FEV_1/FVC signifies *obstructive* disease of the air passages. If either of these indices is markedly abnormal, more rather than less time should be spent in preparing the patient for operation.

The preparation consists in teaching the patient to expel his sputum more effectively.

Two or three times a day the patient is instructed by a physiotherapist in a routine of breathing exercises, in which he learns to expand all parts of his chest, and is subjected to postural drainage and percussion. Postural drainage results from the patient adopting a series of post-ures so that gravity is invoked to drain various segments and lobes of the lungs in turn. During each period in one position, the physiotherapist applies vibratory percussion to the chest wall in the appropriate area, in order to loosen the sec-retions so that they will the more readily drain out. This process should be continued until the physiotherapist feels that the respiratory pas-sages are as free of sputum as it is possible to get them. Another facet of preparation is to send some sputum for bacteriological examination so that the sensitivities of the organisms can be demonstrated. This knowledge can be invaluable later if chest complications follow surgery, so that the appropriate agents can be selected if antibiotic treatment is indicated.

Recent acute bronchitis

Chronic bronchitis causes postoperative compli-cations by the excessive production of mucus in the respiratory passages (p. 224). Patients with acute bronchitis are liable to continue producing excessive quantities of mucus for 2 or 3 weeks after the illness has subsided. Elective surgery should therefore be postponed for at least this length of time, and preferably 1 month.

It is always a problem to know whether a com-mon cold constitutes an indication to postpone routine operation. If the patient says that usually his colds tend to 'go to the chest', it is wise to postpone, and in all cases the author prefers to err on the side of caution.

Abnormal shadow in chest x-ray

It is imperative to exclude open tuberculosis (i.e. the patient who is exhaling tubercle bacilli in his breath) for obvious reasons concerned with the contamination of anaesthetic apparatus and the spread of infection. Operation must be post-poned till three specimens of sputum have been examined by staining techniques. In the absence of open tuberculosis, the most likely cause for an abnormal shadow is carcinoma of the bronchus, but there are many other possibilities. The deci-sion whether investigation of the chest lesion or carrying on with the elective procedure for which the patient was admitted should take precedence depends upon the nature of the known disease. If the chest is to be investigated first, further radiographic studies are undertaken — lateral and oblique views, more penetrated films, tomo-grams can all be helpful. A tissue diagnosis may be achieved by needle biopsy through the chest wall if the lesion is peripheral, or via a bronchoscope for lesions closer to the hilum. The possibility that the shadow might be caused by an enlargement of a lymph gland should be con-sidered, and appropriate investigations of the reticuloendothelial system performed (p. 211). Mediastinoscopy, or ultimately thoracotomy, may be required to produce a diagnosis. The principles of management of a carcinoma of the bronchus confirmed by biopsy are lobectomy or pneumonectomy, according to the size and site of the tumour, and provided that spread has not already occurred directly or by lymphatic or blood-borne metastasis, to neighbouring struc-tures making operation technically impossible, or to distant parts.

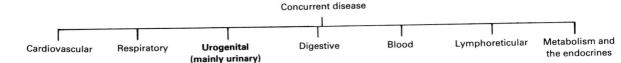

Concurrent disease

| Cardiovascular | Respiratory | Urogenital (mainly urinary) | Digestive | Blood | Lymphoreticular | Metabolism and the endocrines |

Urogenital

Abnormalities of the genital system will probably manifest themselves as disorders of the external genitalia or of the secondary sexual characteris-tics. These are unlikely to interfere with anaes-thesia and operation, and their investigation can usually be safely deferred. They are further con-sidered elsewhere (p. 160). The important

abnormalities of the urinary system are chronic renal failure and chronic retention of urine.

Chronic renal failure

This is usually diagnosed from a high blood urea concentration, and should be confirmed by measuring creatinine clearance if the high urea is an entirely unexpected finding in a patient who otherwise seems fit. If the blood urea is not too high (under l3 mmol/litre, 80 mg/100 ml), it can be worth getting an IVP: above that level the ordinary IVP will probably not show any contrast in the renal tract due to the poor concentrating ability of the kidneys, but an infusion urogram (in which the contrast material is injected intravenously not as a single bolus but as a long-continued infusion) may succeed in showing the anatomy of the renal tract. This can, however, further depress renal function, and ultrasound is preferably the first investigation to be tried.

The important cause to exclude is chronic retention of urine, since if this condition is present the patient should be treated by prolonged drainage from the bladder and in most cases the renal failure is cured. If the patient is passing some urine and the bladder is not palpable, chronic retention is not present.

In the absence of chronic retention, and provided that the uraemia is not so severe as to contraindicate the routine surgery contemplated, it is reasonable to proceed with the operation and defer further investigation of the kidneys till later. If the operation to be performed is laparotomy, the chance of getting biopsies of the kidneys is naturally taken. Many cases of chronic renal failure are accompanied by hypertension, and the effect of this factor during and after the operation must be remembered (p. 205). The other point is to ensure that the patient does not become fluid-deplete, thereby adding a pre-renal to the renal element of his uraemia.

Chronic retention of urine

This subject is considered in Chapter 15. From the present standpoint, the important consideration is whether the kidneys have been damaged by the back-pressure. If there is clear-cut evidence of renal failure, then an attempt is made to improve renal function by prolonged catheter drainage of the bladder; priority is then given to correcting the cause of the retention, usually some form of bladder neck obstruction. The urinary tract takes precedence under these circumstances over all other elective surgery, because experience shows that this policy gives the best results. If there is no renal failure, and the symptoms of difficulty with micturition are not too great, it is best to proceed with the elective operation. Before the operation, however, the patient should be encouraged to practise the difficult art of passing his urine into a bottle while lying in bed. Such practice is useful prophylaxis against his developing complete retention in the early postoperative period.

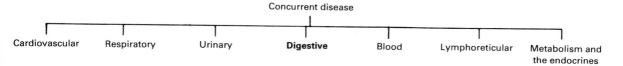

Concurrent disease

| Cardiovascular | Respiratory | Urinary | **Digestive** | Blood | Lymphoreticular | Metabolism and the endocrines |

Digestive

Evidence of poor nutrition (weight loss, muscle wasting, anaemia, specific features of the avitaminoses) are important in their own right, since they may adversely affect wound healing, and also because they may be due to serious disease of the digestive tract rather than to an inadequate diet.

Symptoms or signs of intra-abdominal disease should always be fully investigated if the intended operation is a laparotomy, so that the surgeon may be in a better position at the time of the operation to assess the various abnormalities present and carry out the best treatment. For example, it is awkward to find gallstones unexpectedly and to have to call for the services of a radiographer without prior warning so that peroperative cholangiography can be done.

Clinical jaundice, or abnormalities of hepatic function shown by biochemical tests, should always be fully investigated before routine surgery. Cholestatic jaundice significantly affects operative morbidity and even mortality through its effect upon blood clotting, and anaesthetic agents may have severe and untoward side-effects on a damaged liver. Bear in mind the possibility that the patient is a carrier of hepatitis B. Is he a member of the well known risk groups — drug addicts, homosexuals, patients requiring frequent transfusions, or natives of countries such as China where hepatitis B is rife.

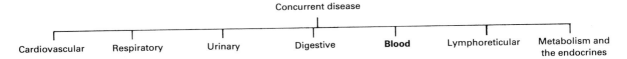

Blood

The important considerations are haemostasis and thromboembolism.

Faulty haemostasis

The surgeon relies so completely on the normal mechanisms of haemostasis to stop the bleeding he produces that he may come to overlook their importance. It is vital that the least hint of a bleeding diathesis should lead the resident to ask a haematologist to carry out a battery of screening tests for faulty haemostasis. The important disorders of blood coagulation are haemophilia and Christmas disease. In both, the platelet count and the bleeding time and prothrombin time are normal, but the clotting time and the thromboplastin generation time are prolonged. Refinements of the last test permit the differentiation between the two diseases. In haemophiliacs there is a deficiency of antihaemophilic globulin AHG, in Christmas disease of factor IX, the Christmas factor. AHG is labile, and therefore only present to an appreciable extent in the plasma of freshly shed blood. It can be preserved by immediately freezing the plasma and, recently, powerful preparations of this substance have become available in the form of cryoprecipitates of fresh whole blood. Surgery is possible in haemophiliacs if their concentration of AHG is made normal by suitable infusions of cryoprecipitate immediately before surgery, followed by topping-up doses to keep the AHG concentration higher than 40 per cent of normal until the wound is securely healed and all stitches have been removed (about 2 weeks). Christmas disease is managed along similar lines, but fortunately factor IX is stable so there is less difficulty in preparing concentrates and ordinary stored dried plasma may be adequate.

All patients about to undergo a general anaesthetic and who are of the Negro or Arab races or hail from the borders of the Mediterranean should have their blood screened for sickle cell disease. This disease results from the inheritance of an abnormal gene from both parents (the possession of only one gene characterizes the sickle cell trait, which is harmless), and the consequent presence of haemoglobin S in the erythrocytes.

As a result the erythrocytes are abnormally sensitive to hypoxia, reacting by becoming crescent shaped. They are then particularly liable to become rapidly haemolysed. The anaesthetist must be warned that the patient has sickle cell disease, so that he can take particular care to prevent hypoxia at all stages of the anaesthetic.

For jaundice and haemostasis, see p. 125.

Thromboembolism

The presentation, aetiology and management of thromboembolism are discussed on p. 233. Clearly, if a patient presents for elective surgery with clinical manifestations of the disease and the diagnosis is confirmed by appropriate investigations, the operation must be deferred for several weeks or months. The important consideration before elective operation is prophylaxis. Predisposing factors towards thromboembolism include the contraceptive pill, neoplastic disease, chronic cardiac disease especially congestive heart failure, peripheral vascular disease including varicose veins, and blood dyscrasias. Some operations are particularly liable to thromboembolic complications, notably operations on the hip and pelvic operations. In the light of the presence and strength of such factors, a decision must be taken about prophylaxis.

Several methods of prophylaxis of deep venous thrombosis are available: agents reducing the coagulability of the blood, such as small-dose heparin injections, dextran infusions; and agents reducing stasis in calf veins by mechanical measures, namely intermittent calf compression or calf-muscle electrical stimulation, or graded compression by special elastic stockings. The former group are slightly more effective, but increase the risk of postoperative bleeding and so are contraindicated if such bleeding would be dangerous, for example after intracranial operations. A decision to use heparin, or other agents affecting blood clotting, should not be undertaken lightly. It should be remembered that such measures do not completely prevent deep venous thrombosis, that it is usually not the thrombosis itself which matters but the pulmonary embolism it may give rise to, and that only one study so far has claimed to show that small-dose heparin reduces the incidence of post-operative pulmonary embolism. By contrast, the mechanical measures seem to be safe. The author at present uses graded compression elastic stockings as routine prophylaxis.

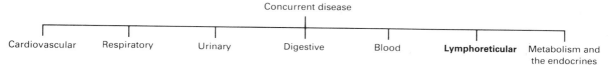

Lymphoreticular system

A history of allergic diseases such as hay-fever, asthma and urticaria should be noted, together with any known allergens so that they can be avoided. With the widespread use of antibiotics for relatively trivial illnesses, sensitivity to the common antiobiotics is common. A permanent record of known sensitivities must be kept in the patient's notes.

A more difficult problem is posed by any clinical suspicion that the patient has a reticulosis.

The grounds will probably be enlarged lymph nodes, or a palpable spleen or liver. See p. 114 for further details of investigation and management, but it is usually reasonable to biopsy the lymph nodes under the same anaesthetic under which the elective operation is performed. But if the patient is a male homosexual or has had multiple blood or blood product transfusions (e.g. for haemophilia), think of AIDS (p. 274).

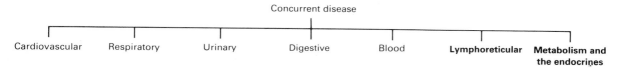

Diseases of metabolism and the endocrines

The routine preoperative assessment may lead to a clinical suspicion of any of the disorders in this category; they commonly present with few symptoms and signs and these are correspondingly readily ignored by the patient and even by

his attending physician. The conditions of diabetes mellitus, thyrotoxicosis and adrenal dysfunction are emphasized because these are the ones most likely to produce disasters if not properly handled before the patient is anaesthetized for his routine operation.

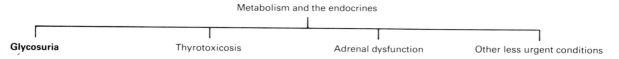

Diabetes mellitus

Trauma, including that of anaesthesia and a surgical operation, has a diabetogenic effect and this, in combination with the long period of fasting demanded routinely of the patient before and after his operation, is very likely to produce diabetic coma in an uncontrolled diabetic. The coma may readily be misinterpreted as sleepiness following the anaesthetic, and the danger of this situation is apparent. Therefore, the least suspicion of diabetes, even a trace of sugar in the

sample of urine tested routinely on arriving in the ward, must lead to sufficient investigation to prove or disprove the diagnosis.

In all cases of diabetes, the advice of a physician should be sought. If the impending operation is not at all urgent, there is no great problem: the disease is brought under control with some combination of diet and hypoglycaemic agents, and it is unusual for the operation to have to be deferred longer than a week. The problem arises when the operation is urgently required, especially when the indication for operation is sepsis, since the diabetes may be impossible to control until the septic focus has been drained. Some combination of glucose and insulin in an intravenous infusion is likely to be needed, together with frequent monitoring of the blood glucose concentration.

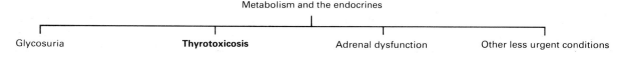

Thyrotoxicosis

Anaesthesia and operation may induce a thyrotoxic crisis, and are therefore contraindicated in a thyrotoxic patient. Where there is no hurry to perform the surgery, the decision whether to treat the thyrotoxicosis itself by medical, radiotherapeutic or surgical treatment can be taken along the usual lines (p. 41). If there is some urgency, the quickest way of controlling the thyrotoxicosis — 10 days of potassium iodide solution followed by subtotal thyroidectomy — will be indicated. The nasty problem, fortunately rare, is when a thyrotoxic patient requires an emergency operation. Iodide by intravenous injection and propranolol to block the effects of T3 and T4 at the periphery are the best that can be done.

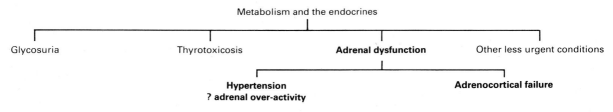

Adrenal dysfunction

The potentially lethal effects of certain disorders of the adrenal glands in combination with surgical operations depend upon the influence of these disorders on arterial blood pressure. There is a group of three conditions producing hypertension — Cushing's syndrome, Conn's syndrome and phaeochromocytoma — while adrenal failure — Addison's disease, adrenal suppression by steroid therapy — produces hypotension. The first group produce their ill-effects by exposing the patient to the increased risk of complications of hypertension, cardiac, neurological, vascular or renal, during and after the operation, while the second group may result in death via intractable peripheral circulatory failure if the true cause — lack of cortisol — is not appreciated.

Cushing's syndrome results from raised levels of plasma cortisol, persisting throughout each 24 hours without any evidence of the normal diurnal rhythm. Apart from hypertension, the main clinical features of the syndrome are obesity of the trunk (but not of the limbs), a moon-like facies due to oedema of the face, purple striae in the skin overlying accumulations of fat, a thin skin, a tendency towards bruising, a predisposition towards infection, especially of the skin, weakness of the muscles and backache due to osteoporosis. In the female, amenorrhoea and hirsutism occur.

If the syndrome is suspected, the advice of a physician should be sought because the investigation of such a case demands complicated endocrinological tests. Meanwhile, however, x-rays of the skeleton and of the pituitary fossa should be undertaken, and the clinician should pay attention to any clue which suggests the appearance of a carcinoma somewhere other than in the adrenals.

The skeletal x-rays are to confirm osteoporosis. Hypercortisolaemia can be due to exogenous steroids (this should have been established by the history), to a functioning adenoma or carcinoma of the adrenal cortex, or to hyperfunction of the adrenal cortex under the stimulus of excessive production of adrenocorticotrophic hormone (ACTH). The last-named may originate in the anterior pituitary from a functioning tumour that enlarges the pituitary fossa, or 'ectopically' in one of a number of malignant lesions that may occur in diverse regions of the body (e.g. carcinoma of the bronchus).

Without going into details, the endocrinological studies aim first to establish hypercortisolaemia, secondly to distinguish between pituitary-dependent and pituitary-independent disease. Cortisol levels are measured in venous plasma on several occasions at about 9 a.m. and midnight: patients with Cushing's syndrome do not necessarily have a raised morning level, but are distinguishable from normal in that the normal circadian rhythm, with very low levels at midnight, is missing. Pituitary dependence is investigated by various tests which increase or decrease the output of ACTH by the pituitary and assess whether there is any resultant change in adrenal activity. Metapyrone, for example, stimulates pituitary ACTH secretion, while dexamethasone suppresses it. The adrenal activity can be quantified both by plasma cortisol measurements and by measuring the output of various metabolites of corticosteroids in 24-hour urine collections. If the results suggest pituitary independence, the pattern of urinary metabolite secretion may point to carcinoma rather than adenoma of the adrenal. An ectopic site of production of ACTH is suggested by very high levels of plasma cortisol, and an associated marked disturbance of plasma electrolyte concentrations (potassium below 2.5 mmol/litre, bicarbonate above 35 mmol/litre).

The differential diagnosis between bilateral adrenal hyperplasia, single and bilateral adenomas, single and bilateral carcinomas, is aided by ultrasound, CT-scan, tomography, arteriography or venography, while selective catheterization of adrenal veins to yield blood samples from different sites for the measurement of cortisol concentration is particularly valuable. Nevertheless, if operation upon the adrenals (rather than upon the pituitary or upon a neoplasm elsewhere) is indicated, both adrenals must be exposed by the surgeon.

Conn's syndrome is basically the combination of hypertension and hypokalaemia due to the hypersecretion by the adrenal, not of cortisol but of aldosterone (or, occasionally, certain other hormones such as corticosterone). The cause of the hypersecretion may be an adenoma or carcinoma of the adrenal or hyperplasia of the zona glomerulosa where aldosterone is manufactured.

The diagnosis, like that of Cushing's syndrome, is difficult to make, and expert advice should be obtained. Measurements of aldosterone levels in the plasma, or of its secretion rate in the urine, are sensitive to the patient's rate of intake of sodium, and it is essential to stablize the sodium intake before making the measurements. Thus on a sodium intake of 100 mmol/day, the normal range of aldosterone output in the urine is 70–200 μg/day. Diagnosis is aided by finding a *low* level of renin in the plasma. This distinguishes primary hyperaldosteronism from the common differential diagnosis of a patient with some other cause for hypertension who has been treated with diuretics that have produced sodium depletion, a consequent *increase* in renin production, and a *secondary* hyperaldosteronism. The effect of spironolactone, which blocks the sodium-retaining *action* of aldosterone on the kidney tubules, may also assist diagnosis.

When the diagnosis has been established, the remarks about the differentiation between hyperplasia, adenoma and carcinoma by radiological studies, and about the importance of exposing both adrenals at operation, apply to this condition as well as to Cushing's syndrome.

Phaeochromocytoma is a tumour of the adrenal medulla, or of similar chromaffin tissue in a large variety of other sites. Whether its oncological behaviour is benign or malignant, its clinical importance can be gauged by the fact that, if untreated, it invariably proves fatal. The tumour secretes an excess of catecholamines, adrenaline or noradrenaline or both, and these agents produce hypertension that is fixed or paroxysmal. The condition is by no means uncommon — more than 1000 cases are reported each year in the United States — so all patients with hypertension should be screened for this condition, no matter how likely it seems that they belong to the 'essential' hypertension group.

The diagnosis depends upon measuring high levels of catecholamines in the plasma, or (and much more easily) high outputs of the metabolites of catecholamines in the urine. Vanillylmandelic acid (VMA) used to be the popular metabolite to measure, but the results obtained by the estimation of metanephrine are more specific and this is now the method of choice. Tests dependent on the effects upon the hypertension of either stimulation (e.g. by histamine or tyramine) or suppression (by adrenergic-blocking drugs such as phentolamine) have been abandoned because they are dangerous, especially the former group.

Phaeochromocytomas are derived from tissue of the embryonic neural crest, and may therefore occur not far from the mid-line anywhere from the skull to the perineum. Only 2 per cent occur in the skull, neck and thorax, and these sites should be investigated routinely by x-rays if search in the more usual areas has failed. In the abdomen, most tumours occur in the adrenals, particularly in the right adrenal, and so it is reasonable to ask for an ultrasound and for an intravenous pyelogram with tomography since these investigations may demonstrate a tumour on one or both sides. More elaborate investigations such as arteriography, venography and venous sampling have been employed, but they may stimulate a dangerous paroxysm of hypertension. In any case, since the tumours are multiple in at least 20 per cent of cases, no matter what the localizing investigations show, the surgeon must search the whole length of the abdominal cavity in the mid-line posteriorly, down to the bladder and the pelvic floor.

Finally, it should be remembered that the incidence of familial phaeochromocytoma is high, and the relatives of the patient may be offered screening tests.

Adrenocortical failure may present with a very insidious picture of muscular weakness, lethargy, and a tendency to hypotension that may only become manifest when the patient stands up. In all cases of adrenocortical failure, cortisol secretion is inadequate, but in a proportion of cases there is also a deficiency of aldosterone.

The two main types are inadequate stimulation by ACTH due to disease of the hypothalamus or pituitary (e.g. a non−secreting pituitary neoplasm), and primary adrenocortical failure, which may be due to tuberculosis or autoimmune disease (Addison's disease) or suppression by exogenous steroid therapy. Tests to establish the diagnosis of adrenocortical insufficiency, and to differentiate the primary and secondary forms, are analogous to those used in the investigation of Cushing's syndrome (p. 212). Plasma cortisol levels tend to be low and to show no circadian rhythm, but it is much more important that they do not rise after stimulation with exogenous ACTH. Plain x-rays of the abdomen may show calcification in the area of the adrenals in patients with tuberculous adrenalitis, while x-rays of the pituitary fossa are required in the search for a pituitary tumour. Adrenal and other antibodies should be measured, because other forms of autoimmune disease often coexist.

Apart from the treatment of any primary cause, a patient with adrenocortical failure is managed by substitution therapy with a glucocorticoid (cortisone or cortisol), together with a mineralocorticoid (e.g. fludrocortisone) for those who need it.

It is most important to stress that any patient who has received corticosteroid hormones during the previous 5 years should be assumed to have adrenal glands that are suppressed to some extent and therefore likely to be unresponsive to the stress of anaesthesia and surgery. There is no need to investigate their adrenal function if there are no relevant symptoms or signs; the important principle is to give cortisone or cortisol in a regular dose starting 12 hours before operation, and continuing for a few days afterwards to cover the period of stress. An average regime might be 100 mg cortisol 12-hourly for 2 days, then tailed off quite rapidly over the next 2 days.

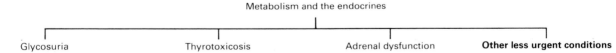

Metabolism and the endocrines

| Glycosuria | Thyrotoxicosis | Adrenal dysfunction | **Other less urgent conditions** |

Less urgent disorders

Endocrine diseases with possible adrenal effects include disorders of the hypothalamus/pituitary such as gigantism and acromegaly, galactorrhoea due to excessive release of prolactin, and hypopituitarism, including dwarfism; and disorders of the male or female gonads that may be primary, or themselves secondary to pituitary or adrenal cortical dysfunction. With regard to the patient admitted for a routine surgical operation, the important consideration is to ensure that adrenocortical production of cortisol and the response to stress are normal. In that case there is usually no contraindication to performing the operation and completing the investigations of the endocrine abnormality afterwards.

The other endocrine gland which may require investigation is the parathyroid, usually because a blood sample taken for routine analysis is reported to have an abnormal calcium concentration. This problem is discussed on p. 344.

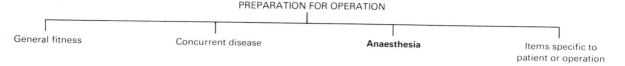

Anaesthesia

Topics of particular importance to the anaesthetist are drugs and the state of the upper alimentary tract — apart from various matters such as blood transfusion and the prevention of chest problems, which are discussed on pp. 202 and 207.

Drugs

The anaesthetist tries to get the patient to arrive at the operating theatre in a relaxed frame of mind, and sleepy, so that his natural anxieties are allayed. The premedication injection, usually given about 1 hour before the operation, is therefore an opiate, tranquillizer or sedative. An anticholinergic drug such as atropine is combined with this to reduce secretions of the respiratory tract, in an effort to reduce the likelihood of postoperative pulmonary segmental collapse (p. 224). If the patient has a general anaesthetic, this is probably induced by a barbiturate, and maintained by an inhalational gas mixture together with intravenous supplements of other drugs such as narcotics and relaxants and sometimes specific agents to reduce blood pressure. This is complex polypharmacy, and the anaesthetist must ensure that the patient has not in the past reacted adversely to any of the drugs to be used, and that the patient is not receiving any therapy which would react adversely with the anaesthetic agents.

The problems of treatment with corticosteroid drugs, hypotensive agents and the contraceptive pill have already been mentioned. A history of a heavy intake of alcohol should be viewed with suspicion. Such patients often require larger doses of anaesthetics than usual, but they tend to be particularly sensitive to agents which might have adverse effects upon the liver, such as halothane, presumably because they already have a subclinical interference with liver function. Full details of any narcotics and tranquillizers taken are also important.

Upper alimentary tract

During an inhalational anaesthetic, an anaesthetist has to perform various manipulations in the mouth and throat such as forcing the mouth of the unconscious patient open with a gag, intubating the trachea under vision with a laryngoscope or blind via the nostril, and so on. If the patient has loose teeth due to chronic gingivitis, there is obviously a risk that he will lose one during these manipulations, with a possibility even of subsequent inhalation. Even if this does not happen, the mechanical disturbance of the teeth within their loose, infected sockets may result in a bacteraemia or septicaemia, and small particles of debris from the sockets are more likely to be inhaled and cause a severe inflammatory reaction in the lungs.

For this reason the resident should pay particular attention to oral sepsis in his patients, and attention by a dentist may well be necessary in pronounced cases, even if this means putting off the operation for a few days.

The anaesthetist will insist that the patient has nothing to eat or drink for at least 4 hours, and preferably 12 hours, before the operation. The reason is that stomach-emptying rate is notoriously unpredictable, and particularly under the emotional stress engendered by an impending surgical operation it may be very slow. Induction of anaesthesia often provokes retching, and if the stomach is full there may be vomiting of its contents which, since the induction has paralysed the cricopharyngeal sphincter, may well give rise to inhalation of the vomitus into the respiratory passages with a resultant very severe illness of pulmonary oedema and segmental collapse (Mendelson's syndrome).

Flow-chart 18.1   *PREPARATION FOR OPERATION*

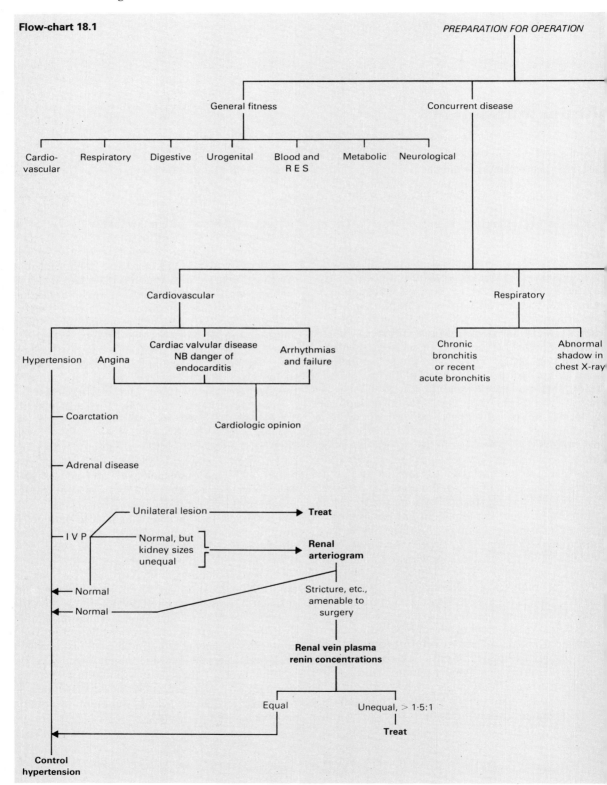

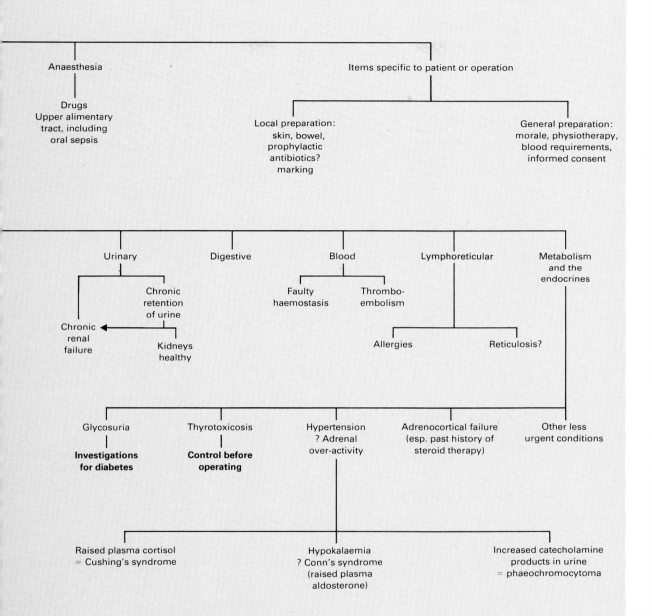

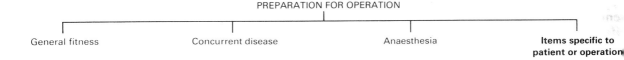

Items specific to patient or operation

Local preparation

The skin

Naturally, the skin of the area to be incised should be as clean as possible. Most surgeons rely on making sure that the patient is socially clean by insisting on a bath the day before operation, perhaps using a powerful agent with detergent and antibacterial properties such as hibitane. Some surgeons still require that the operation area should be specially cleansed and wrapped in sterile towels shortly before the operation.

The bowel

Operations on the bowel should be performed in circumstances where the bowel is as empty as possible. An important cause of breakdown of an anastomosis in the large bowel is the disruptive pressure of hard faeces. The small bowel is bound to contain some liquid, but even in operations on the small bowel it is nevertheless important that the large bowel is empty so that intra-abdominal manipulations are easier for the surgeon, and there is less likelihood of severe constipation, or even obstruction, after the operation. As a routine before laparotomy it may be enough to give an effective purgative on the day before operation, but in the case of operations on the large bowel sterner measures are necessary. Some surgeons rely on repeated enemas, others on a regime of magnesium sulphate repeated every 2 hours until copious diarrhoea is produced. Other regimes include washing out the bowel from above with a continuous instillation into the stomach of the osmotically active agent mannitol, or more simply of saline. Surgeons also differ as to whether an attempt should be made to sterilize the large bowel before operations upon it. Probably the majority do, using little-absorbed antimicrobial agents such as phthalylsulphathiazole, streptomycin, or neomycin by mouth.

Prophylactic antibiotics?

There are certain well defined indications for this form of treatment; to prevent bacterial endocarditis during operations on patients with deformed heart valves, for example (but see p. 206), or to prevent clostridial infections in patients undergoing above-knee amputations. For most operations on infected or potentially infected regions such as the intestine or biliary tract, a short (24—72 hour) course of antibiotics active against both anaerobes and aerobes is commonly advised.

Visible marking

It is the duty of the resident to mark clearly on the patient with some form of indelible ink the side of operation (in the case of lateralized lesions) and the affected digit in appropriate cases. More detailed marking may be required in special cases; in patients with varicose veins, for example, the general course of the veins and the sites of suspected perforators may be mapped.

General preparation

Remember the importance of maintaining the patient's *morale*. Patients awaiting an operation are likely to be apprehensive, and it is well documented that disorders of blood coagulation, for example, are commoner in excessively anxious patients. Remind him of the importance of pre-operative *physiotherapy* — breathing exercises to help prevent chest problems, leg exercises to help prevent thromboembolism.

Give consideration to the question whether blood should be ordered. If blood has been cross-matched, make certain that all relevant documentation has been performed; in some hospitals, for example, the patient must wear a special wristlet with the details of the cross-matched bottles written on it.

The nursing staff should ensure that in relevant cases the patient's bowel is empty, and in all cases that he empties his bladder before the pre-medication is given.

Ensure that the patient understands the situation in which he is likely to find himself when he regains consciousness: details of intravenous infusions, drains, likely restrictions on food and drink, etc.

Informed consent

Remember to obtain the patient's informed consent, not only to the procedure that is envisaged but also to any alternative that is reasonably likely. Explain the possibility of common complications peculiar to the operation (e.g. facial nerve paresis after parotidectomy).

Conclusion

After all the points in this Chapter have received due attention, the resident may, with a clear conscience, put the patient's name on the operating theatre list!

Further reading

Bauer, J.J., Gelernt, I.M., Salky, B.A. and Kreel, I. (1985). Is routine postoperative nasogastric decompression really necessary? *Annals of Surgery* **201**, 233–6.

Browse, L.N. (1977). What should I do about deep vein thrombosis and pulmonary embolism? *Annals of the Royal College of Surgeons of England* **59**, 138–42.

Gunning, A.J. (1976). Surgery in the haemorrhagic diatheses. In: Current Surgical Practice, Vol. 1, pp. 34–46. Ed. by G.J. Hadfield and M. Hobsley. London, Edward Arnold.

Hughes, E.S.R. (1972). Asepsis in large bowel surgery. *Annals of the Royal College of Surgeons of England* **51**, 347–56.

Mills, I.H. (1974). Primary hyperaldosteronism. *Clinics in Endocrinology and Metabolism* **3**, 593–608.

Palmer, K.N.V. and Sellick, B.A. (1952). Effect of procaine penicillin and breathing exercises in postoperative pulmonary complications. *Lancet* **i**, 345–7.

Plumley, P.F. (1966). A simple regime for preparation of colon before large bowel surgery. *British Journal of Surgery* **53**, 413–14.

Sellors, T.H. and Hobsley, M. (1963). Coarctation of the aorta. Effect of operation on blood pressure. *Lancet* **i**, 1387–91.

Smiddy, F.G. (1976). *The Medical Management of the Surgical Patient*. London, Edward Arnold.

Steinbeck, A.W. and Theile, H.M. (1974). The adrenal cortex (excluding aldosteronism). *Clinics in Endocrinology and Metabolism* **3**, 557–91.

Treasure, T. (1983). Coronary artery by-pass surgery. *British Journal of Hospital Medicine* **33**, 259–263.

Wolf, R.L. (1974). Phaeochromocytoma. *Clinics in Endocrinology and Metabolism* **3**, 609–21.

Chapter 19

The Early Postoperative Period

The time a patient spends in hospital after an operation under general anaesthesia falls usefully into three periods: the period of unconsciousness or semi-consciousness, then the rest of the first 48 hours, and finally the period after 48 hours. The second and third are discussed in detail in this Chapter. The period of disturbed conscious-ness is dominated by the considerations applying to the care of an unconscious subject (p. 282), although the care of intravenous drip treatment and drainage tubes, particularly those of the suction variety or the sealed drainage after thoracotomy, also requires attention.

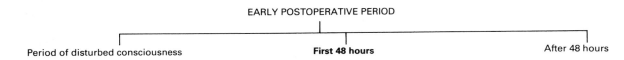

EARLY POSTOPERATIVE PERIOD

| Period of disturbed consciousness | **First 48 hours** | After 48 hours |

The first 48 hours

Once the patient is fully conscious, and provided that there is no other reason for doubting his competence to maintain his own airway, the chief items requiring attention during the first 2 days are drains, fluid and electrolyte balance, retention of urine, shock, fever and chest complications.

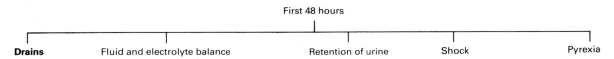

First 48 hours

| **Drains** | Fluid and electrolyte balance | Retention of urine | Shock | Pyrexia |

Drains

The resident should make sure that he understands why the surgeon has used a drain. The possible reasons are: to prevent the formation of a haematoma; to prevent the pocketing of pus in a wound where infection is already established or is considered likely to eventuate; to form a track from the site of an anastomosis in the gastro-intestinal tract so that if a leak occurs the irritant contents of the tract are directed to the exterior rather than permitted to flood the peritoneal cavity; and to drain the pleura after thoracotomy (p. 226). Of these various types, drainage to prevent a haematoma is unique in that the drain is nearly always removed during or at the end of the first 48 hours, while drains for other reasons are kept in place longer. Therefore only drains to prevent a haematoma will be considered here, while other sorts of drain are dealt with on pp. 225, 226 and 228.

Drainage to prevent a haematoma

Indications Since a drain constitutes a potential route of contamination of the wound by micro-organisms from the exterior, drainage to prevent a haematoma should not be undertaken lightly. The specific indication is that the tissues of the wound are very vascular, so that an ooze from capillaries may be expected even though all obvious bleeding points from arteries and veins have been secured. Common sites that routinely require drainage for this reason include the neck, the breast, and the groins and scrotum, but the surgeon may feel that an individual operation at some other site may require this precaution because bleeding during the operation has been unexpectedly heavy.

Prophylaxis   Prevention is better than cure, and the best outcome is that the drain inserted should produce no blood and should be removed after 24 hours. At the end of any operation, but particularly after one upon a highly vascular area, the surgeon must ensure that the patient's systolic blood pressure, which was probably depressed during the operation, has been returned to its normal level. Important measures required are to return the patient to the horizontal position (if the operation has been conducted with a head-up tilt), and to ask the anaesthetist to reverse any hypotensive effects of his anaesthetic agents or of any blood loss, if necessary by the appropriate intravenous volume replacement.

Mode of drainage   *Open* drainage, usually by a corrugated rubber or plastic drain, leads to the exterior any blood collecting in the wound, to be absorbed in dressings. The advantage is that blockage is unlikely, since the draining force is capillary attraction along the gutters of the corrugated drain, and there is no tube to block. The disadvantage is that the blood-soaked dressings are an open invitation to infective organisms. Although this danger can be minimized by applying a colostomy bag around the drain site, closed drainage via a tube into a closed receptacle is usually favoured. One cannot rely upon gravity for the draining force, and some form of apparatus to apply suction to the drain is used: continuous suction from a pump, a previously evacuated glass container, or a rubber bulb that can be squeezed before connection to the drain so as to produce suction (e.g. Canny–Ryall's syringe).

Care of drainage   With *open* drainage, it is important to ensure that the outer layer of dressings does not become blood-soaked. Redressing the wound may be necessary at frequent inter-

vals so that there is always an outer layer of gauze, gamgee or cotton wool that is clean and dry, and therefore likely to be an effective barrier against infection. With *closed* drainage, the most important consideration is to avoid blockage of the tube. The most dangerous period is while the patient is in the recovery room, because the attendant nursing staff have naturally to give prime consideration to maintenance of the airway. Allowing the drainage tube to become kinked is a potent source of trouble because the blood blocked in the drainage tube clots.

Management of failure   Should a swelling be noted in the wound despite drainage, then in the case of closed drainage every effort should be made to unblock the tube. If this fails, or if open drainage (or no drainage at all) has been used, there is a choice of three methods of management: conservative, aspiration, or surgical re-exploration. A conservative policy may be adopted if the swelling is small and not expanding and if the patient's general condition is good. If the haematoma is large enough to suggest that healing will be seriously delayed but the other conditions are satisfied, it is worth trying aspiration, but this procedure is often unsuccesful because the collection of blood is often organized. If aspiration fails, of if the swelling is expanding or is causing interference with the blood supply of the skin, or if infection seems likely (as after appendicectomy), or if the bleeding is producing shock, there is no alternative to reopening the wound, evacuating the blood, securing any bleeding points found, and closing the wound again.

Duration of drainage   If blood loss via the drain is negligible, the drain can be removed 24 hours after the operation. If there has been an appreciable loss of blood, the drain is removed when it is certain that the trend is towards a reduction in blood loss, and when the blood loss is less than 30 ml in the previous 12 hours.

For the special case of bleeding via the urethra, see p. 228.

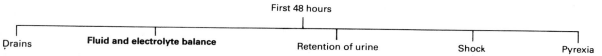

	First 48 hours			
Drains	Fluid and electrolyte balance	Retention of urine	Shock	Pyrexia

Fluid and electrolyte balance

Indications

After many operations there is no contraindica-

tion to the patient drinking as soon as he is conscious, and eating as soon as he feels like it. This is the most desirable regime after operation, but cannot always be achieved.

There are two main contraindications to oral feeding *ad lib.* — the protection of a suture line in the upper alimentary tract, and the threat of paralytic ileus or mechanical obstruction. Often both contraindications coexist.

Protection of an anastomosis

A large volume of fluid passing along the lumen of the alimentary tract in a region where an anastomosis has been performed obviously poses a threat to the integrity of the suture line. In the case of the oesophagus and stomach, it is possible to aspirate the secretions of the tract above the anastomosis through a nasogastric tube, thereby reducing the flow through the anastomosis. In the oesophagus, peristalsis induced by swallowing may be a disruptive force and can be minimized by forbidding ingestion for 4 days, a common regime after oesophageal anastomoses.

Precautions against intestinal obstruction

Paralytic ileus (p. 312) is particularly likely after abdominal operations in which the intestines require much handling or the alimentary tract has to be opened, and also after certain other operations such as any upon the kidneys, even when the peritoneum has not been opened. Mechanical obstruction (p. 313) may be produced by oedema of the tissues at an anastomosis and, particularly when the anastomosis is high enough (the gastroduodenal region), proximal decompression by nasogastric suction can keep the patient comfortable and free from abdominal distension, nausea and vomiting.

The regime

When normal oral feeding is contraindicated, intravenous feeding is instituted. During the first 48 hours only water, sodium and possibly potassium require consideration, and rational therapy is aided, in this as in all cases of intravenous feeding, by dividing the patient's needs into basal requirements, the replacement of abnormal losses, and the replacement of existing deficits.

Basal requirements each 24 hours in a temperate climate are 2–3 litres of water, 80 mmol sodium and 80 mmol potassium. In the first 24–48 hours after a surgical operation, the metabolic response to trauma is evident and from the present viewpoint this consists of an inability of the kidney to excrete extra water and extra sodium and a tendency to excrete more potassium than normal. The change in handling of water is usually said to be due to a stimulation of antidiuretic hormone (ADH), and also to the sodium retention, while the sodium/potassium changes are presumed to be due to alterations in corticosteroid hormone production, especially aldosterone. This classical description is probably not true, according to the most recent evidence, and the true mechanism remains shrouded in mystery. Whatever the mechanism, it is wise to limit water intake, in the first 24 hours at least, to 2 rather than 3 litres. A sodium load of 80 mmol does not seem to tax unduly the excretory powers of the postoperative kidney, and so 80 mmol/24 hours can be given on both the first and second days. The temptation to give potassium to replace the excess urinary loss should be resisted. Urine output may be very low during this period so that potassium given intravenously accumulates in the plasma; alterations in the sodium pump mechanism under the influence of changes in corticosteroid secretion allow sodium to leak into, and potassium to leak out of, the cells; and the excess urinary losses are very small anyway in relation to total body potassium. So for all these reasons added potassium may produce dangerously high levels in the plasma with the risk of cardiac arrest. Basal requirements may thus be summarized as 2 litres of water and 80 mmol of sodium on the first day and this can be conveniently given as 0.5 litre normal saline (160 mmol/litre, 9 g/litre), 1.5 litres of dextrose solution (228 mmol/litre, 50 g/litre). On the second day the dextrose solution can be increased to 2.5 litres if a regime of 3 litres/24 hours is to be adopted; or, more elegantly, the change is made when the urine output is observed to rise and its specific gravity to fall.

Abnormal losses from the alimentary tract — vomiting or nasogastric tube aspirations, diarrhoea, fistula fluid — are collected and measured accurately and replaced volume for volume by normal saline. The assessment is normally performed every 12 hours, but may be necessary more frequently if losses are occurring rapidly. Occult losses such as fluid sequestrated in loops of distended bowel or in a peritoneal exudate are much more difficult to deal with since their volume can only be estimated. Haematocrit and plasma protein estimations can be particularly useful in such cases (p. 315).

Pre-existing deficits should have been largely replaced before the operation (p. 268).

Anything by mouth?

For reasons already stated, nothing to be swallowed should be given to a patient with an oesophageal anastomosis for about 4 days, but his mouth is washed out at frequent intervals to promote comfort and prevent such complications of oral sepsis as ascending parotitis (p. 48). In most patients, however, there can be no contraindication to letting them have 30 ml water by mouth each hour. This volume is small compared to that secreted by the upper alimentary tract in an hour, even if the operation is one such as vagotomy or gastrectomy which has reduced the rate of secretion from an important part of the tract. While there is a nasogastric tube in the stomach so that its contents can be emptied an hour later, before the next drink of water, there is no danger of a massive accumulation of liquid in a poorly emptying stomach with a risk of copious vomiting and aspiration pneumonia (so-called gastric ileus or acute dilatation of the stomach). The advantage from the viewpoint of the patient's morale is obvious, but a further advantage is that this regime can form the basis of a technique for deciding rationally when intravenous treatment can be stopped and oral feeding commenced. When a 12-hour balance shows that less has been aspirated from the stomach than has been swallowed, the water dose can be increased to 60 ml hourly and the period between aspirations lengthened to 2 hours. When a positive oral balance has been demonstrated on this schedule, 90 ml water is given hourly and the aspiration interval lengthened to 3 hours. A positive oral balance at this stage is the signal to take down the intravenous infusion because 24 × 90 ml is about 2 litres and, therefore, an adequate oral intake.

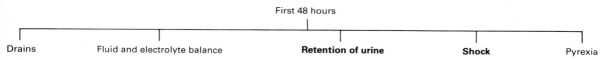

First 48 hours

Drains | Fluid and electrolyte balance | **Retention of urine** | **Shock** | Pyrexia

Retention of urine

See p. 228.

Shock

The first warning that the patient is becoming shocked is usually given by the routine nursing chart of pulse and blood pressure. Such charts are usually plotted hourly while the patient is still drowsy from his anaesthetic, or while he is receiving a blood transfusion (see below), and so for most patients this covers the period of the first 24 hours when the risk of reactionary haemorrhage is greatest.

Bleeding is the commonest cause of shock in the early postoperative period, but the possibility of other causes such as cardiogenic, vasodilator, or reductions in circulating blood volume due to loss of constituents other than blood should be borne in mind (see Chapter 22). A determination of haematocrit may be invaluable, and it is therefore good practice to measure haematocrit shortly after a major operation to establish a baseline. Remember that a blood transfusion does not immediately raise the haematocrit because the haematocrit of bank blood with its high fraction of anticoagulant solution is only about 35 per cent.

Reactionary haemorrhage (rare after the first 24 hours) is treated conservatively by blood transfusion in the first instance, unless the onset is so sudden and catastrophic as obviously to require immediate re-exploration. In most cases conservative management suffices, although operation may become necessary either to secure the bleeding point or to evacuate the resultant haematoma (p. 279).

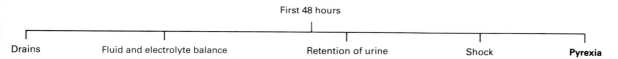

First 48 hours

Drains | Fluid and electrolyte balance | Retention of urine | Shock | **Pyrexia**

Pyrexia

The two common causes in the first 48 hours are blood transfusion and pulmonary segmental collapse.

If the fever starts during a blood transfusion or within 2 hours of the end of a transfusion, it is wise to assume that the blood is responsible. This remark applies even if there is some evidence of respiratory embarrassment (e.g. dyspnoea or cyanosis) because these can be produced by transfusion reactions. The transfusion should be stopped immediately, and samples of the blood remaining in the bottle and of the patient's blood, and also the whole transfusion apparatus, should be sent immediately for urgent haematological assessment of possible incompatibility, or of infection of the stored blood. In the majority of cases neither of these factors will be found present, and if there is no evidence to suggest any other cause of pyrexia one assumes that the cause is the pyrogenic property of blood itself. This is an obscure subject: the mechanism may involve antigens in the formed elements of the transfused blood other than the erythrocytes. It is known, however, that antihistamines added to stored blood do not reduce the incidence of pyrogenic reactions, that the reactions are very common if one looks for them, and that the individual susceptibility of the recipient is an important factor so that subsequent blood transfusions are also likely to produce fever.

Occasionally, other causes of pyrexia which are commoner later than the first 48 hours are encountered; but if blood transfusion is not responsible the most likely origin is the chest.

Postoperative chest complications

Pulmonary segmental collapse occurs more commonly in the first 48 hours than later, and the most frequent first evidence is the sudden onset of marked pyrexia. In many cases, examination reveals dyspnoea, cyanosis and twitching of the alae nasi due to laboured respiration.

There may be abnormal physical signs in the chest — deviations of the trachea to the affected side, dullness, reduced air entry — and added sounds in the affected region. More often there are few or no signs, and it must be stressed that in the early stages the chest x–ray may be normal.

The basic cause is blockage of a bronchus by inspissated secretions of the epithelium lining the upper respiratory tract and the tracheobronchial tree.

Aetiology

There are three groups of factors.
Reduction in the ability to expectorate mucus is mostly due to limitation of the power of coughing by the pain of the surgical wound. Thoracic and abdominal, particularly upper abdominal, wounds are prone to this complication while operations on the head and neck and extremities are relatively immune. The power of a cough is related to the volume of air taken into the chest immediately prior to the expulsive act, and it is this preliminary inhalation which is particularly limited by pain. Other possible factors are depression of the cough reflex centre by the continuing effects of anaesthetic agents, and by narcotics given to relieve pain after the operation, and depression of the ciliary apparatus of the respiratory tract by the same influences.

Increased viscosity and volume of the mucus are probably less important except when there is a bronchorrhoea as in patients with chronic bronchitis or recent acute bronchitis. The starvation required before a general anaesthetic may have an influence, and the preoperative atropine used to reduce the volume of sputum also increases its viscosity so that its effect may not be entirely beneficial.

Bronchospasm reduces the calibre of the air passages and correspondingly increases the liability to blockage and the force needed for effective expectoration. Patients with chronic bronchitis often have an element of asthma. There are also reflex arcs producing bronchoconstriction in response to the stimulation of stretch receptors in the peritoneum lining the upper abdomen, and it is possible that this is a factor in making the upper abdominal operation particularly likely to produce this complication.

Management

The mainstay of treatment is mechanical aid to dislodge mucous plugs so that they can be more readily expectorated. The physiotherapist employs postural drainage, arranging the patient's position so that in turn the various affected bronchopulmonary segments are given vertical, gravity-assisted drainage, in association with vibratory and slapping percussion to the overlying chest wall. Adequate pain relief before these manoeuvres is essential if the best results are to be obtained. Sputum can be made less tenacious, and constricted bronchioles can be relaxed, by the prephysiotherapy inhalation of appropriate aerosols containing detergent and sympatholytic agents. In most cases, such treatment is rapidly successful. Some clinicians add systemic antibiotics as a routine, and it is a wise precaution to send sputum for culture and sensitivity at the first evidence of any chest problem. If there is no rapid improvement within 48 hours, or if the clinical picture is unusually severe, antibiotics should be instituted immediately and the possibility of more rigorous mechanical treatment considered. This more rigorous treatment consists of the passage through the nose of a catheter into the bronchi so that the plugs can be directly aspirated, or even a period of endotracheal intubation and artificial ventilation. The decision to institute such treatment requires experience, but the underlying principles are that severe localized segmental collapse (e.g. of a single main bronchus), with correspondingly low arterial oxygen tension, requires direct aspiration while a patient who is becoming exhausted by the effort of trying to expel his secretion from all areas of the lung has a rising arterial carbon dioxide tension as well and requires assistance with his ventilation. In the special case of massive collapse of one lung or a major lobe, bronchoscopy may be needed to achieve efficient clearing of the obstruction.

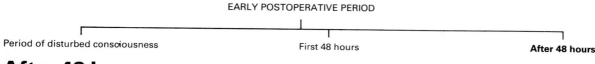

EARLY POSTOPERATIVE PERIOD

Period of disturbed consciousness   First 48 hours   **After 48 hours**

After 48 hours

The main problems are: fluid and electrolytes and nutrition in general; drains of various sorts other than those for reactionary haemorrhage; drains at special sites such as the pleura, the bladder, and fistulae; pyrexia; and thromboembolism.

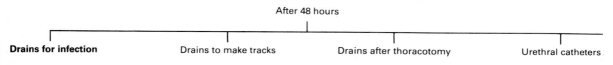

After 48 hours

Drains for infection   Drains to make tracks   Drains after thoracotomy   Urethral catheters

Drains for infection

In wounds with established infection, drains are left in place till the margins of the wound are granulation tissue without sloughs and the cavity is limited to the immediate neighbourhood of the drain. The drain is then shortened daily by 2–5 cm till it comes out. It is important to ensure that the drain by its presence is not impeding rather than facilitating drainage, and that no pocketing is occurring in regions of the wound remote from the drain.

Where a drain was inserted to reduce the risk of infection in a contaminated wound, if no sign of infection develops within 5 days it is usually safe to remove the drain.

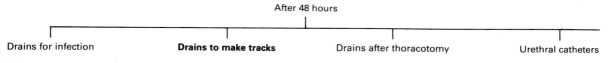

After 48 hours

Drains for infection   **Drains to make tracks**   Drains after thoracotomy   Urethral catheters

Drains to make tracks

The prime indication is the presence of a suture line in the gastrointestinal tract in circumstances in which the operator thinks that a leak is a real possibility. Such leaks could result in a flooding of the peritoneal cavity with infected and highly irritant bowel contents and an ensuing generalized peritonitis. The idea of a drain is to guide the leaking fluid away to the exterior.

Leakage at a suture line in the alimentary tract rarely occurs before the fourth day, and in oesophagus or colon it may be delayed until about the twelfth day. By the fourth day one hopes that adhesions have formed all round the drain, to omentum and neighbouring loops of small bowel, thereby forming a track from the suture line to the exterior. Corrugated rubber or plastic is the best material for such drains, as the corrugations provide channels not easily obliterated by any particulate matter that there may be in the leaking fluid, and there is a strong capillary force attracting the discharge to the exterior.

The time relationships mentioned show that drains in this category must be maintained in position for at least five days (by which time a reasonably firm track has probably formed) and possibly up to twelve, depending on the site of the suture line and the degree of risk associated by the surgeon with the individual circumstances of the case. Most are removed about the seventh day. In the case of an oesophageal anastomosis, the risk of leakage is so high that one usually insists on radiological evidence that the anastomosis is intact (with a small swallowed meal of an opaque nature, such as sodium diatrizoate; Gastrografin) before removing the drain (see next section).

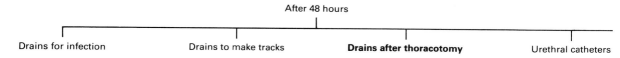

After 48 hours

Drains for infection   Drains to make tracks   **Drains after thoracotomy**   Urethral catheters

Drains after thoracotomy

The basic physiology is so important that it is repeated here. The pleural cavity is the potential space between the parietal pleura, which is adherent to the inside of the chest wall, and the visceral pleura, which is adherent to the surface of the lung; the two pleural layers are continuous at the root of the lung. The elastic recoil of the lung produces a force tending to separate the two layers of pleura as the lung tries to collapse, but this is resisted by the surface tension of the thin layer of liquid which occupies the pleural space.

When a hole is made in the chest wall into the pleural cavity, the film of liquid is broken, the surface tension destroyed, and the lung collapses. A small tear may be made in the pleura by accident during surgery on the chest wall (e.g. biopsy of the internal mammary lymph nodes), in the abdomen (e.g. adrenalectomy), or in the neck (e.g. cervical sympathectomy). The surgeon should inform the anaesthetist immediately, so that the latter can take steps to keep the affected lung expanded by intermittent positive pressure ventilation. Indeed, in operations where such a possibility arises the anaesthetist always uses a cuffed endotracheal tube against this possibility. If the hole in the pleura is small and there is no question of any damage to intrathoracic structures, the only precautions that need be taken are for the anaesthetist to keep the lung well expanded while the structures superficial to the pleura are closed (it is unnecessary to suture the pleura itself), and to get a chest x-ray a few hours after the operation to check that the lung has remained expanded.

The situation is quite different if the chest has been opened deliberately by a larger incision, as part of a surgical operation. Reactionary haemorrhage from intrathoracic structures is likely, and, even if the operation has not involved cutting the lung itself, that organ is very likely to have been damaged by the manipulations of retraction, etc. In consequence, one must expect a leak both of blood and of air from the alveoli of the damaged area of lung, into the pleural cavity. It is thus essential to drain the pleura.

Tubing of very large (1–1.5 cm) bore, made of plastic or rubber is used. Since air tends to collect at the top of the pleural cavity and blood at the bottom, two tubes may be used. In most cases it suffices to have a single tube which runs downwards from the apex of the lung to exit through the chest wall between the lower ribs posterolaterally: there is a large hole in this tube about 0.5 m from its top end, and the tube is adjusted so that this hole drains blood from the base of the chest. Changes in position of the patient will facilitate drainage of both air and liquid from the whole cavity.

To prevent air being sucked into the chest by the negative intrathoracic pressure of inspiration, and consequent collapse of the lung, it is necessary to fit the drain with a non-return valve. The type usually used in routine hospital practice is the underwater seal (Fig. 19.1). The drain dips a few centimetres under the level of water in a bottle. When the intrapleural pressure rises a few centimetres because of coughing, movements, or the accumulation of blood or air, the pleural collection drains into the bottle with visible bubbling in the case of air. However, when the intrapleural pressure drops below atmospheric, the level of water in the tube rises a few centimetres but the seal remains unbroken.

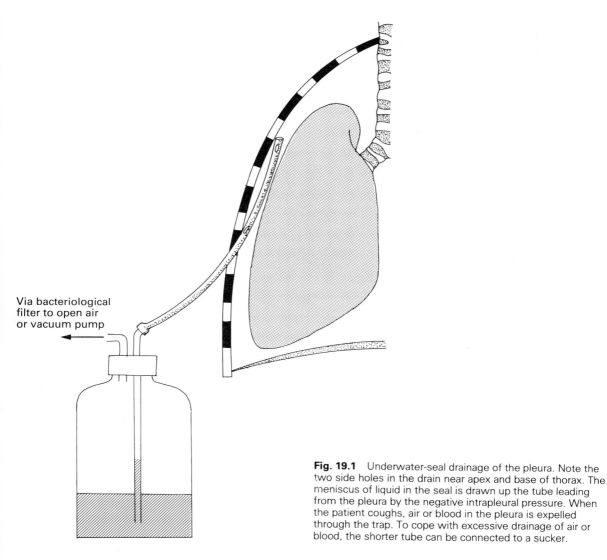

Fig. 19.1 Underwater-seal drainage of the pleura. Note the two side holes in the drain near apex and base of thorax. The meniscus of liquid in the seal is drawn up the tube leading from the pleura by the negative intrapleural pressure. When the patient coughs, air or blood in the pleura is expelled through the trap. To cope with excessive drainage of air or blood, the shorter tube can be connected to a sucker.

Via bacteriological filter to open air or vacuum pump

A large pair of artery forceps is routinely kept close by the underwater seal. This is used to clamp the tube before undertaking any manoeuvres such as moving the patient for bed-making that might result in an accidental breaking of the seal. It is, of course, critical that the system does not become blocked by external mechanical pressure or clots of blood within the tube: stripping the (clamped) tube downwards between finger and thumb usually clears clots.

The up-and-down movement of the water meniscus in the drain, dependent on the respiratory swing of intrathoracic pressure, becomes damped down in 2 or 3 days as the lung expands to press against the tube. The volume of liquid which drains from the chest is measured by its accumulation in the bottle, and a chest x-ray is taken daily. When the lung is fully expanded in the x-ray, when any air leak from the lung has sealed as demonstrated by the disappearance of the swing and the absence of any bubbling for at least 24 hours, and when the liquid collecting rate has dropped to an acceptable level (say, less than 100 ml in 24 hours), the drain may be removed. The exception to this statement is when the operation has included an oesophageal anastomosis; the risk of leakage persists for 12 days, and it is wise to maintain drainage for something approaching that period.

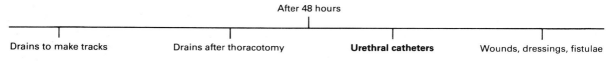

After 48 hours

Drains to make tracks   Drains after thoracotomy   **Urethral catheters**   Wounds, dressings, fistulae

Urethral catheters

Whatever the indication for catheter drainage of the bladder in the postoperative period, the standard technique of management is that the urine drains via a closed system into a plastic bag. The closed system has replaced open drainage because of the high risks of ascending infection with the latter. In some systems it is not even necessary to change the bag when it is full, or when its contents are to be measured, since it is fitted with a tap which permits transfer of its contents to a second container.

Further protection against infection is given by using non-irritant plastic material for the catheters (the old-fashioned red rubber is particularly irritant), and by ensuring that the size of catheter is correct: it should be large enough to prevent slipping in and out along the urethra, a very damaging process, yet not so tight as to obstruct the orifices of the urethral glands. Some units use a mechanical barrier soaked in a bactericidal liquid at the point where the catheter enters the urethra. The most important protection against infection remains the care taken to maintain sterility when the catheter was introduced. The author does not use prophylactic antibiotic or chemotherapy, though some units do.

The decision of when to remove the catheter depends upon the reason for its introduction. If the operation has involved a suture line in the bladder itself, and the catheter is a prophylactic measure against leakage of urine through this wound, then the drainage should be maintained 10 days. If the operation has been one such as prostatectomy in which there is likelihood of considerable reactionary haemorrhage along the lower urinary tract, then the catheter is left in place until bleeding has slowed so much that the urine draining is only tinged pink with blood. If the catheter is meant to circumvent an expected temporary interference with micturition, such as

may be produced by dissection in the region of the autonomic nerve supply to the bladder during excision of the rectum, 5 days is usually sufficient to enable the bladder to recover its tone. Finally the catheter may have been introduced simply so that urine output could be checked as an indicator of an adequate cardiac output during an operation in which a large loss of blood occurred or had been anticipated, and in these circumstances the catheter can be removed as soon as the circulation is stable and there are no reasons for expecting a considerable further haemorrhage, i.e. after 24 hours.

Acute retention is a relatively common phenomenon in the early postoperative period, whether because a long period of drowsiness allows the bladder to become over-stretched and a latent tendency to outflow obstruction in a middle-aged or elderly man becomes manifest, or because of psychological disturbances associated with local pain (for example, after herniorrhaphy), or distaste of the use of a bottle in bed, in younger patients. If the usual conservative remedies of an injection of morphine, the sound of running water, and lying in a warm bath do not help, urethral catheterization may prove necessary. The catheter is usually removed after 24 or 48 hours, but in older men normal micturition may not be established and it may be necessary to proceed to prostatectomy.

When a decision has been made to remove a catheter, this should be implemented early in the morning: if the patient is not going to be able to micturate, it is better to learn this and deal with the problem during the day, rather than having to face a possibly difficult situation during the night. A useful technique to establish confidence in the patient that he will be able to pass his water is to clamp the catheter for a few hours beforehand, and to encourage the patient to urinate as the catheter is being withdrawn.

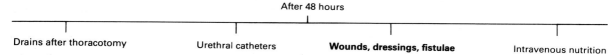

After 48 hours

Drains after thoracotomy   Urethral catheters   **Wounds, dressings, fistulae**   Intravenous nutrition

Wounds, dressings and fistulae

Clean' wounds

Surgical incisions made under full aseptic precau-

tions, and in circumstances in which bacterial contamination is not expected, require only minimal attention. For the first 24 hours the break in the skin is a possible portal of exogenous infection, and it is necessary to cover the wound with some impervious layer, whether a conventional dressing or an artificial skin produced by the hardening of an applied liquid film such as collodion. The less bulky the dressing the better: evaporation of surface moisture must be encouraged to prevent the tissues from becoming macerated and, hence, permeable to micro-organisms. Stitches or clips are removed at a time depending upon local blood supply and the factor of any tension acting to distract the wound edges. For an incision in the skin crease in the neck, a very vascular area, 3 or 4 days suffice; for a vertical incision in the leg, 10 days is advisable.

Contaminated wounds

Traumatic wounds that contain dead or foreign material and have not been surgically explored till more than 4 hours have elapsed, and surgical wounds in which the large bowel has been opened or an infected region of the tissues drained, should be assumed to be potentially infected. One approach to this problem, the use of prophylactic antibiotics, has its adherents, and there is no doubt of its value in certain situations; e.g. the use of penicillin to prevent tetanus and gas gangrene when mid-thigh amputations are performed for ischaemic disease, or of rectal suppositories of metronidazole before appendicectomy to reduce the incidence of infection in the subcutaneous layer of the wound. Another approach, drainage of the wound, has little to recommend it because only the tissues in the immediate vicinity of the drain are adequately drained. The author finds that the technique of leaving the skin and subcutaneous tissues open for 5 days — standard management for traumatic cases — is also valuable for others in this category of wound. A large occlusive dressing is applied to soak up any exudate, and provided the moisture does not reach the exterior this dressing need not be disturbed till the fifth day. An alternative technique is to accept that some infection is inevitable and use daily dressings moistened with an antiseptic. If there is no infection at this stage, the wound may be closed (delayed primary suture); however, this step is frequently unnecessary if the wound lies in the skin crease. If infection does occur, it is usually mild and only superficial.

Infected wounds

A frankly infected wound consists of an interrup-tion in the skin communicating with a granulation-lined cavity containing pus. The essential of management is to obtain free drainage, and this means making sure that the hole in the skin is of adequate dimensions, that any particulate debris in the cavity is removed, that any granulation-lined track (a sinus) extending from the main cavity is incised, and that gravity is invoked to increase drainage. Regular irrigations are useful, and dressings must absorb the discharge efficiently to prevent soaking through to the outer layer and must be changed frequently enough to prevent this happening. These dressings should not be packed tightly into the wound as this might actually prevent healing. It is particularly important not to allow the skin to heal over a residual cavity which is bound to break down again.

Fistulae

A fistula is an abnormal communication between two body cavities, or between a body cavity and the external surface. The latter type, or external fistula, concerns us here.

In the field of general surgery, any postoperative fistula encountered is likely to originate in the gastrointestinal or urinary tract. The first suggestion of a fistula is therefore the appearance at the abdominal wall, either through a wound or along a drain track, or at some point near the wound, of fluid that looks like faeces or urine. There is usually no doubt about urine, with its characteristic appearance and smell; a faecal leak, however, may be simulated by fluid from an internal collection infected with *E. coli*. The simplest way of confirming a faecal fistula is to give the patient an oral dose of methylene blue; the dye is readily recognized in the effluent, and the length of time that elapses between ingestion and appearance is a rough measure of the distance along the alimentary tract of the origin of the leak. If necessary, confirmation of a urinary fistula can be obtained in a similar fashion by an intravenous injection of indigo-carmine, a dye excreted by the kidney within a few minutes.

The liquid reaching the exterior may not constitute the total volume of leak; the remainder may be spreading in the abdomen, producing a spreading peritonitis. This disaster may be recognized by the development of shock (from the exudation of protein-rich material from the capillaries of the inflamed peritoneum), or the symptoms and physical signs of peritonitis. In these circumstances, laparotomy in order to seal or exteriorize the leak is mandatory.

A fistula from the gastrointestinal tract is a very serious condition. Liquid escaping along the track would normally be reabsorbed further down the gut: this loss of what is effectively normal saline can kill the patient unless it is measured and replaced (p. 222). Moreover, the secretions of the alimentary tract are there mainly for their digestive properties, and they are as capable of digesting the skin of the abdominal wall as they are of digesting food. The essentials of management are therefore to intubate the fistula and apply aspiration, thereby accurately collecting the whole volume lost and minimizing the contact of the liquid with the patient's skin, and to protect the skin by the application of various impervious materials such as karaya gum, buffer jelly or Stomahesive. The higher in the digestive tract is the origin of the fistula, the greater the volume of the intestinal secretions lost and the more digestive their properties. Thus a small fistula from the left side of the colon will normally heal if the patient is kept on fluids only by mouth for a few days, but a leak from the upper small intestine demands that the volume of intestinal secretions be cut down by reducing the stimulatory effect of food. Feeding the patient on a so-called 'elemental' diet (i.e. a synthetic mixture of nutrient materials that are completely absorbed) may be sufficient for fistulae from the distal small bowel, but for the really high-level ones it is vital to stop all oral feeding and to maintain nutrition by the intravenous route (next section).

The surgeon should bear in mind certain factors that militate against the healing of a fistula: obstruction in the relevant tract distal to the point of origin of the fistula; the presence of a foreign body, or of chronic disease such as tuberculosis, Crohn's disease or carcinoma; or, in long-standing cases, the growing of epithelium from the skin along the track to meet epithelium from the body cavity. Such factors, if found, must be dealt with before the fistula can be expected to heal. Otherise, the management is to reduce the flow of secretions through the track as already described, and to let the strong natural tendency towards healing do the rest.

After 48 hours

| Urethral catheters | Wounds, dressings, fistulae | **Intravenous nutrition** | Pyrexia |

Fluid and electrolytes: nutrition

Potassium

The same principles of fluid and electrolyte balance apply as in the first 48 hours (p. 222), but there is no contraindication to adding potassium once the urine output has increased to above 750 ml/24 hours. If the patient is doing well and it seems likely that he will be taking all his liquid orally by the third or fourth day, there is no need for potassium. If there have been no complications, or if paralytic ileus shows no sign of relenting, potassium should be started. A reasonable ration is 80 mmol/24 hours. A sudden rise in plasma potassium concentration can produce cardiac arrest, so it is wise to insist that the rate of administration should never exceed 20 mmol in 1 hour. Potassium is usually given by adding a small volume of strong solution of potassium chloride to a half-litre or litre container of some standard liquid for intravenous infusion. This practice is dangerous both because of the possibility of a dangerously rapid rise in plasma potassium concentration if the container is not well shaken to achieve good mixing and also because of the danger of introducing infection. Suitable sodium/potassium mixtures have recently become commercially available. An excellent mixture for routine use contains 80 mmol of sodium and 80 mmol of potassium in 2 litres of water, the whole made isotonic with glucose.

It is worth noting here that the plasma potassium concentration is only a rough guide to overall potassium balance. The partition of potassium between the cells and the extracellular compartment is affected by several factors which may be altered during the postoperative period; acid-base balance, the activity of the sodium pump and the adrenocortical steroid hormone response to trauma. Misleading high plasma concentrations may also be an artefact resulting from haemolysis in the blood sample due to faults in the technique of taking the blood, e.g. withdrawing it from the vein too rapidly through too fine a needle. For these reasons it is a good rule to check any unexpected plasma reading by an independent technique — the ECG: both deficiency and excess of potassium produce characteristic changes.

Energy and protein

The postoperative period is characterized by a negative balance of energy (joules or calories) and nitrogen. The negative protein balance can be reduced, but probably not entirely prevented, by a large intake of energy.

The negative nitrogen balance is an embarrassment to the patient, who requires large quantities of amino acids to build the new tissues of his healing wound. At the same time there is a loss of nitrogen in any exudate poured out into the wound, especially if infection occurs, and an acceleration of catabolism of protein resulting from starvation, decubitus and the adrenocorticosteroid response to trauma.

When the patient is able to start eating again as soon as 3 or 4 days after the operation, the problem is likely to be of only theoretical importance. If, however, oral feeding is contra-indicated for a much longer period, for example by a high small bowel external fistula (p. 230), it becomes essential to feed the patient intravenously. The essential requirement is the amino acids, but infused amino acids are wastefully burned unless the patient receives a sufficient supply of energy from carbohydrate or fat at the same time. Up to a point, moreover, the greater the intake of energy the less protein breakdown occurs in the body.

The problem is that both amino acids and simple carbohydrates such as glucose are small molecules and correspondingly osmotically active: to give the patient sufficient of these foods within the reasonable limits of the daily water intake, 2–3 litres, would require grossly hypertonic infusions which would rapidly produce thrombophlebitis at the usual sites of injection into superficial veins. It is true that fat consists of large molecules with a small osmotic effect, but a balance must be obtained between carbohydrate and fat if the latter is not to cause ketosis.

To solve these problems, hypertonic or otherwise irritant liquids are injected directly into the innominate vein or superior vena cava, where they are so rapidly diluted by the rapid flow of blood as to be rendered innocuous. There are various routes whereby the cavae can be reached: the basilic at the elbow, and the jugular and the subclavian veins in the neck. The author finds the subclavicular route to the subclavian vein the most generally satisfactory.

With care, the same caval line can be maintained for several weeks or even months. The most important complication is infection which, travelling along the catheter from the puncture site in the skin, produces septicaemia. To prevent septicaemia, it is important that such lines should be inserted only under full aseptic precautions, that the point at which the catheter passes through the skin is protected by an efficient bactericidal dressing that is frequently changed, and that the point of puncture of the skin should be as far as possible from the point at which the catheter enters the vein. Should the patient at any stage develop a high temperature, it should be assumed that the cause is septicaemia. The catheter is removed and its tip sent for culture; likewise, samples of blood taken by venepuncture elsewhere are cultured. Usually the temperature drops within a few hours of removing the catheter, but if it does not, antibiotic therapy should be started while awaiting the report on the culture and sensitivity of the samples sent.

With regard to the details of the fluids administered, there are many regimes which can deliver 8–14 MJ (2000–3000 kcal) and 70–100 g amino acids, in 2–3 litres of water. While the amino acids are run in, the energy required to save the amino acids for synthesis rather than catabolism is simultaneously infused. The source of energy is either carbohydrate or alcohol, separately or in combination, or else a suspension of fat. The latter must be given separately by a Y-connection; the former substances are given either separately or as a mixture with the amino acids. When fat is used, a sample of venous blood should be taken daily, centrifuged, and the plasma inspected for lipaemia, a sign that no further fat suspension should be given. If concentrated glucose solutions are used, all urine samples should be tested for glucose: insulin given on a sliding scale according to the degree of glycosuria can help to get the glucose into the cells and thereby prevent an osmotic dehydration which can result in coma or death.

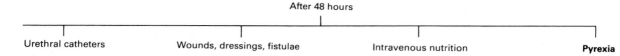

After 48 hours

Urethral catheters   Wounds, dressings, fistulae   Intravenous nutrition   **Pyrexia**

Pyrexia

The causes of pyrexia that are common during the first 48 hours may still be operating at a later time. However, the necessity for blood transfusion is probably past and it is relatively unusual for a postoperative atelectasis to occur for the first time at this stage. The two major causes are infection and thromboembolism.

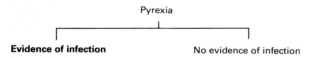

Pyrexia

Evidence of infection   No evidence of infection

Infection

The first place to look for the cause of the temperature is the wound. The third day would be rather early for infection to be manifest, but any time between the third and tenth day is possible. The first sign may be an erythematous flare around stitch holes, or a region of pain and tenderness without any visible sign of inflammation. When pus forms, the line of the incision itself becomes soft in contrast with the surrounding induration. As soon as it becomes clear that infection has been established and pus has formed, free drainage must be established (p. 229).

After laparotomy (and very rarely after operations at sites remote from the abdomen), infection may become established in various recesses of the peritoneal cavity. The commoner sites are the pelvis and the subphrenic spaces. In all cases of suspected infection, blood should be sent for a white count. A high leucocyte count with a polymorpholeucocytosis supports the diagnosis of infection, though a normal white count does not exclude the diagnosis. Ultrasound is particularly good at demonstrating intraperitoneal collections of liquid.

A pelvic abscess characteristically irritates the rectum and produces a form of diarrhoea in which the patient passes mostly mucus. Whether or not this sign is present, a rectal examination should be done as a routine: a boggy indurated swelling in the pouch of Douglas clinches the diagnosis. Provided that there is no evidence of septicaemia, antibiotics are withheld. The abscess usually drains itself into the rectum (or vagina in the female), though occasionally it becomes necessary to interfere by pushing a pair of sinus forceps into the fluctuant mass through the rectal wall at the tip of a proctoscope.

A subphrenic abscess can be a very difficult clinical problem. All cases of unexplained pyrexia after operation should have the appropriate radiological investigations, but the difficulty particularly arises where the onset is very insidious and the only clinical abnormality is a patient who fails to thrive as well as he should. There may be some abnormal physical signs: the chest may move less well on the affected than on the unaffected side, and there may be dullness and reduced air entry at the lung base due to either collapse/consolidation or a pleural effusion, or both. A bulging in the flank, or below the costal margin anteriorly, is a very late sign, and the condition should have been diagnosed by then.

The important evidence is from imaging techniques. If ultrasound is not available, or in the rare cases in which it is unhelpful, one might have to rely on CT-scanning (much more expensive). There are also older techniques. On screening, the diaphragm on the affected side moves poorly, or not at all, when the subject sniffs, and the horizontal interface between liquid and gas in the abscess is seen below the diaphragm. In this respect, the similar shadow in the stomach can be confusing, and the best way to make sure whether there is a separate gas/liquid-filled cavity is to take a lateral film in the erect position when the subject has just swallowed a mouthful of a radio-opaque meal. Simultaneous liver/lung scans may demonstrate an abnormal gap between the organs.

Such techniques establish whether the cavity is on the left side or right, and whether it is near the front or the back, and this evidence decides the correct route for needle drainage and replacement with antibiotics. This is usually performed under ultrasound control and repeated as often as necessary. Very occasionally, open surgical drainage is required.

If a urethral catheter has been passed on the patient, a likely cause of postoperative pyrexia is urinary infection. It is often said that the pyrexia of cystitis is unusual in that there is little increase in the pulse rate compared with the rise in temperature. The patient usually complains of frequency of micturition and a burning dysuria during the act, but even if these clinical features are absent it is wise to send a mid-stream specimen of urine for bacteriological examination in any case of postoperative pyrexia for which there is no obvious cause.

Finally, the possibility of septicaemia, which may occur on its own or as a complication of any of the foregoing focal infections, must be remembered. In any patient with suggestive clinical features such as headache, shock or rigors, or in any patient in whom the investigations outlined in the previous paragraphs have drawn blank, blood samples should be sent for culture.

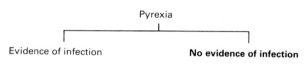

Thromboembolism

There is no doubt that thrombosis in the veins of the lower limb or pelvis can be associated with pyrexia. The presence of pyrexia should therefore lead to a careful search for other clinical evidence of deep venous thrombosis. The usually accepted signs of deep venous thrombosis are localized pain or tenderness in the calf or along the course of the femoral vein in the thigh, oedema, cyanosis, engorged superficial veins, or a raised skin temperature of the affected limb particularly in its distal regions, and pain in the calf when the patient's foot is forcefuly dorsiflexed by the examiner — Homans' sign.

Unfortunately, these clinical signs are grossly unreliable. Homans himself, not long after the publication of the paper in which he described his sign, issued a disclaimer of its value in clinical practice, although this second article seems to have been in general ignored. During the last decade, when accurate methods for the diagnosis of venous thrombosis became available, abundant evidence has appeared that the previously accepted clinical signs are often present in the absence of thrombosis, and particularly that the absence of all these signs does not exclude the diagnosis.

Notwithstanding the comments of the previous paragraph, the generally accepted practice at present is that if there is no clinical evidence, the cause of the pyrexia is sought elsewhere, whereas if there are features suggestive of thromboembolism then further consideration is given to this possibility. Exactly what is done depends in the first instance upon the availability of reliable diagnostic tests.

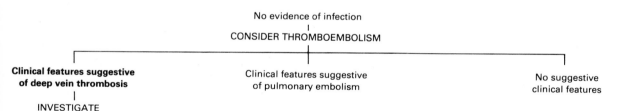

Diagnostic tests The best test in this situation is *phlebography*, because it is the only one that will give a rapid and reliable result anywhere in the lower limb and pelvis. The essence of the technique is that a radio-opaque solution is injected into a vein on the dorsum of the foot, and the contrast is forced into the deep veins by the pressure of a tight cuff at the ankle. Thrombi show up as filling defects in the deep veins. Alternative but less accurate investigation techniques are Doppler ultrasound and radioactive-labelled fibrinogen uptake. Above the knee, the Doppler ultrasound technique gives good results. The ultrasound signal is directed towards the femoral vein in the upper thigh, and the calf is squeezed: if the main venous channels are open, the resultant surge of blood in the femoral vein is picked up on the answering signal reflected back to the source, but if the femoral vein is completely obstructed there is no change in the signal. Below the knee, the radio-iodinated fibrinogen method is effective. An injection of fibrinogen labelled with radioactive ^{125}I is incorporated into the thrombus and results in a local increase in radioactive emission, as detected with an external counter, in the region of the thrombus compared with neighbouring points on the same limb or corresponding points on the opposite limb. A single injection of fibrinogen yields counts that remain above the discriminatory level for about 6 days; the actual counts naturally fall during this period, so for purposes of comparison they are usually expressed as percentages of the count over the heart, which acts as a large pool of un-fixed fibrinogen in the circulation. Readings in the upper thigh are more difficult to interpret than those in the more distal parts of the limb because of interference from the large vascular areas of the pelvic vessels, and also of the urinary bladder into which the label gradually leaks as the fibrinogen is metabolized.

Management of 'clinical' deep venous thrombosis
If the special tests are performed, the diagnosis is either refuted — in which case the patient can be treated symptomatically or some other cause sought; or confirmed. There is no consensus about the treatment of this condition: the possibilities are conservative measures, or an active attempt to destroy or at least limit the clot so as to reduce the risk of pulmonary embolism. Conservative measures include the application of firm elastic bandages or stockings to the leg, thereby forcing blood into the deep veins and increasing the linear velocity of flow in these. Opinion is divided, however, as to whether the patient should be put to bed for a few days in the hope that this will reduce the chance of direct trauma to the leg resulting in the detachment of an embolus, or whether ambulant exercise should be encouraged to increase the rate of blood flow in the veins. The possibilities in the case of active treatment include anticoagulants, fibrinolytic agents, operative thrombectomy, and interruption of the main proximal venous pathway (e.g. the inferior vena cava).

The primary aim of treatment is to prevent pulmonary embolism, a potentially fatal condition. The rationale of anticoagulants is that the initial thrombus is usually attached firmly to the wall of the vein and is unlikely to become detached and embolize, whereas the subsequent formation of propagated soft clot proximally is much more dangerous because this clot is only loosely attached, and it is the formation of the propagated clot which the anticoagulants are supposed to prevent. The rationale of the other methods is obvious. There is some evidence (to this author's mind, far from convincing) that all these methods can reduce the risk of pulmonary embolism, but in deciding on treatment three factors should be borne in mind. First, studies with the fibrinogen technique have shown that,

at least in patients over the age of 40 years, the incidence of deep venous thrombosis after major surgery is about 30 per cent — and the majority of these patients have no symptoms or signs and would therefore in the normal way never be considered for treatment. Secondly, the vast majority of patients with proven deep venous thrombosis come to no harm: indeed, spontaneous reso-

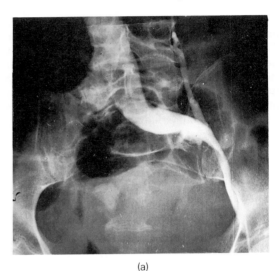

(a)

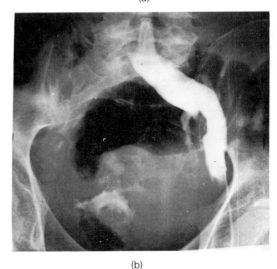

(b)

Fig. 19.2 Spontaneous disappearance of thrombus in deep vein. The patient, a man of 58 years, underwent partial gastrectomy. Radiofibrinogen studies (for reserach) indicated a clot in the left thigh on the fifth postoperative day. A phlebogram confirmed the clot and also showed one in the left iliac veins (a). A repeat phlebogram on the tenth day showed patent iliac veins (b). No treatment had been given, and there had been no symptoms or signs of thromboembolism.

lution of the clot with recanalization of the vein is the usual course of events (Fig. 19.2). Thirdly, the treatments suggested are neither entirely effective nor entirely safe. Anticoagulants can produce haemorrhage, either at the site of the recent operation or indeed 'spontaneously' anywhere in the body, but on the other hand there are many reports of fatal pulmonary embolism despite anticoagulation. Fibrinolytic agents such as streptokinase and urokinase have unpleasant side-effects of pyrexia, bleeding, etc. Thrombectomy is followed by a very high rethrombosis rate and is nowadays rarely performed. Interruption of the inferior vena cava forms the sump of a new stagnant backwater of the circulation, and it has been reported that fresh clot may form immediately proximal to the block.

The real problem is that there is no convincing controlled trial of the efficacy of these remedies at preventing pulmonary embolism in patients with proven deep vein thrombosis. If, after balancing all the pros and cons, a surgeon feels that treatment is indicated, then in Britain the experts recommend thrombectomy (with the Fogarty catheter, p. 351) for fresh, loose clot, full anticoagulation with heparin for one week followed by warfarin for 6 months in patients with older, fixed clot, and interruption of major venous pathway (the superficial femoral vein for preference, unless the clot has extended proximal to this or is present in both legs) if a long fixed clot, unsuitable for thrombectomy, has a proximal loose 'tail' which looks likely to become dislodged as an embolus.

Flow-chart 19.1

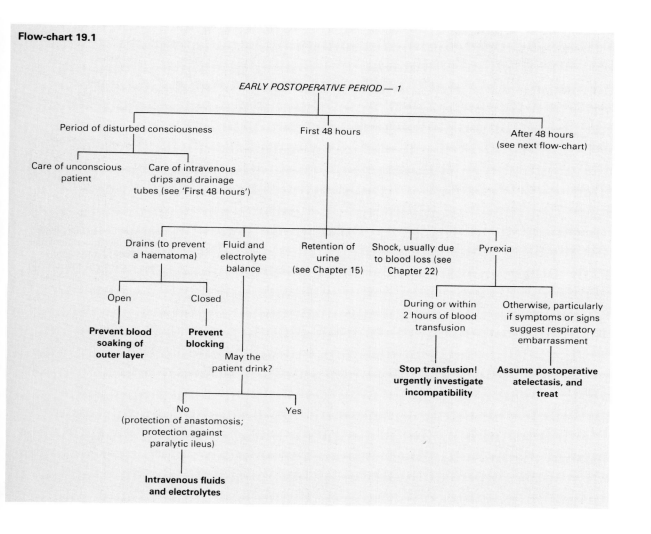

Flow-chart 19.2

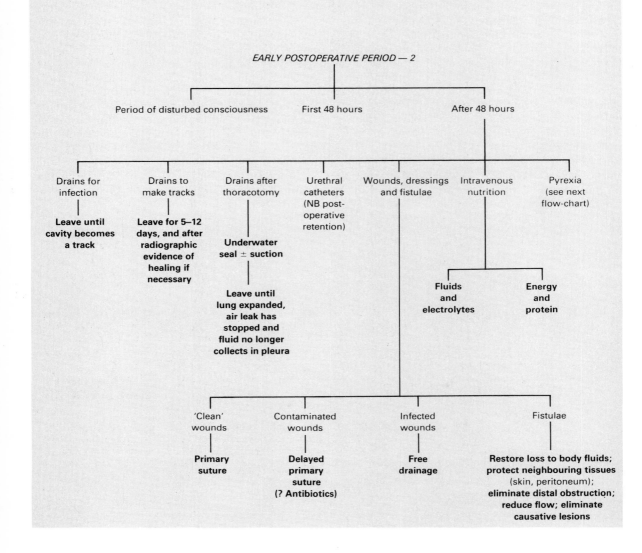

EARLY POSTOPERATIVE PERIOD — 2

Period of disturbed consciousness   First 48 hours   After 48 hours

Drains for infection

Leave until cavity becomes a track

Drains to make tracks

Leave for 5–12 days, and after radiographic evidence of healing if necessary

Drains after thoracotomy

Underwater seal ± suction

Leave until lung expanded, air leak has stopped and fluid no longer collects in pleura

Urethral catheters (NB post-operative retention)

Wounds, dressings and fistulae

Intravenous nutrition

Fluids and electrolytes

Energy and protein

Pyrexia (see next flow-chart)

'Clean' wounds

Primary suture

Contaminated wounds

Delayed primary suture (? Antibiotics)

Infected wounds

Free drainage

Fistulae

Restore loss to body fluids; protect neighbouring tissues (skin, peritoneum); eliminate distal obstruction; reduce flow; eliminate causative lesions

Flow-chart 19.3

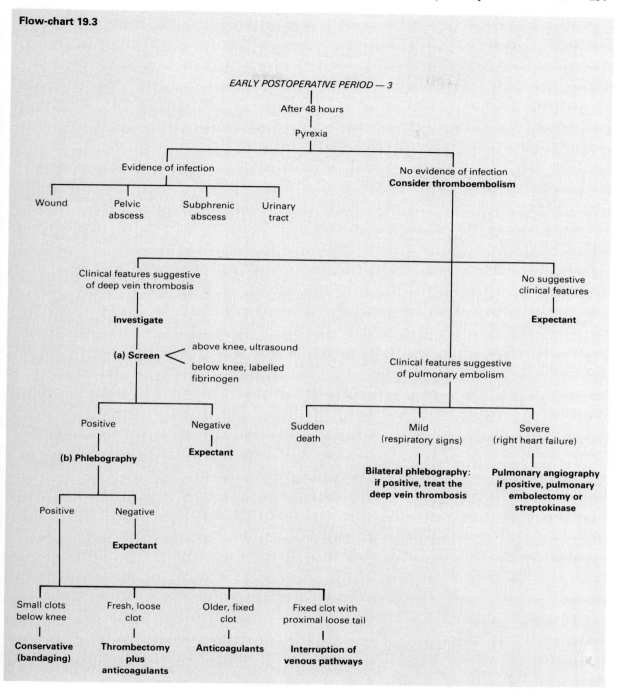

CONSIDER THROMBOEMBOLISM

Clincal features suggestive
of deep vein thrombosis

**Clinical features suggestive
of pulmonary embolism**

No suggestive
clinical features

Management of 'clinical' pulmonary embolism

This is another controversial problem, mainly because of the difficulty of being sure of the diagnosis and because of the dangers of the available treatments. Apart from cases presenting as sudden death, the problem falls into two categories: embolus suspected because of chest symptoms and signs such as dyspnoea, pain and haemoptysis, but without evidence of right heart strain; and patients severely ill with right heart failure manifesting hypotension, raised jugular venous pressure, cyanosis and gallop rhythm. As in the case of venous thrombosis in the legs, the difficulty starts with the diagnosis: techniques such as lung scanning and pulmonary angiography are still only available in special centres, and myocardial infarction is a common cause of the clinical picture with right heart strain, postoperative atelectasis of the clinical picture without right heart strain.

The experts recommend that for the mild group bilateral phlebography be performed, and if that demonstrates clot in the veins of the leg or pelvis the situation should be treated by anticoagulants or thrombectomy or vein interruption as descri-

bed in the previous section. For the ill patient, observation for a few hours is advised, together with appropriate measures such as oxygen; should the patient deteriorate, the only active treatment possible is pulmonary embolectomy, best done on full cardiopulmonary bypass and always preceded by a pulmonary angiogram to confirm the diagnosis. If such investigation and treatment is impossible, or if the patient neither deteriorates nor improves, the effect of streptokinase may be tried. If the patient recovers, further management is as for the mild group.

There is a syndrome of recurrent small pulmonary emboli which ultimately produce the clinical picture of severe pulmonary hypertension. It is particularly for this situation that a technique has been invented for inserting a sieve in the inferior vena cava by a percutaneous technique. The sieve is inserted at the end of a long catheter which passes through the cavae (and right atrium). It is then opened like an umbrella to impact in the inferior vena cava above its bifurcation and the catheter is withdrawn. The technique is safe and seems to be effective.

Further reading

Alberti, K. G. M. M. (Ed) (1975). Parenteral nutrition: a clinical conversation. *Clinical Trials Journal* **12**, Suppl. 1.

Browse, N. L. (1977). What should I do about deep vein thrombosis and pulmonary embolism? *Annals of the Royal College of Surgeons of England* **59**, 138–42.

Chitwood, W. R., Lyerly, K. K. and Sabiston, D. C. (1985). Surgical Management of Chronic Pulmonary Embolism. *Annals of Surgery* **201**, 11–26.

Evans, M. and Pollock, A. V. (1985). A score system for evaluating random control clinical trials of prophylaxis of abdominal surgical wound infection. *British Journal of Surgery* **72**, 256–60.

Hobsley, M. (1958). Chlorpheniramine maleate in prophylaxis of pyrexial reactions during blood transfusions. *Lancet* **i**, 497–9.

Kyle, J. (Ed) (1984). *Pye's Surgical Handicraft*, 21st edn. Bristol, Wright, P. S. G.

Lee, H. A. (1975). Intravenous nutrition. *Annals of the Royal College of Surgeons of England* **56**, 59–68.

Nassos, T. P. and Braasch, J. W. (1971). External small bowel fistulas. *Surgical Clinics of North America* **51**, 687–92.

Nicolaides, A. N. (1975). *Thromboembolism*. Lancaster, M. T. P.

Ochsner, A. and Groves, A. M. (1933). Subphrenic abscesses: an analysis of 3372 collected and personal cases. *Annals of Surgery* **98**, 961–9.

Palmer, K. N. V. and Sellick, B. A. (1953). The prevention of postoperative pulmonary atelectasis. *Lancet* **i**, 164–70.

Sturridge, M. F. and Treasure, T. (1985). *Belcher's Thoracic Surgical Management*. London, Baillière Tindall.

Wilkinson, A. W. (1973). *Body Fluids in Surgery*, 4th edn. Edinburgh and London, Churchill Livingstone.

Part II

Emergencies

Chapter 20

The Severely Injured Patient

Disease produced by trauma is highly prevalent in our violent world. Even where there is no war in progress at the moment, the motor car takes its toll, and so, too, do industrial and household accidents. Mortality rates are high, and though household accidents are common in the elderly, the age group of patients mostly affected is young: this combination enhances the gravity of the problem.

At first sight, the variety of both the traumatic agent and the way in which the body can be damaged is so enormous that it might be thought impossible to cover the whole subject in a single chapter, even though various aspects of trauma are deferred to the subsequent four chapters. However, it is proposed to concentrate on principles rather than details; to formulate rules of wide general applicability to the whole range of possible injury situations rather than to try to describe those situations. Obviously, this chapter is not a textbook of traumatology. Nevertheless, in complicated cases the life of the patient depends on the ability of his medical attendant to dissect away the irrelevancies and find immediately the right solution to the urgent problems besetting the patient. In these circumstances, a clear grasp of principles should stand the doctor in good stead.

Before enunciating any principles of management, it will be useful to consider what is meant by the phrase *severely injured patient*. Clearly, severity is not concerned simply with the bulk of tissue damaged. It is true that a burn is an example of a type of injury where the effects are largely strictly related to the area of tissue destroyed, but there are many forms of injury for which this parallelism does not hold. For example, a patient may have a score of superficial lacerations over a wide area of the outer aspect of the thigh, and he is in discomfort but he is not in danger; on the other hand, in another patient a tiny puncture of the lung and the consequent development of a tension pneumothorax threatens his life. Viewed in this way, it becomes clear that a severe injury is most usefully thought about as one which threatens life.

This line of thought leads logically to what may be stated as the first, and paramount, principle in the management of the severely injured patient: *save life*. This principle may appear to be so obvious as hardly to be worth stating, but the value of stating it explicitly will become manifest shortly.

The second great principle is concerned with the quality of life to be offered to the survivor. Clearly, the ideal is that the patient's wounds should be completely healed, and that he should be restored to a state of normality with regard to both structure and function. Thus this second principle may be expressed as: *repair damage*. A corollary of this principle, so important that it should be included in the statement of the principle itself, is that from the moment that the patient is first seen, every effort must be made to prevent further damage occurring. The second principle may therefore be expanded to: *limit damage; repair damage*.

There remains a third consideration. The complexities of modern scientific medicine, and the marvels which can be achieved by way of ingenious investigations and powerful remedies including surgical skill, must not be allowed to obscure the fact that one of the physician's duties is to relieve suffering. The third principle may therefore be stated as: *relieve symptoms*.

It is worth pointing out that these three principles sum up the management of *every* patient, not just of those suffering from trauma. However, the statement of these principles in this explicit fashion, summarizing the three areas of *action* required by the doctor, are particularly useful in cases of severely injured patients because they lead to three further principles of what one might call *philosophy* — principles, that is, which guide the doctor in making decisions as to the best way to achieve the three basic goals.

When a doctor is faced with a severe case of multiple trauma, many things which the patient needs to have done for him may spring to the doctor's mind. The latter has to decide not only what has to be done, but also in what order they should be done, because not everything can be done at once. Indeed, there will be some occasions when two procedures may each individually appear desirable, but are mutually incompatible. The doctor has to assign priorities at every stage of management, and this task is enormously simplified by the consideration that saving life must take precedence over repairing damage, and that both predominate over the relief of symptoms. Whenever there is a problem of deciding priorities, the doctor must assign the competing factors to their various categories, and the application of this first guiding principle usually indicates the correct manner of proceeding.

The second guiding principle follows directly from the first: if priorities are to be assessed, it is quite clear that only one person can act as assessor. Frequently, several doctors and medical auxiliaries work simultaneously on a seriously injured patient: an anaesthetist may be maintaining the airway, a house-surgeon taking a sample of blood, another surgeon starting an intravenous infusion, and a nurse pressing a pack over a bleeding artery. It is imperative that, no matter how many experts in various fields are rendering their assistance, only one person should make the decisions about priorities. Exactly who that person should be is of much less importance, provided that everyone knows who it is.

The third guiding principle is again an obvious deduction from the first two. The decisions with regard to priorities need to be right. Unless one wishes to rely upon luck, it is therefore necessary that each decision is made in the light of the most complete and accurate information about the patient and his injuries that can be gathered at that moment.

Before considering the application of these three principles of action and three philosophical guides in greater detail, it is convenient to subdivide the management of a severely injured patient into four geographical stages — the sites at which the doctor is looking after his patient. These four geographical stages are: (1) *in the field*, i.e. at the site of an accident or on the battlefield, etc.; (2) *in the hospital, the emergency room or casualty department;* (3) *in hospital*, during *definitive treatment*; and (4) *convalescence and rehabilitation*. In urban conditions, stages (1) and (2) may be virtually the same. This subdivision simplifies the description because the comparative emphasis to be laid on each of the three primary principles of action varies during these four stages. The complete management of a patient with serious injuries — from the time of injury to the moment when he takes his place in society restored to his previous activities and abilities, or at least to a state as near his previous one as possible — may occupy several months or even years. The relative priorities of the three principles remain immutable: but in the early stages the doctor finds himself thinking most of the time about saving life while in the later stages the threat to life has largely receded and the doctor is concerned most of the time with symptoms.

In the field

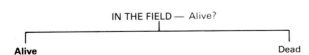

IN THE FIELD — Alive?

Alive   Dead

Saving life

A human being dies when his brain dies. A brain dies when its structure is destroyed by local trauma, direct or indirect. Nothing can be done about direct trauma, but an injury needs to be violent indeed to reach directly the brain within its bony citadel. On the other hand, the presence of the rigid skull causes the brain to be vulnerable to the indirect trauma of the rotational and vibrational stresses which produce the clinical picture of concussion, and of the effects of raised intracranial pressure produced by bleeding within the skull and interference with the free circulation of cerebrospinal fluid. Nothing active can be done about concussion: either the injury is too severe to be compatible with recovery or it is not.

Apart from the effects of local trauma, the brain can also be affected by remote factors, i.e. ones that do not act upon the brain itself. The life of cerebral cells depends upon a supply of oxygen and glucose, since anaerobic metabolism is not possible even for short periods. Irreversible changes take place if the lack of oxygen and glucose lasts for a short period of time, probably not much longer than 3 minutes. In patients who have undergone injury there is unlikely to be any shortage of glucose in the blood. One must always bear in mind the possibility that an unconscious patient may not have fallen by accident and sustained cerebral concussion, but rather have become unconscious because of some such reason as hypoglycaemia and therefore fallen. Nevertheless, in the vast majority of cases the vitality of the brain is threatened by lack of oxygen rather than by lack of glucose. The supply of oxygen reaches the brain via the circulating blood, and therefore the threat to life may be analysed in terms of failure of oxygenation of the blood, and failure of the cerebral circulation, including cardiac arrest (Chapter 21). For a further discussion of brain damage, see Chapter 24.

Alive

|

CHECK AIRWAY

Failure of oxygenation (anoxia)

Oxygenation of the blood depends upon the presence of adequate oxygen in the atmosphere, a patent airway between the atmosphere and the pulmonary alveoli, effective ventilation to achieve movement of gas between the atmosphere and the pulmonary alveoli, and effective exchange of the respiratory gases between the alveoli and the alveolar capillaries. These aspects must be methodically checked, and any deficiencies corrected if possible.

For example, the patient is removed from the *atmosphere* of the collapsed mine where the oxygen has been used up, or from the water where he has drowned. His *airway* is next cleared: false teeth or other foreign material are removed digitally from his mouth and pharynx, the jaw is pulled forwards to control the tongue, and when other considerations allow he is turned into the prone position with his head on one side. Properly equipped first-aid teams carry artificial airways and nasopharyngeal tubes. Rarely, external pressure on the trachea (throttling) will need relieving.

Ventilation is checked. If the patient is not breathing spontaneously, artificial ventilation is started, probably by mouth-to-mouth ventilation. If the patient is breathing, are the ventilatory efforts adequate, or is he cyanosed? The ventilatory excursions of the chest wall are observed, and any external pressure (for example by the crushing effect of masonry or car wreckage) removed.

Airway clear

|

Patient not breathing and/or cyanosed   Patient breathing, not cyanosed

Respiratory gas exchange between the alveoli and the alveolar capillaries depends upon two physiological processes: diffusion and distribution. *Diffusion* is the passage of the gases in solution across the alveolar membrane. Disorders of diffusion are rare: occasionally, exposure to a noxious gas such as chlorine produces pulmonary oedema with a disturbance of diffusion. Naturally, the patient should already have been removed from such an atmospheric environment. *Distribution* expresses the balance between air supply and blood supply in the various regions of the lung. Pneumothorax and tension pneumothorax result in collapse of the lung, with destruction of aeration but preservation to some extent of blood supply. They may escape diagnosis if a stethoscope is not available, but there is no mistaking a sucking wound of the chest wall: through a large wound in the chest wall, air is noisily sucked into the pleural cavity with each inspiration. Not only is the ipsilateral lung collapsed, but the pressure of air in the pleural cavity may displace the mediastinum to the opposite side and embarrass the opposite lung and kink the great vessels with reduction of the venous return to the heart. The only available first-aid measure is to attempt to limit the movement of air into the pleural cavity by an occlusive pad and bandage constructed from the cleanest materials at hand. Finally, distribution may be obviously impaired by a flail chest injury. If a large section of chest wall is functionally detached from the remainder by the breaking of several ribs in more than one place, the act of inspiration causes that segment of chest wall to be sucked inwards by the negative intrathoracic pressure instead of moving outwards with the rest of the chest wall. The expansion of the ipsilateral lung is thereby limited. Careful observation of the movements of the chest wall should lead to the diagnosis: the first-aid treatment is to limit at least the outward movement of the flail segment during expiration by an occlusive pad and bandage.

Failure of the cerebral circulation

The cerebral circulation may become inadequate because of *local* factors, i.e. those affecting the cerebral circulation alone, or because of *general* factors, i.e. those affecting the circulation as a whole.

Local factors comprise obstruction to the carotid arteries or obstruction to the jugular veins in the neck (strangling). The constricting agent must be removed immediately.

General factors are far more common. They comprise the cessation of the heart beat and reduction of cardiac output by factors local to the heart such as cardiac tamponade (bleeding into the pericardium) or by diminution of the circulating blood volume. In the first-aid situation, cardiac tamponade is unlikely to be diagnosed, and diminution of the circulating blood volume is necessarily synonymous with haemorrhage because no other fluid can be lost quickly enough from the circulation to produce an immediate threat to life. This leaves for consideration cardiac arrest and haemorrhage.

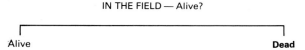

Cardiac arrest (see Chapter 21) should always be thought of as cardiorespiratory arrest because spontaneous ventilation ceases very soon after the heart stops beating. Arrest is diagnosed by absence of the carotid pulse or, if a stethoscope is available, by absence of the heart sounds. It is unlikely that any first-aid measures will succeed unless at least three helpers are present: one to perform mouth-to-mouth ventilation, one to perform external cardiac massage, and one to summon aid. Occasionally, a heart that has been stopped by a sudden savage insult such as electrocution will start again if the precordium is struck a sharp blow with the flat of the hand.

Usually, the cause of the arrest is damage to the heart itself as a result of exsanguination or local trauma, and this is likely to be irreversible. Death can be difficult to diagnose, especially if the casualties who are clearly still alive, and requiring urgent treatment, are numerous. A portable ECG with three leadless electrodes can be useful in this situation.

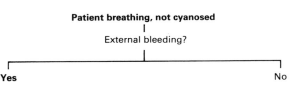

Haemorrhage is the commonest threat to the adequacy of the cerebral circulation in trauma. External haemorrhage is obvious, and should be stopped by firm pressure at the bleeding point, using the cleanest technique that is found to succeed. Direct pressure is far more effective than pressure over the proximal pressure points (i.e. points where the main artery proximal to the site of haemorrhage crosses a bone against which it can be easily compressed). Direct pressure is also far safer than a tourniquet, which crushes the tissues locally and may result in gangrene of the distal tissues if it is left applied longer than three hours. However, a tourniquet is still occasionally useful.

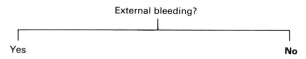

Internal haemorrhage cannot be seen, but its likelihood can be deduced from the signs of shock. This subject is considered in Chapter 22. For the present, we may note that, fortunately, the cerebral circulation is not too sensitive to a reduction in blood volume: the cerebral blood flow is maintained, despite a falling total cardiac output, by a variety of compensatory measures which modify the regional distribution of the blood.

If signs of shock are present, measures to attempt to maintain the cerebral circulation should be undertaken: the patient is kept still, lying down in a horizontal position and with the legs raised, and he is not allowed to be too warm. Note that the horizontal position is preferable to inclining the body so that the head is lower than the heart, while cutaneous vasodilatation shunts much-needed blood through the skin so that it is better to keep the patient cool rather than warm. An intravenous infusion is started, and opiates (p. 248) given if these are available.

Limiting and repairing damage

The most important measure of the few available under this heading in the field is that the source of trauma, if still acting, should be removed. Action under this heading has already been advised for various aspects of preserving life: further examples are switching off the current in a case of electrocution, and washing the reagent out of a chemical burn.

One of the chief factors causing further damage in a wound is infection. Open wounds should be covered with the cleanest dressing handy. Fractures are splinted because movement of the bone ends relative to each other increases the damage to local tissues, both directly and by aggravating haematoma formation.

Treating symptoms

Little can be done in the field. The splinting of fractures comes under this heading because limiting the movement of the bone ends reduces pain. The relief of pain by drugs, even supposing that suitable drugs happen to be available, is too difficult a matter for generalizations. This topic is considered in the next paragraph. The most important measure is reassurance of the patient, particularly about the severity of his injuries, about the length of time that it will take to get him to hospital, and about informing his relatives about him.

Pain relief

Some of the decisions about priorities in the field are extremely difficult. The question of relief of pain by drugs such as morphine is a typical example. Certainly no one who may have an intra-abdominal injury should be given an opiate, because the drug may mask the signs of peritonitis or intraperitoneal haemorrhage and thereby delay surgery when the patient is seen in hospital. Cases with head injury will be likely to be unconscious, or at least dazed, immediately after the trauma, and so the well known contraindication to morphine in head injuries is less troublesome. In other patients it may be considered right to give morphine, but the doctor should make certain that the dose, route and time are communicated to the medical staff of the hospital to which the patient is sent. In shocked patients with a sluggish peripheral circulation, drugs injected subcutaneously or intramuscularly may be only slowly absorbed, and slow injection by the intravenous route is preferable.

A particularly useful agent for controlling pain in the field is a gas mixture of equal parts of oxygen and nitrous oxide (Entonox). Inhalation of this mixture provides excellent pain relief without producing unconsciousness.

Difficult problems may arise in relation to moving the patient. Movement increases shock, hence the well worn phrase 'Splint them where they lie'. Yet there may be reasons demanding that the patient should be moved, either to remove him from a source of danger or to enable a more complete diagnosis or treatment of other injuries to be achieved. The question of transport is particularly important if there is a possibility of injury to the back. A patient lifted inexpertly by shoulders and heels has his spine forced into flexion, and an unstable fracture-dislocation of the cervicothoracic spine may then crush the cord, producing paraplegia, quadraplegia or even death, depending on the level of the injury. A well trained ambulance team, or a stretcher-bearer party of the armed services, are extremely adept at coping with such problems in the field. If such experienced aid is available, the doctor without particular expertise may be well advised to leave the decisions to them.

There is no doubt that the period in the field, at the site of the accident or injury, is the most dangerous for any severely injured patient. The proportion of deaths occurring in this period is very high, and it is at least arguable that many of these might be prevented if expert medical help and equipment could be made available on the spot. The diagnosis and management of such injuries as tension pneumothorax and cardiac tamponade, which are usually left until the patient arrives in the casualty department after the added trauma of the journey, could in theory be better treated on the spot by bringing the emergency surgical team to the patient. Such a philosophy is difficult to implement because of logistics and technical problems of the mobility of the surgical team. Nevertheless, a start has been made in this direction in several places, notably Japan, West Germany and in two localities in the UK, while paramedical personnel are now frequently being trained to carry out such procedures as putting up intravenous infusions.

Hospital: emergency

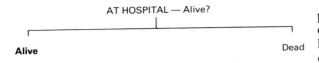

AT HOSPITAL — Alive?

Alive   Dead

Saving life

The accent remains on this principle when the

patient arrives in the casualty department. In essence, the procedure to assess the threats to life and deal with them is the same that has been described for the situation in the field. The difference now is that plenty of hands are available together with sophisticated apparatus and techniques of measurement.

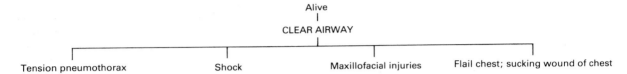

Alive

CLEAR AIRWAY

Tension pneumothorax   Shock   Maxillofacial injuries   Flail chest; sucking wound of chest

As always, *maintenance of the airway* is the first consideration, and if after the removal of obstructions in the mouth and pharynx any doubt remains, the anaesthetist present usually elects to use endotracheal intubation to ensure a patent airway. As the guardian of the airway, the senior anaesthetist present is normally in overall charge at this stage. This step is also important in the management of *cardiac arrest*, but that subject is considered in Chapter 21. *Pneumothorax* is diagnosed by auscultation and a portable chest x-ray, the latter being a mandatory investigation in all severely injured patients. It is treated by aspirating the pleural cavity through an intercostal needle or a small intercostal tube inserted in the eighth intercostal space in the mid-axillary line, and connected to an underwater seal and suction drainage (Chapter 19). *Haemopneumo-*

thorax is diagnosed by the x-ray appearances and treated similarly. The disturbances of ventilation/perfusion ratios produced by a *sucking wound of the chest wall*, and by a *flail chest*, are rapidly brought under control by endotracheal intubation and intermittent positive pressure ventilation. The flail chest may need no other treatment than the continuance of artificial ventilation until sufficient healing occurs so that the chest wall moves in one piece again. The sucking wound can also be controlled by intermittent positive pressure ventilation for an hour or so, but requires definitive surgery to restore the integrity of the pleural cavity by closing the wound. *Maxillofacial injuries* may also threaten the airway by haemorrhage or excessive mobility of the tongue, and endotracheal intubation or tracheostomy may be required.

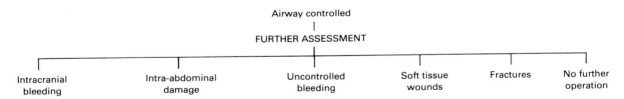

Airway controlled

FURTHER ASSESSMENT

Intracranial   Intra-abdominal   Uncontrolled   Soft tissue   Fractures   No further
bleeding   damage   bleeding   wounds   operation

Haemorrhage is the next consideration, but the management of blood loss is described in Chapter 23. A good intravenous infusion line is set up at one or, preferably, at two sites as soon as possible. *Head injury*, and the possibility of *intracranial haemorrhage* are discussed in Chapter 24.

The final threat to life comes from *intraperitoneal injury*, and this aspect is dealt with in Chapters 25 and 28. The treatment of this by

laparotomy may well merit the highest surgical priority after the airway and relief of tension pneumothorax.

The management of these threats to life may have been all done in the casualty department, or may have necessitated transfer to the operating theatre for an emergency operation. During such an operation, the opportunity will probably be taken (unless the general condition of the patient precludes this) to carry out any operative treatment under the general heading of limiting and repairing damage. In either case, once the threats to life have been controlled the patient is sent to the recovery room or surgical ward and the emphasis switches to definitive treatment. Nevertheless, in the casualty department certain measures to limit and repair damage, and to treat the patient's symptoms, may be undertaken.

Limit and repair damage

When some progress has been made towards resuscitating the patient, consideration can be given to this, the second main principle of treatment. The prophylaxis of infection is the dominant factor. Obvious dirt or other foreign material should be picked out of wounds, and the original dressings, which were the cleanest available at the site but probably not sterile, changed for proper sterilized dressings. Once the life-threatening haemorrhage from a wound has been stopped, a more careful diagnosis of the structures injured can be undertaken, both clinically and by special investigations. In clinical terms, the casualty surgical officer asks himself which bones, arteries, tendons and nerves may have been damaged, and looks for appropriate signs of interruption or partial damage of these structures. Occasionally, damage to a vein such as the inferior vena cava may require consideration. Fractures may be obvious, especially if compound, or if displacement, angulation or shortening have occurred; or they may be suspected on the grounds of localized bone tenderness or of bone pain on attempted use. Signs of ischaemia — reduced or absent peripheral pulses, and pallor and objective coldness of the tissues — are sought distal to the wound, while cutaneous sensation and the movements of muscles are also tested. The degree of contamination of the wound is assessed, and any loss of skin noted. At this stage, radiology can assist in the diagnosis of fractures and of foreign bodies in wounds.

In the light of all this evidence about the wound, how it was caused, how much destruction of tissue has resulted, how much contamination with dead or foreign material has occurred, how much time has passed since the injury, and what structures have been damaged, a decision is made whether the wound can safely be repaired immediately — probably under local anaesthesia

— or whether a formal operation will be required with full anaesthesia when the patient's general condition allows. Also at this stage, a decision should be made as to whether antibiotics should be used prophylactically, and whether any immunological protection should be invoked against specific diseases.

The use of antibiotics in the prophylaxis of wound infections is a vexed question, and there is a wide range of surgical opinion between the extreme views of always using antibiotics and of never using them in these circumstances. No evidence has ever been produced that prophylactic antibiotics can influence the rate of wound infection in really clean incised wounds, such as those made by a scalpel during a surgical operation, in which tissue destruction is minimal and no infected tissue planes have been opened. On the other hand, the factors of heavy soiling, widespread tissue destruction, and a long incubation period since the injury occurred might influence the surgeon to try prophylaxis.

It is particularly important that penicillin should be given (to patients without a history of penicillin sensitivity) if the local factors in the wound suggest anaerobic conditions that might favour the growth of *Clostridium tetani*. A deep punctured wound is a case in point. Such patients should be started on a course of active immunization with tetanus toxoid immediately, or if already immunized they should be given a booster dose of toxoid. Routine anti-tetanus serum (ATS) injections are dangerous because they are raised in the horse and a potent source of anaphylactic reactions, and are probably no more effective than antibiotics administered immediately. For similar reasons, penicillin or ampicillin have also replaced the appropriate antiserum as prophylaxis for gas gangrene.

Treating symptoms

In the hectic period spent resuscitating a patient in the casualty department there is little time for symptomatic treatment. Nevertheless, all handling of injured parts should be as gentle as possible, and this applies just as strongly if the patient is unconscious as it does if he is conscious and able to complain of pain; rough handling undoubtedly increases traumatic shock. In cases when the patient is conscious, it is particularly important to make as full an explanation to him at all stages of what is happening — as full, that is, as is consistent with reassurance in what is perhaps a critical situation. The use of opiates can be considered on a more logical basis at this stage than in the field, since the amount of information about the nature and extent of the patient's injuries is now much greater. The comfort of a hot or cold drink must still of course be withheld if there is any likelihood of surgery being necessary within the next few hours, or there is any possibility of intra-abdominal injury.

Recapitulation

1. Life-threatening conditions are diagnosed and treated as rapidly as possible, the aim being to produce a stable circulation and respiratory gas exchange.

2. If an emergency operation is needed to correct life-threatening conditions, operative procedures of lesser urgency can be fitted in at the same time, when the patient's condition permits.

3. If an emergency operation is not needed, the patient's wounds are assessed completely and a decision made whether they can be simply treated immediately or whether definitive surgical operation is necessary.

4. After resuscitation, followed either by an emergency operation or by simple measures to promote healing, the patient is transferred to an intensive care area or to a surgical ward for further observation and the planning of definitive treatment.

Hospital: definitive

Saving life

By this stage the threat to life has receded. It is still possible for a relapse to occur, due to incomplete correction of a fault at an earlier stage, or for an entirely new life-threatening condition to occur as a complication that might follow any trauma including a surgical operation (see Chapter 19). Nevertheless, the accent is now upon the second principal aim.

Limiting and repairing damage (see flow-chart, p. 252)

There are many principles which must be borne in mind if the patient is to get the best chance of complete restoration of structure and function. Apart from their number, there is no difficulty in stating or understanding these principles, and they are described shortly. (They may, of course, be much more difficult to carry out in practice than to state in theory.)

The real difficulty arises in cases of multiple trauma and consists of the assessment of priorities: which injuries must be dealt with early, which can be left till later, and, most important of all, if one injury contraindicates surgery and another demands it, which must take precedence? It is in this situation that the importance of a team leader to weigh decisions becomes manifest. The writer believes that it is unusual for one person to be the correct choice as team leader in both the casualty and the definitive surgical situations. In the casualty department the

leader should be particularly well versed in the management of the life-threatening conditions. In the definitive stage, the decisions being taken have not the urgency of those in casualty, but nevertheless they might greatly influence the quality of life of the patient when recovery is as complete as can be achieved — several months hence. In the nature of things, it is unlikely that the expert in resuscitation can also follow up his patient in routine out-patient clinics for months on end: his place is with the next seriously ill patient needing immediate resuscitation. At the definitive stage, therefore, the leader of the team should be a general surgeon as a rule, though in particular cases where the injuries are concentrated in the chest, or in the skeletal apparatus, or in the urinary system, he might be a thoracic or orthopaedic or urological surgeon.

Examples of situations in which the assessment of priorities is difficult are given later. The principles of repairing damage are stated below.

1 Prevent infection

All foreign material and dead tissue must be removed, and jagged, devitalized edges of the wound excised. After any reparative procedures have been undertaken (see principle 3, below) the wound must be closed with skin coverage. Dead space must be obliterated by suitably placed sutures that bind the deeper layer to the next superficial, or by suction drainage.

However, if it is anticipated that there will be a considerable serous or bloody accumulation in a wound, and it is feared that drainage tubing may readily block, free drainage by guttered material acting by capillarity may be preferable. In either case, the drainage system should be enclosed in some way at the exterior to prevent ascending infection. Care should be taken to ensure that the arterial blood supply to the wound is as free as possible. Constricting bandages must be avoided at all costs. In particular, the possibility of damage to a neighbouring major artery demands full exploration: never accept a diagnosis of 'arterial spasm' following trauma in explanation of any evidence of ischaemia. Venous drainage must also be facilitated, since an impaired venous ' outflow results in an unnecessary exaggeration of the inevitable post-traumatic oedema; the resultant stagnant condition of the circulation and waterlogging of the tissues facilitate the growth of any micro-organisms that may have escaped the toilet of the wound. Increased tissue oedema also has a deleterious effect on the local arterial blood supply at arteriolocapillary level. For all these reasons, unrestricted venous drainage must be encouraged and this is another reason why tight bandages should be avoided at this stage, desirable though they might have been as a first-aid measure. The other important measure, where practicable, is elevation of the part so that gravity can assist. Within the wound the sutures used to coapt cut edges of deeper layers should be inserted and withdrawn in large bites, well away from the free edges, and tied without undue tension; the same considerations apply to the skin wound. Buried suture materials should be either fine absorbable material (chromic catgut causes less tissue reaction than plain catgut and so chromic is preferable, but a synthetic absorbable material may be considered) or, if greater strength is needed, an inert non-absorbable material like monofilamentous nylon.

Sometimes the likelihood of infection is so great, either because the contamination is so heavy or because it occurred longer than 6 hours previously, that the above policy is modified. The figure of 6 hours has been derived from the clinical observations of surgeons in the armed forces in both the First and Second World Wars: the incidence of infection in wounds treated as above by *direct primary suture* rises steeply if the operation takes place longer than 6 hours after the injury. Gross contamination may be inferred from the direct evidence of heavy soiling and considerable tissue destruction; it should also be assumed to have occurred if a body cavity with a heavy population of pathogenic bacteria, such as the colon, has been breached.

The policy in such cases is known as *delayed primary suture*. A minimum of buried sutures is used to repair deeper layers, and the skin and subcutaneous fat are left entirely open. Fat is a rather poorly vascularized tissue and, therefore, especially prone to infection. The theory underlying this technique is that with the superficial tissues open there is no chance of post-traumatic oedema raising tension in the subcutaneous layer and thereby encouraging infection. The risk of further infection entering from without is appreciable, but less than the known risk from the heavily contaminated wound; one attempts to minimize this risk of entry of infection by suitable occlusive dressings. In practice this policy works well in such cases: any infection that occurs is mild and superficial, but often the wound remains clean. The delayed primary suture may then be performed on the third to fifth day, or if a mild infection ensues it is allowed to settle and a *secondary suture* performed about the tenth day.

2 Promote healing

All the measures described under principle 1, above, may be said to promote healing. The other important considerations are rest, both local (i.e. of the injured part) and general (i.e. of the patient as a whole), and *nutrition*. The factor of nutrition includes not only the general nutritional status in terms of calories and proteins, but also the more specific healing properties associated with adequate oxygenation of blood containing a normal concentration of haemoglobin, and a normal supply of vitamin C and other growth factors. The rapid correction of anaemia plus a generous balanced normal diet is the best and usual way to achieve these conditions, but there may be problems with the diet after severe trauma. They are no different from the nutritional problems which may arise after elective major surgical procedures, and are considered in Chapter 19.

3 Restoration of structure and function

The restoration of structure does not necessarily restore function, but at least it is a good start.

The most satisfactory restoration of structure is achieved by *direct apposition* of the cut edges of the injured structure after the devitalized margins have been suitably trimmed. If that is not possible, either because the gap is too great or because the structure has been so disorganized and devitalized by the trauma that it must be removed, consideration is given to whether it can be removed without jeopardy to the patient or whether it needs replacement. In making this decision, more weight should be given to the functional rather than to the anatomical aspect, though cosmetic considerations naturally arise. If it is decided that the patient can do without the structure, e.g. a ruptured spleen, it is removed and the wound closed. However, if it is decided that the structure must be replaced, then the possibilities are that it should be replaced by a *rearrangement* of the patient's own tissues (e.g. nerve- and tendon-transplantation, or an autogenous skin graft to achieve skin cover), by a *homologous graft* from another human donor, by a *xenograft* from another species (e.g. an animal bone graft), or by a *prosthesis*. Which procedure is used, and whether it is done at the time of the original operation or deferred till a later date, are questions requiring great expertise and judgement.

Treating symptoms

Little need be said about symptomatic measures. Each patient and each symptom must be treated as an individual problem, and the demands of the more important life-saving and healing principles conflict less often with symptomatic treatment than was the case at earlier stages.

Priorities

The possibility of a conflict of priorities can be illustrated by some examples.

If a patient has suffered a head injury, it is important that he should not be given a general anaesthetic because anaesthesia may increase brain damage and may mask the development of life-threatening intracranial complications (however, anaesthesia may be needed to control fits; see Chapter 24 for the use of hyperventilation to reduce cerebral oedema, and for the indications for making burr holes). On the other hand, if he also has open injuries elsewhere that are not amenable to operation under local anaesthesia, the surgeon would like to operate within six hours of the infliction of the wound. This conflict is easy to resolve: the question of the wound is related to the repair of damage, the question of the head injury to the preservation of life, and the latter takes precedence. The next two problems are more difficult as the alternatives in each case are of the same general level of priority.

The best results with suturing a cut motor nerve are obtained when the repair is performed immediately. On the other hand, should the wound be heavily contaminated, it may be feared that infection will occur and jeopardize the integrity of the suture line in the nerve. It can be a fine decision, but in cases of doubt the surgeon will probably deal with the rest of the wound on its merits, mark the ends of the nerves by stitches, and prepare to explore the wound again when all infection has subsided a few weeks later.

A compound fracture of the tibia and fibula may be extremely unstable, so that reasonable alignment and coaptation of the bone ends, necessary to promote healing and prevent angulation and shortening, may best be achieved by a metal plate screwed to the bone segments. On the other hand, the open wound may be heavily contaminated, and the last thing the surgeon wants to do is leave a large foreign body in the wound to promote infection with its risk of the serious complication of osteomyelitis. There is no right answer to this question; what is actually done will depend on the experience and judgement of the surgeon and the exact circumstances of the case.

Rehabilitation

The principles of rehabilitating the convalescent patient, no matter whether the illness from which he suffered was traumatic or of some other variety, are simple to state but much more difficult to execute.

First, the patient is taught to make the best functional use of whatever structures are left to him. Secondly, he is given apparatus to extend or magnify his residual capacity. Thirdly, he is shown how to reorder his life, both his work and

Flow-chart 20.1

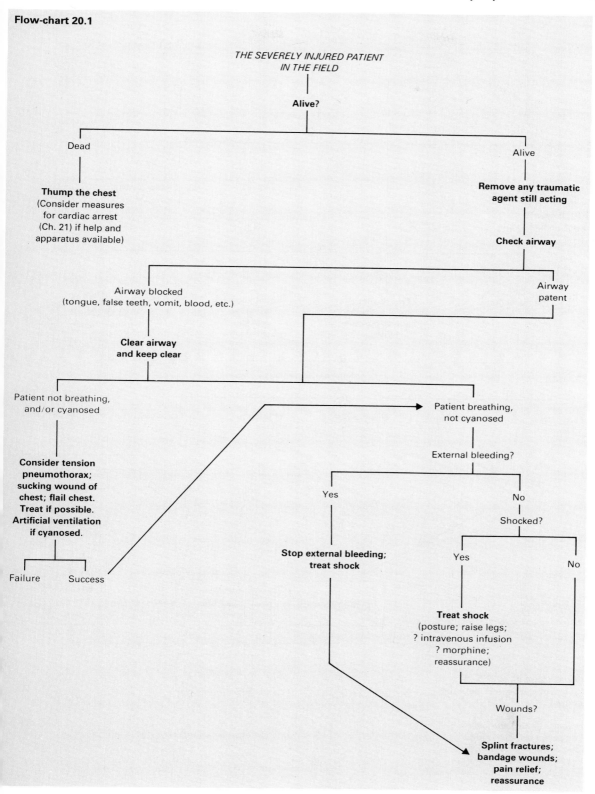

THE SEVERELY INJURED PATIENT
IN THE FIELD

Alive?

Dead

Alive

Thump the chest
(Consider measures
for cardiac arrest
(Ch. 21) if help and
apparatus available)

**Remove any traumatic
agent still acting**

Check airway

Airway blocked
(tongue, false teeth, vomit, blood, etc.)

Airway
patent

**Clear airway
and keep clear**

Patient not breathing,
and/or cyanosed

Patient breathing,
not cyanosed

External bleeding?

**Consider tension
pneumothorax;
sucking wound of
chest; flail chest.
Treat if possible.
Artificial ventilation
if cyanosed.**

Yes

No

Shocked?

Failure

Success

**Stop external bleeding;
treat shock**

Yes

No

Treat shock
(posture; raise legs;
? intravenous infusion
? morphine;
reassurance)

Wounds?

**Splint fractures;
bandage wounds;
pain relief;
reassurance**

Flow-chart 20.2

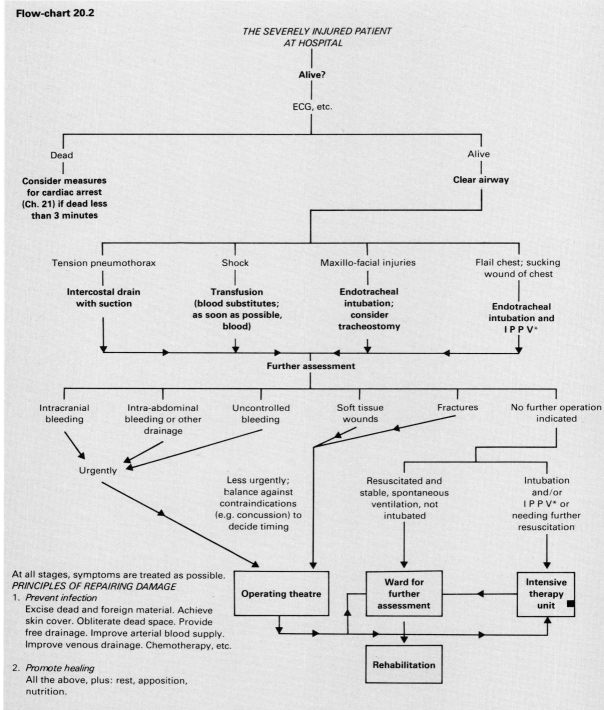

*THE SEVERELY INJURED PATIENT
AT HOSPITAL*

Alive?

ECG, etc.

Dead

**Consider measures
for cardiac arrest
(Ch. 21) if dead less
than 3 minutes**

Alive

Clear airway

Tension pneumothorax

**Intercostal drain
with suction**

Shock

**Transfusion
(blood substitutes;
as soon as possible,
blood)**

Maxillo-facial injuries

**Endotracheal
intubation;
consider
tracheostomy**

Flail chest; sucking
wound of chest

**Endotracheal
intubation and
I P P V***

Further assessment

Intracranial
bleeding

Intra-abdominal
bleeding or other
drainage

Uncontrolled
bleeding

Soft tissue
wounds

Fractures

No further operation
indicated

Urgently

Less urgently;
balance against
contraindications
(e.g. concussion) to
decide timing

Resuscitated and
stable, spontaneous
ventilation, not
intubated

Intubation
and/or
I P P V* or
needing further
resuscitation

At all stages, symptoms are treated as possible.
PRINCIPLES OF REPAIRING DAMAGE
1. *Prevent infection*
   Excise dead and foreign material. Achieve
   skin cover. Obliterate dead space. Provide
   free drainage. Improve arterial blood supply.
   Improve venous drainage. Chemotherapy, etc.

2. *Promote healing*
   All the above, plus: rest, apposition,
   nutrition.

3. *Restoration of structure and function*
   By direct apposition if possible.
   If impossible, and the structure is
   necessary, replace it by rearrangement
   of the patient's tissues, by donor graft,
   or by prosthesis.

Operating theatre

**Ward for
further
assessment**

**Intensive
therapy
unit**

Rehabilitation

* I P P V = intermittent positive pressure ventilation

his hobbies, so as to modify them to his limited capacities. Finally, he is encouraged to make the best of his abilities, whether natural or artificially aided, and to adjust to his new life.

The details of the first principle lie in the domain of the physiotherapist and the occupational therapist; the second in that of the rheumatologist or expert in physical medicine who is also concerned in all the other principles; the third depends on a variety of people, laymen such as, in the United Kingdom, the disablement resettlement officers of the Department of Health and Social Security, medical auxiliaries such as health visitors, doctors at rehabilitation centres, and employers willing to retrain the victim of major trauma. The important point to remember is that the fourth principle, while owing much to all the other individuals concerned and to the patient's family and friends, is peculiarly the province of the surgeon who looked after the patient in hospital and the general practitioner. The first because of the special relationship that inevitably develops between an ill patient and his medical attendant, and the second because he is the doctor who usually knows the patient best; both have much to offer the patient in the field of encouragement and exhortation to yet greater efforts.

Further reading

Calne, R. Y. (Ed.) (1983). *Liver Transplantation.* London and New York. Grune and Stratton.

Dudley, H. A. F. (1976). The principles underlying the management of the seriously injured patient. In: *Current Surgical Practice*, Vol. 1, pp. 15-21. Ed. by G. J. Hadfield and M. Hobsley. London, Edward Arnold.

Gray, R. C. and Coppel, D. L. (1975). Intensive care of patients with bomb blast and gunshot injuries. *British Medical Journal* i, 502–4.

Hughes, S. (1983). *The Basis and Practice of Traumatology.* London, William Heinemann Medical Books Ltd.

Kyle, J. (Ed.). (1984). *Pye's Surgical Handicraft*, 21st edn. Bristol, Wright, P. S. G.

Morris, P. J. and Tilney, N. L. (Ed.) (1984). *Progress in Transplantation* Vol. I. Edinburgh, Churchill Livingstone.

Sevitt, S. (1974). *Reactions to Injury and Burns.* London, Heinemann Medical.

Snook, R. (1974). *Medical Aid at Accidents.* London, Update.

Templeton, J. and Wilson, R. I. (1983). *Lecture Notes on Trauma.* Oxford, Blackwell Scientific Publications.

Chapter 21

Cardiorespiratory Arrest

Cardiorespiratory arrest is the cessation of respiration and circulation; as a result of the lack of circulation to the brain the respiratory centre is damaged and within 1 minute ventilation ceases.

The maximum length of time for which the brain can survive at normal temperature without a supply of oxygenated blood is between 3 and 4 minutes; after this interval, the cerebral changes are irreversible and the patient is dead. This fact emphasizes the extreme importance of the condition, and the necessity for very rapid and effective management. It is interesting that the acceptance of this situation as an extreme emergency has led to descriptions of its management that follow the pattern of dealing with the presentation, just as advocated for every situation in this book. Because such descriptions are readily available, only a concise account is given in this chapter.

Cardiorespiratory arrest is recognized by cessation of the heart beat and unconsciousness. Suspicion is usually first aroused by the inability to feel peripheral pulses such as the radial; this suspicion should be checked with the carotid or femoral artery. Ventilatory movements need not be completely absent: there may be ineffectual gasping movements, but the patient usually becomes cyanosed. After 1 minute the pupils dilate and later they become unresponsive to light: if this stage persists for more than 1–2 minutes, the patient is unlikely to recover as a sentient being, so every effort must be made to get the heart going before this happens.

The efficiency of management of such an urgent condition necessarily depends upon the facilities available to the attendant physician. The management under ideal circumstances is described first, and notes are then added about how this management can be adapted to less than ideal circumstances.

Management in ideal circumstances

The ideal place to deal with a patient whose heart has stopped is the operating theatre. Not only is it likely that all the apparatus required will be readily available, but there will also probably be several trained people present to perform the multiplicity of tasks entailed.

Usually the senior anaesthetist present takes command and undertakes artificial ventilation while the surgeon institutes cardiac massage, starting with a blow to the precordium which sometimes suffices to get the heart going again. Theoretically, a third person is deputed to note the passage of time. Others are requested to get any apparatus, drugs, etc., required by the anaesthetist in his attempts to get the heart going again. An intravenous infusion line is needed as soon as possible, if one is not running already, and the patient's legs are elevated to increase venous return.

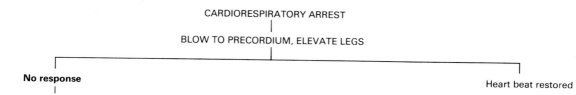

CARDIORESPIRATORY ARREST

BLOW TO PRECORDIUM, ELEVATE LEGS

No response

EXTERNAL CARDIAC MASSAGE

Heart beat restored

Cardiac massage

The essence of cardiac massage is that the heart is squeezed rhythmically and firmly, with a brief period of rest between each squeezing action. Blood is forced out of the heart by the squeezing action, into the aorta since that is the only direction permitted by the heart valves. Reliance is placed on the elastic recoil of the walls of the heart chambers to induce refilling from the great veins during the brief pause before the next squeeze.

The exact technique used depends on the circumstances. If the chest is already open, the surgeon compresses the heart between the palms of both his hands. If the abdomen is open, effective compression may be obtained between one hand pressing on the heart through the diaphragm, and the other depressing the anterior chest wall as described in the next paragraph.

If neither the chest nor the abdomen is open, *external* cardiac massage is performed. The surgeon lays his dominant hand flat on the patient's sternum and the chest wall immediately to the left of the sternum, and backs it up with his other hand. He exerts pressure on the region, particularly with his thenar and hypothenar eminences, producing a depression of the anterior chest wall through a range of 3–5 cm. The counter-pressure to this manoeuvre is provided by the rigid resistance of the operating table below the patient's back. The cycle of pressure/relaxation is repeated about 60 times per minute. For children, fingers only are used.

Cardiac massage is useless unless it is effective in maintaining a circulation, at least to the brain. The anaesthetist checks the efficacy of the massage by feeling for pulsation in the carotid or femoral arteries, and by observing the pupils: the latter should remain reasonably contracted, or if they had been dilated they must be seen to become smaller. If these criteria cannot be satisfied with external cardiac massage being undertaken, the internal form must be instituted or the patient will die.

The pressure exerted on the chest wall in external cardiac massage must be effective but not excessive: fractured ribs or sternum, with resultant damage to the underlying lungs or pericardium, is not an uncommon complication.

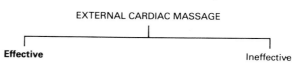

EXTERNAL CARDIAC MASSAGE

Effective

Ineffective

Artificial ventilation

If the patient has not already undergone endotracheal intubation, the anaesthetist clears the airway, inserts a cuffed endotracheal tube and maintains mechanical ventilatory movements by intermittent positive pressure, applied through his anaesthetic apparatus. Evidence of the adequacy of this ventilation is provided by the disappearance of *central cyanosis* — i.e. cyanosis of the mucous membranes, lips, tongue, etc., that does not disappear with the application of local friction. If the ventilation is inadequate, there must be an obstruction to the airway, an impediment to expansion of the chest wall, some factor producing collapse of one of both lungs, or pulmonary embolism or other serious disease of the lungs.

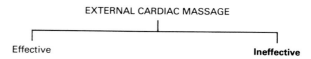

EXTERNAL CARDIAC MASSAGE

Effective

Ineffective

Passage of time

The surgeon and anaesthetist must judge whether an adequate cerebral circulation has been achieved within the required period of 4 minutes, or whether there has been necessarily a longer delay so that there is no point in pursuing the resuscitatory efforts.

The decision to stop resuscitation is so important — literally a matter of life and death — that there is a considerable natural reluctance to accept the inevitability of the situation, and efforts are often prolonged considerably beyond the critical time interval. The experience of the clinician in charge is usually a decisive factor in this situation. Twenty minutes can be considered a maximum unless hypothermia is present.

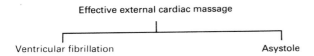

Diagnosis of the type of arrest

The heart may fail to produce a cardiac output of blood either because it is truly arrested — *asystole* — or because its action is grossly irregular and uncoordinated — *ventricular fibrillation*. The anaesthetist asks for electrocardiographic leads to be attached to the patient, and an electrocardiograph distinguishes between these two possibilities. Naturally, if the chest is open the difference between asystole and ventricular fibrillation can be seen with the naked eye, but it is still important to start ECG monitoring as the period shortly after an episode of cardiac arrest may be associated with various arrhythmias that may require exact diagnosis and specific management.

Measures to restart the heart

A single blow to the precordium, at the beginning of cardiac massage, may be sufficient to restart the heart when the period of arrest has been very short. Usually, it will be necessary to use other aids. It is important not to lose sight of the principle that the cause which gave rise to the arrest in the first instance must be corrected, but even after such correction has been achieved other measures may be necessary, and the choice of these measures depends largely on the type of arrest.

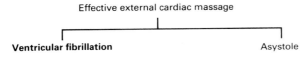

Ventricular fibrillation

The procedure required in these circumstances is electrical defibrillation. The defibrillating electrical shock is applied to the ventricles by large flat plates, attached to a source of electrical current that can be activated to produce a shock of short duration. One or a few shocks with direct current at 50–100 J is usually sufficient to stop the heart completely. In refractory cases one can gradually raise the current to 400 J or try alternating current. Recovery from the asystole may be spontaneous, or may require aids as discussed below for the management of primary asystole. A potent cause of failure of the electrical defibrillator is low temperature: when the cardiac temperature falls below 26°C the likelihood of developing ventricular fibrillation progressively increases, so that the possibility of stopping fibrillation at a low cardiac temperature becomes remote. Warming any blood or other fluid being transfused, and also the inspired air, is the quickest way of correcting this fault. Once normal rhythm has been restored, prophylactic lignocaine 100 mg intravenously and later mexiletine orally may successfully suppress any tendency to recurrence.

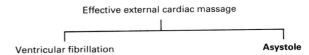

Cardiac asystole

Many agents have been known to set the heart beating again. Personal preferences vary with regard to the order in which these agents should be used, but the list contain atropine (2 mg), adrenaline (10 ml, 1 in 10 000 solution), and calcium (as 10 ml of 10 per cent calcium chloride solution).

Other measures

Maintenance of the circulation through cardiac massage is facilitated by having the circulation full, and rapid intravenous infusion of blood (if available and already cross-matched) or other liquids designed to expand the circulation is an important measure. The infusate should, if possible, be warmed to 37°C, for reasons mentioned in the section on ventricular defibrillation.

Potent causes of depression of cardiac muscle include (Table 21.1) disturbances in blood gas tensions (hypoxia, hypercarbia), metabolic acidosis and a lowered extracellular concentration of potassium or calcium. Adequate artificial ventilation should correct the first error, and appropriate injections of alkali, potassium or calcium may be tried if there is reason to suspect the

Table 21.1 Cardiorespiratory arrest

Aetiology predominantly cardiac	Aetiology predominantly peripheral	Aetiology predominantly respiratory
Coronary ischaemic disease	Exsanguination	Anoxia:
Cardiac tamponade	Plasma or saline lack	Upper airway obstruction
Air embolism	Widespread vasodilatation:	Insufficient oxygen in inspired
Potassium excess or deficiency	Deep general anaesthesia	gas
Electrocution, cold immersion,	High spinal block	Inhalation of vomit
'vagal inhibition'	High epidural block	Untreated respiratory failure:
Excess catecholamines:	Drug overdose	Drug overdose
Fright	Profound hypothermia	Deep anaesthesia
Iatrogenic	Anaphylaxis	Failure to remove carbon dioxide
Profound hypothermia	Septicaemia	from anaesthetic closed circuit
Drug overdose		Drowning
Septicaemia		Severe pulmonary disease
		Pulmonary embolism
		Fat embolism
		Phosgene inhalation

Note that many factors (e.g. drug overdosage) overlap the boundaries of the main aetiological classification.

other factors. Sodium bicarbonate is often given in concentrated solution (1 mmol/ml: 84 g/litre) 50–100 mmol intravenously as a standard measure, on the grounds that no matter how short the period of arrest has been, some metabolic acidosis must have developed as a result of inadequate tissue perfusion.

The measure is often dramatically successful, but it probably acts by expanding the circulation through its osmotic effect dragging fluid from the interstitial space into the vascular compartment as well as by its alkalinizing effect; sodium bicarbonate does not penetrate rapidly into cells, and it is the acidosis within the cardiac cells that is the cause of the arrest. Overloading the circulation by its osmotic activity is a real danger, and the absolute maximum dose of sodium bicarbonate in an adult is 200 mmol. Care must be taken with the injection because this concentrated alkaline solution is intensely irritant if it extravasates. The extracellular concentration of calcium may be low due to excessive parathyroid hormone secretion or to rapid transfusion of citrated blood because citrate chelates calcium ions. So-called 'citrate intoxication' is particularly a problem if hypothermia prevails, because citrate is normally metabolized in the liver by reactions that are particularly sensitive to temperature.

Ventricular fibrillation is an extreme degree of hyperexcitability of cardiac muscle, and predisposing factors (Table 21.1) tend to be the opposite of those producing asystole: in other words, they consist of hypercarbia, metabolic alkalosis, potassium excess and calcium excess. Hypercarbia may result from under-ventilation of an anaesthetized patient, and potassium excess from rapid transfusion of old bank blood; the other factors are less commonly encountered.

More heroic measures may be contemplated, depending on the circumstances of the case and, in particular, upon the prospect of ultimate recovery afforded by the combination of a young patient, a hitherto healthy myocardium, and a potentially temporary or reversible cardiotoxic factor. The circulatory functions of the heart and the gaseous exchange mechanism of the lungs can be taken over by an extracorporeal artificial circulation incorporating a pump-oxygenator if the appropriate facilities are available. Meanwhile, the heart is allowed to rest in the hope that, after a variable period, it will recover its contractile function. Occasionally, the ventricles recover co-ordinated contractile function but the left ventricle in particular remains too damaged to maintain an adequate cardiac output and systemic arterial pressure. In these circumstances, left ventricular function can be aided by various temporary mechanical devices such as a balloon passed into the aorta via an arteriotomy and expanded rhythmically and synchronously with diastole by an electrical triggering mechanism actuated by the R-wave of the electrocardiogram. Thus coronary flow is aided by raising the diastolic pressure and then lowering the resistance in systole.

Flow-chart 21.1

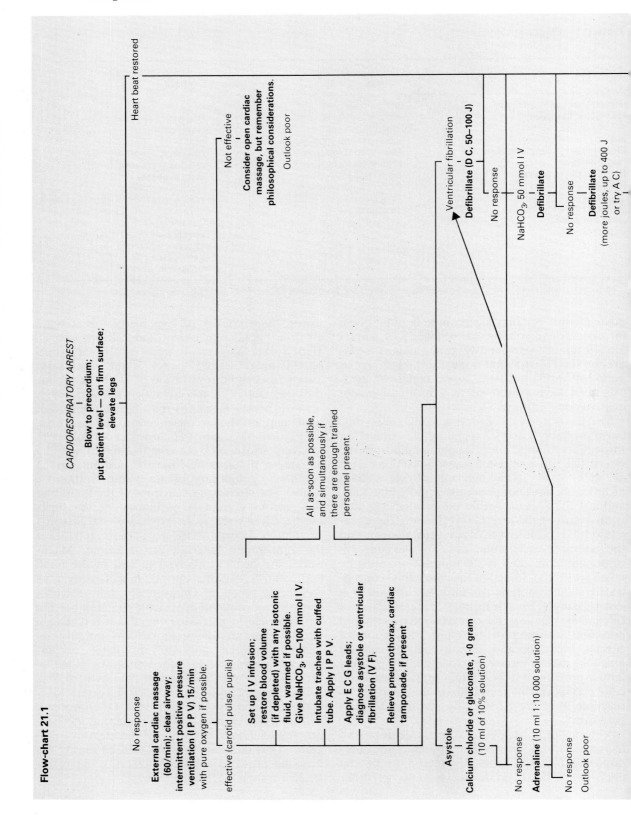

CARDIORESPIRATORY ARREST
Blow to precordium;
put patient level — on firm surface;
elevate legs

Heart beat restored

No response

External cardiac massage (60/min); clear airway; intermittent positive pressure ventilation (I P P V) 15/min with pure oxygen if possible.

effective (carotid pulse, pupils)

Not effective

Consider open cardiac massage, but remember philosophical considerations.

Outlook poor

All as soon as possible, and simultaneously if there are enough trained personnel present.

Set up I V infusion; restore blood volume (if depleted) with any isotonic fluid, warmed if possible. Give NaHCO₃, 50–100 mmol I V.

$$\text{Give NaHCO}_3, 50\text{–}100 \text{ mmol I V.}$$

Intubate trachea with cuffed tube. Apply I P P V.

Apply E C G leads; diagnose asystole or ventricular fibrillation (V F).

Relieve pneumothorax, cardiac tamponade, if present

Ventricular fibrillation

Defibrillate (D C, 50–100 J)

No response

NaHCO₃ 50 mmol I V

Defibrillate

No response

Defibrillate (more joules, up to 400 J or try A C)

Asystole

Calcium chloride or gluconate, 1·0 gram
(10 ml of 10% solution)

No response

Adrenaline (10 ml 1:10 000 solution)

No response

Outlook poor

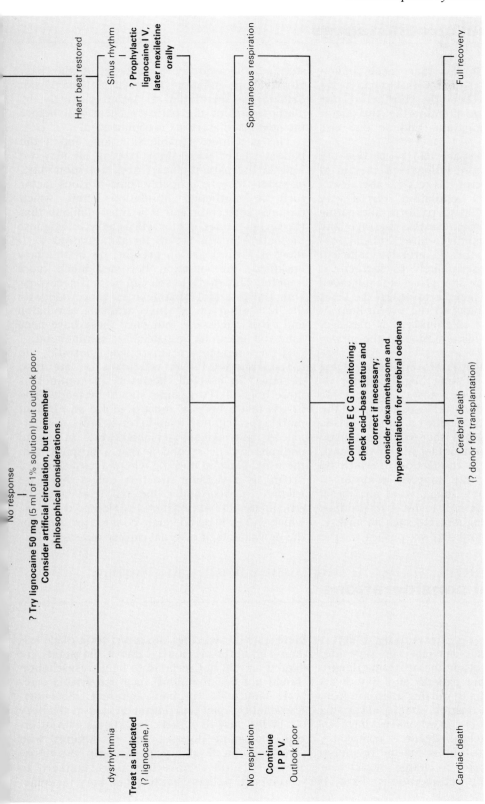

Less than ideal circumstances

What can be done in less than ideal circumstances to manage a patient with cardiac arrest can best be approached by considering the problem in the extreme situation that the doctor has no specialized apparatus and no one else there to help him.

External cardiac massage can be carried out for some minutes before fatigue sets in, but at the same time the doctor has to clear the airway and institute artificial ventilation. For a very short time it is feasible to perform alternating brief periods of external cardiac massage and mouth-to-mouth or mouth-to-nose artificial ventilation, but clearly this is grossly inefficient resuscitation and most unlikely to succeed. It follows, therefore, that the best a single-handed doctor can hope to achieve is to restart the heart *immediately*, with a blow to the precordium or with a few seconds of external cardiac massage, and then to transfer his attention to the airway and ventilation.

The situation is much improved if the doctor has available a self-inflating bag respirator or even an artificial (Brook) airway suitable for ventilatory resuscitation. The essence of the latter is, on the patient's side, a curved plastic mouthpiece which hooks the patient's tongue forwards and helps to maintain his airway, and, on the doctor's side, a connection to which he can attach a bag he can squeeze in order to insufflate the patient's lungs with air, or a mouthpiece into which he can blow to produce the same effect. Having inserted such an airway, the usual routine followed is six pushes on the sternum followed by a squeeze of the bag. However the inflation of the lungs is achieved, deflation is permitted to occur passively by elastic recoil of the patient's chest wall before the next insufflatory act is commenced.

This is a more tenable situation, and if the patient's heart soon starts beating all may we well. If the patient's heart does not soon start, however, there is probably some noxious factor such as ventricular fibrillation acting which requires correction and it is most unlikely that the single-handed doctor will be able to diagnose the nature of this factor, let alone correct it. If there is a third person present, no matter how unskilled, the situation becomes much more hopeful. This third person can help, if necessary, with the essential preliminaries concerned with the institution of effective artificial ventilation and cardiac massage, but once those have been achieved he can be despatched to summon aid.

If the emergency occurs outside hospital, the chances are that the aid will arrive too late to be effective. In hospital, however, the outlook is more hopeful. Two points should be made. The first is that a hospital must organize an efficient mobile resuscitation team in terms both of experienced and skilled personnel and of useful equipment. The second is that a hospital bed, the usual place in hospital where a cardiac arrest occurs, is a yielding structure unless there are fracture boards under the mattress, and the patient should be transferred rapidly to the floor, which will provide adequate counter-pressure for the movements of external cardiac massage.

Philosophical considerations

The instinct of a doctor is always to try to defeat death. External cardiac massage can save life, but used in hospital outside the operating theatre it is distressing to other patients and may divert much-needed medical and nursing attention from other patients. Resuscitation should always be attempted in any patient in whom no diagnosis has been made or whose death is completely unexpected. Before instituting the full regime in other patients the doctor in charge should bear in mind the following considerations. First, if there is doubt whether the arrest took place less than 4 minutes previously, and if the pupils are dilated and do not respond to light, resuscitation should not be attempted since irreversible cerebral damage is probably present. Secondly, resuscitation may be contraindicated in the very old or the very ill patient, in patients with incurable malignant disease, and in patients with severe chronic disability, particularly respiratory disease. Thirdly, resuscitation is unlikely to succeed in patients with pulmonary oedema, with severe chronic chest disease, and with chest deformities such as kyphoscoliosis. Notwithstanding the foregoing, one cannot make strict rules. Where doubt exists, the patient must be given the benefit of the doubt.

When resuscitation fails, death may be due to failure of the heart or to failure of the brain. In the latter circumstance, the possibility should be considered that the patient's kidneys, liver or heart might be suitable for transplantation.

Further reading

Briggs, B. D., Sheldon, D. B. and Beecher, H. K. (1956). Cardiac arrest: study of a thirty-year period of operating room deaths at Massachusetts General Hospital, 1925–1954. *Journal of the American Medical Association* **160**, 1439–44.

Calne, R. Y. and Williams, R. (1977). Orthotopic liver transplantation: the first 60 patients. *British Medical Journal* **1**, 471–6.

Harrison, M. J. G. (1976). The diagnosis of brain death. *British Journal of Hospital Medicine* **16**, 320–23.

Mattar, J. A., Weil, M. H., Shubin, H. and Stein, L. (1974). Cardiac arrest in the critically ill. II. Hyperosmolal states following cardiac arrest. *American Journal of Medicine* **56**, 162–8.

Rowlands, D. J. (1976). Cardiac arrest. *British Journal of Hospital Medicine* **16**, 310–19.

Worthley, L. I. G. (1976). Sodium bicarbonate in cardiac arrest (letter). *Lancet* **4**, 903–4.

Chapter 22

The Diagnosis of Shock

The concept of shock has grown gradually, and very haphazardly, out of observations on wounded soldiers in the First World War. Partly in consequence of this, there has been a tendency for the subject to be dominated by the impression that shock is something which follows external physical violence. Yet the clinical state produced by a variety of other disturbances may have important features in common with those occurring after trauma, so the concept of shock has been extended to cover these disturbances.

The result at the moment is that the term 'shock' is applied to such a wide variety of clinical states that some authorities question whether the word should ever be used by itself, or whether it can only have real meaning if used in conjunction with some adjective such as traumatic, hypovolaemic (*syn.* oligaemic), etc.

The importance of seeking whether any specific meaning, in clinical terms, can be given to the concept of shock is that it would act as a unifying basis for the protean manifestations encountered in patients shocked for various reasons. This unifying concept should be of great help in the recognition that a patient was suffering from shock, no matter what the cause. The point is that the shocked patient is dangerously ill: shock is a condition that threatens life. Early recognition and prompt treatment are mandatory, and it must be a great help to the clinician if, instead of trying to recognize one of almost a dozen different varieties of clinical syndromes based on shock, he can train himself to concentrate in the first instance on the crucial decision, is this patient shocked? If the answer to this question is 'Yes', the clinician knows he must proceed with speed to dissect out the essential aetiological factors from the large number of possibilities and try to put them right.

Recognition of shock

Haemorrhagic shock

It is reasonable to start our search by considering the type of shock which is best understood — that due to blood loss. Provided that the blood loss is not too great and that the period of exsanguination is not too long, the restoration of the blood volume by the transfusion of blood equal in volume to the loss dramatically restores the patient to health. Countless experimental studies in animals have supported and amplified the human studies.

The clinical condition in severe cases is unmistakable. The patient is agitated, withdrawn or even comatose. The skin is pale, cold and sweaty. The peripheral veins are empty. The pulse is rapid and shallow, and the systemic arterial blood pressure is low. Respirations are rapid and shallow (air-hunger). The capillary circulation is defective: the blanching of the nail-bed produced by the examiner's digital pressure on the finger-nail takes a long time to disappear after the pressure is relaxed. The urine output is reduced or ceases altogether.

Yet this typical clinical picture is by no means always seen in all its details, even in undoubted cases of shock due to blood loss. Arterial hypotension is often considered to be the most typical finding in shock, yet at least in the earlier stages a patient may have an apparently normal blood pressure. The reason for this is twofold: first, if the patient's usual blood pressure is, say, 150/100 mmHg, then a recorded blood pressure of 110/70 mmHg may be hypotension for him even though it is within the normal range. Secondly, compensatory circulatory adjustments may keep the blood pressure high till a late stage. Even the pulse rate can be misleading: in elderly patients especially, it is quite common to find that the pulse rate does not increase in the earlier stages of shock, and in such cases the final breakdown of circulation with complete collapse of the patient may appear to occur with catastrophic suddenness.

The one physiological fact that one can rely on in a patient with blood loss is that the cardiac output must be less than normal. The various circulatory changes described above are clearly secondary to this cardinal feature of reduced cardiac output. Variations in the precise clinical features of an individual patient represent variations in the circulatory response to the primary insult. It follows that it is unwise to rely on these circulatory responses as an accurate indication of the primary abnormality.

To proceed further, one must ask what the consequences are of a reduction in cardiac output and, in particular, which of those consequences threaten life.

Reduced tissue perfusion

A reduction in cardiac output must result in a reduction in the flow of blood through the tissues. It is known that different tissues and organs have very different sensitivities to a reduction in arterial blood supply. An arterial tourniquet may safely be left in position on the lower limb for 45 minutes, on the upper limb for 60 minutes, while a kidney pedicle may be clamped for 30 minutes. Such insults damage the tissues, as can be demonstrated by the accumulation of the abnormal metabolites of anaerobic metabolism, particularly lactic acid, in the affected region. However, the damage is not irreversible, provided that the period of ischaemia is not maintained beyond the stated times.

The skeletal and connective tissues of the scalp, face, neck and trunk probably have a sensitivity similar to those of the limbs. Precise figures for many of the other viscera are difficult to establish. In some, the presence of a double blood supply at different pressures and containing oxygen in different concentrations (e.g. lungs and liver) is a complicating factor. After the brain and nervous tissue in general, the order of decreasing sensitivity is usually stated as heart and liver, but the position of the lung is debatable. Damage to viscera other than the brain in shock states is considered further on p. 270. There is no doubt, however, that the most sensi-

tive organ is the brain. Brain cells cannot use anaerobic metabolism, and are therefore exquisitely sensitive to a lack of the blood supply that brings them oxygen. If the circulation is completely arrested for 3 minutes, irreversible changes occur in the brain.

Cerebral manifestations: the common factor

If we accept a reduction in cardiac output as being the primary defect in haemorrhagic shock, then the most certain clinical manifestation to result must be a disturbance of cerebral function. It is true that cerebral blood flow remains remarkably little affected as cardiac output falls, within certain limits. The phenomenon known as *autoregulation* ensures that the cerebral blood vessels dilate as the cardiac output falls, thereby attracting a greater proportion of the output to the brain. Yet no one who is adjudged on other grounds to be in a state of shock is ever entirely normal in cerebral function.

A wide spectrum of disturbance can be recognized, depending on the severity of the interference with cortical blood supply. The mildest features are sleepiness and a suggestion that the patient is withdrawing from intellectual contact with his environment. Later, restlessness and agitation predominate. Finally, delirium and a clouding of consciousness, proceeding to coma, supervene.

The concept may now be stated that all patients with shock, no matter how produced or how variable the details of the clinical picture may be, share the common primary factor of reduced tissue perfusion, and that the most sensitive manifestation of this factor is cerebral dysfunction. This concept has important practical consequences. Even if it were possible for a reduction in cardiac output to be so well compensated in terms of cerebral blood flow that no disturbance of consciousness ensued, it would follow that no *immediate* threat to life existed. It is true that organs such as heart, lungs, liver and kidneys might be suffering, but the power of recovery of these organs after a period of relative ischaemia is so much greater than that of the brain that the urgency of the situation is much less. Thus the recognition of cerebral dysfunction remains of paramount importance.

Quite clearly, a reduction in cerebral tissue perfusion is not the only possible cause of a disturbance of consciousness. The differential diagnosis of such a disturbance must now be considered.

Causes of cortical dysfunction

Consciousness may be disturbed by direct trauma to the brain or by indirect effects of trauma — concussion, extradural haemorrhage — or by any condition that raises the intracerebral pressure. The blood supply to the brain may be reduced despite a normal cardiac output, by local factors, either in the neck or within the skull – e.g. cerebrovascular accidents, subclavian steal syndrome.

One must remember, also, that what the brain needs for its metabolism is not the blood itself so much as the oxygen and glucose contained within it. Thus hypoxia and hypoglycaemia should both be considered as possible causes of disturbance of consciousness. Also, since cerebral metabolism can be readily poisoned by a variety of agents, one needs to consider drugs with a specific cortical action, uraemia and acid — base imbalance among several other metabolic possibilities.

Finally, there is always the possibility of a psychiatric cause.

If, after a thorough review of the preceding possibilities, the practitioner feels that he can safely exclude them, then the patient should be regarded as shocked, and the next step is to determine the type of shock so that logical treatment can be instituted.

The foregoing considerations lead to the following definition of shock.

Shock is a clinical state characterized by a disturbance of conscious level, and produced by a variety of mechanisms which act via the final common pathway of a generalized reduction in tissue perfusion sufficient to reduce the cerebral blood flow.

Difficulties

Before going on to the differential diagnosis of the cause of shock, due regard must be given to a number of difficulties that may arise once a disturbance of conscious level has been noted.

Many of the conditions, other than a generalized reduction in tissue perfusion, which can impair consciousness can themselves be produced by shock. Thus, severe hypotension results in anuria, which in turn causes both uraemia and metabolic acidosis. Again, a prolonged reduction in perfusion of the lungs is the probable cause of the syndrome known as 'shock-lung': the pulmonary tissue becomes oedematous and multiple infarctions occur, respiratory gas exchange is impaired, and hypoxia ensues. In other words, even if one finds an alternative cause for cerebral dysfunction, one must still look for signs of circulatory disturbance — *any* circulatory disturbance, not just those of haemorrhagic shock, because in some shock states quite different signs of an altered circulation develop, as we shall see in the next section. If any evidence of circulatory dysfunction is present, it is safer to assume that shock is the primary aetiological factor, and to treat that vigorously.

The other important difficulty arises when the patient is already unconscious for a perfectly well understood and valid reason, but where the possibility of shock is also present. The classic example is the patient who is brought in unconscious after a road traffic accident with an obvious head injury, and has a doubtfully lowered blood pressure and quickened pulse rate. Is he bleeding into the peritoneal cavity from a ruptured spleen or some such lesion? This situation illustrates the value of cerebral symptoms as a sensitive indicator of shock. In the absence of the indicator, one is driven to rely on the circulatory signs to diagnose shock. Clearly operation should be avoided if possible, to avoid aggravating the brain lesion or masking the development of intracranial bleeding (see p. 285), yet intraperitoneal bleeding, if it is present, threatens life. Further comments on this problem may be found in Chapter 24.

Differential diagnosis

Central venous pressure

Cardiac output falls either because the heart is too weak to pump out all the blood that returns to it, or because the venous return to the heart is reduced. In the first case, the *central venous pressure* (i.e. the pressure in the great veins) rises; in the second case, the pressure tends to fall, although compensatory venomotor tone may keep it within normal limits for a time.

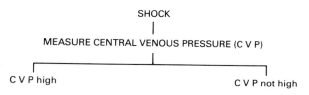

Shock resulting from the first type of disorder is called *cardiogenic*; the simplest term for the second type is *non-cardiogenic*.

The critical discriminant feature between these two types of shock is the central venous pressure (CVP). The CVP can be gauged by simple clinical observations. With the patient semirecumbent (i.e. with his upper half inclined at 45° to the horizontal, his lower half horizontal) the neck veins should in normal circumstances not be visible. If the CVP is sufficiently raised, the neck veins become distended and the CVP can be quantified as the vertical height of the visible column of the blood in the veins above the level of the manubriosternal angle. However, if the patient is severely shocked, it may be unwise to sit him up, thereby tending to lower still further the blood supply to the brain. If the patient is lying supine, the presence or absence of visibly distended veins on the dorsum of the feet may be useful sign: these veins in this position are roughly at the same horizontal level as the left atrium, and in non-cardiogenic shock with a lowered CVP they are usually invisible. Another useful clinical indication is provided by emptying any convenient superficial vein by digital pressure, keeping a segment isolated and empty between two finger-tips, and then removing the distal finger and observing how fast the segment fills, or whether it remains empty for an appreciable time.

Often such simple clinical observations will be adequate. In some circumstances a more accurate measurement will be desirable (for example, in the treatment of internal bleeding, Chapter 23), and this is obtained by passing a catheter from a suitable vein — jugular, subclavian or brachial — into the superior vena cava near its opening into the right atrium. The catheter is attached to a simple manometer filled with saline, and the height of the column of saline noted in comparison with a baseline. The baseline often chosen is the manubriosternal angle, and in that case the normal range is 0–5 cm of saline. With the patient supine, the left atrium is about 5 cm lower than the manubriosternal angle, so the normal range is 5–10 cm saline above the left atrium. The difficulty of knowing exactly where the level of the left atrium is, especially if the patient is not lying flat but on an inclined plane, has led to the introduction of the third intercostal space in the anterior axillary line as the baseline. It is said that this point accurately coincides with the level of the right atrium, no matter what the inclination of the patient to the horizontal might be.

It should be noted that there are two pitfalls in interpreting an actual measurement of CVP. One is the difficulty in establishing the base-line of the right atrium. There is further reference to this problem in Chapter 23. The other is that one assumes the right atrial pressure accurately mirrors the left atrial pressure: it is really the left atrial pressure which tells us whether the systemic cardiac output is reduced by failure of the left ventricle or by failure of the venous return. In a variety of cardiological conditions the two atrial pressures may be very different and to this extent the measurement of CVP may be misleading.

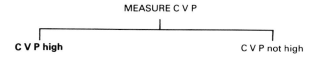

Cardiogenic shock

In a surgically orientated book such as this, it is important to emphasize that a surgeon diagnosing cardiogenic shock should immediately seek the aid of a physician. First, most patients presenting like this have no lesion amenable to surgical treatment, but they need urgent medical measures. Secondly, the diagnosis of the very few surgical conditions which may produce cardiogenic shock requires skills that the surgeon usually lacks. Finally, there is always the possibility, referred to in the previous paragraph, that the right atrial pressure may be difficult to interpret and quite different from the left atrial pressure.

The two conditions of potential surgical importance are now considered.

Cardiac tamponade

The acute form is a surgical emergency. Bleeding occurs into the pericardial sac, usually as a result of trauma but occasionally due to rupture of a dissecting aortic aneurysm into the pericardium. The heart is rapidly and increasingly embarrassed in its action. Filling of both ventricles during diastole is impeded, and the cardiac output falls. The venous pressure rises in both the systemic and the pulmonary circulations: usually only the elevated systemic venous pressure is clinically detectable as the raised CVP.

Normally, the systolic arterial blood pressure falls during inspiration by 5–7 mmHg. In cardiac tamponade, the fall exceeds 10 mmHg — *pulsus paradoxus*. The area of precordial cardiac dullness is increased and the heart sounds are faint to auscultation. Plain x-ray shows widening of the heart shadow, especially in the regions of the pericardiacophrenic angles; screening (fluoroscopy) shows diminished excursions of the borders of the heart.

The diagnosis is made by echocardiography, a technique that is now widely available and can be brought to the patient. Should there be any difficulty in arranging this investigation, the old (and much more dangerous) way of making the diagnosis is by inserting a needle into the pericardial cavity via the fourth left intercostal space, 3–4 cm from the mid-line, and aspirating blood. For treatment, see Chapter 23.

Pulmonary embolus

The sudden obstruction of the right ventricular outflow tract results in a reduced systemic cardiac output and a marked increase in right atrial and central venous pressure but a reduction in left atrial pressure. The diagnosis may be aided by antecedent symptoms and signs related to the peripheral venous system, or by clinical features suggestive of recent small pulmonary emboli with infarction of segments of lung. In the absence of such clinical features, the diagnosis should be considered in any patient with acute cardiogenic shock in whom the cardiological evidence suggests a disproportionate failure of the right side of the heart compared with the left. Such evidence includes a tapping or impalpable apex beat and a right ventricular thrust just to the right of the sternum; on *chest radiography* a prominent pulmonary artery and reduced vascular markings in one or both lungs; and in the *ECG trace*, signs of right axis deviation and right ventricular strain. If the total evidence is sufficiently suggestive, the distribution of the pulmonary arterial blood supply can be further investigated by *scanning* and by *pulmonary angiography*.

The management of pulmonary embolism is considered in Chapter 19, but the importance of getting a cardiological opinion if the condition should be suspected is manifest.

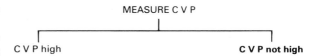

Non-cardiogenic shock

If the CVP is *not* raised, it must be concluded that the action of the heart as a pump is normal. It follows that any reduction in cardiac output must be due to a reduction in the venous return.

The flow of blood in the systemic venous system back to the heart can be reduced in two different ways: by a reduction in the volume of the circulating blood, or by an increase in the volume of the arteriolocapillary bed. The two corresponding forms of shock are classified as *hypovolaemic* or *oligaemic*, and as *shock due to vasodilatation*. The distinction between these two forms of non-cardiogenic shock is not always perfect: the blurring of the boundaries will be discussed later.

Shock due to vasodilatation

The essential feature in the various clinical types of shock due to vasodilatation is that some area or areas of the arteriolocapillary bed, other than the cerebral vasculature, undergo dilatation. In consequence, the distribution of the blood in the circulation is altered though its total volume remains unchanged. Since there is more blood than usual in the arteries and capillaries, there must be less blood in the veins: this accounts for the lowered venous return to the heart, an effect which, if sufficiently severe, results in a lowered CVP. Since the capacity of the peripheral circulation can increase manifold if vasoconstrictor tone is lost, there may be a diversion of blood away from the brain with consequent cerebral manifestations of shock.

C V P not high

Typical clinical picture (vasodilator)   CONSIDER HYPOVOLAEMIA

Typical forms of shock due to vasodilatation are the *vasovagal, anaphylactic* and *sympathetic paralysis* types. They are usually fairly easy to diagnose from their typical clinical features, and their elimination makes it easier to diagnose the remaining forms of non-cardiogenic shock.

Vasovagal shock (syn. syncope, fainting, neurogenic shock) is a condition in which the subject loses consciousness rapidly, within a few seconds of the onset of the disturbance; falls to the ground; and recovers consciousness in a few seconds or minutes. The causative factors are pain, a sudden emotional disturbance, changing rapidly from a sitting or lying posture to the upright (*postural hypotension*), and standing still for a long time. As indicated, the condition is strictly self-limiting, but if the attack lasts long enough for the diagnosis to be seriously in doubt the pulse rate should be counted: it is very low in a vasovagal attack, in the region of 40 beats/minute. Despite the vasodilatation in other areas, the face is always pale.

The mechanism seems to be that any factor which sufficiently reduces venous return — e.g. skin vasodilatation induced by surface heating in a hot bath, visceral dilatation produced reflexly by sudden severe pain, or pooling of blood in the venules of the lower limb when the venous return is impeded by gravity and the calf muscle pump that normally aids venous return is suppressed by standing still — may, in a susceptible subject, produce the typical response. The two main features of this response are: vagal overactivity, produced presumably by stimulation of the vagal centre by a reduction in blood supply; and peripheral vasodilatation, particularly in muscle, produced by some mechanism which remains unknown.

Sympathetic paralysis, by interfering with normal vasoconstrictor tone in the peripheral circulation, renders the patient liable to recurrent attacks of fainting whenever any strain is placed on the peripheral circulation, for example by adopting the erect posture suddenly. The features of this type of shock are therefore identical with those of a vasovagal attack, but due to a definable abnormality of the sympathetic nervous system. Causes of sympathetic paralysis include surgical sympathectomy and ganglion-blocking and adrenolytic drugs. Thoracolumbar sympathectomy used to be performed in the treatment of essential hypertension, but its effect was not permanent. Drugs produce the same effect more reliably: the ganglion-blocking drugs are exemplified by hexamethonium, which is a competitive antagonist to acetylcholine in autonomic ganglia, and phenoxybenzamine, which blocks the *a*-adrenergic receptors in smooth muscle. General anaesthesia paralyses the vasomotor centre.

Anaphylactic shock should be immediately diagnosed by the fact that shock is accompanied by the typical clinical features of bronchospasm and (often) widespread urticaria, following within minutes of a parenteral injection of foreign material. Penicillin and antitetanus serum (ATS) are the most common injections that produce this violent allergic reaction. The disturbance may be so intense as to cause death within a few minutes, but immediate treatment by the injection of 1 ml 1:1000 adrenaline solution by intramuscular injection or 200 mg hydrocortisone intravenously, is usually effective. The combination of the injected allergen with its appropriate cell-fixed antibody (*reagin*) in the tissues results in severe cell damage and the release of histamine. The latter causes the bronchospasm, a profound vasodilatation and an increase in capillary permeability. The vasodilatation is partly responsible for the shock, but the increase in capillary permeability, by permitting a rapid loss of liquid from the circulation, contributes to the shock as well as being responsible for the generalized urticaria.

The remaining types of shock due to vasodila-

tation are not easily recognized, and are left for consideration after the possibility of hypovolaemia has been explored.

C V P not high

Typical clinical picture (vasodilator)

CONSIDER HYPOVOLAEMIA

Hypovolaemic shock

In terms of its major volume-occupying constituents, blood consists of red cells and plasma. Acute losses of red cells alone are not encountered, and so a reduction in blood volume may be due to a loss of whole blood from the circulation (haemorrhage), or a contraction of the plasma volume. However, the plasma is a specialized compartment of the whole extracellular

fluid (ECF), of very similar constitution to that of the ECF: the major difference is that plasma contains protein at a much higher concentration than the ECF. A contraction in plasma volume may therefore be due to a loss of plasma from the circulation, or to a contraction of the whole ECF.

The aetiology and diagnosis of hypovolaemia due to blood loss, plasma loss and extracellular deficits are now discussed.

CONSIDER HYPOVOLAEMIA

Blood loss   Plasma loss   Saline loss   No evidence

Blood loss occurs as the result of trauma, or in consequence of disease of the blood vessel or of neighbouring tissues. Many of the detailed features of haemorrhage are considered in Chapter 23, but from the viewpoint of the differential diagnosis of hypovolaemic shock the essential feature of blood loss is that it has the most dramatic and dangerous effects upon the circulation. The contraction of the circulating volume by a given figure can occur most quickly by the loss of that volume from a large breach in a major blood vessel. Losses of plasma and of ECF take much longer to develop, and the features of shock are milder in consequence. Shock due to blood loss is one of the most urgent emergencies in surgery.

When the blood loss is *external* the diagnosis is obvious; when *internal* or *occult*, the difficulty in diagnosis can be great. If there are circumstances which lead the surgeon to suspect blood loss, the important confirmatory evidence is obtained from the absence of physical signs of extracellular depletion (see below), and from an examination of the blood and urine.

In acute blood loss, since the loss from the circulation is whole blood and there has been no

time for a compensatory shift of fluid to occur from the ECF into the vascular compartment, there is no change in the composition of the residual blood. A venous blood sample is therefore likely to show a normal haemoglobin level or haematocrit (packed cell volume) percentage, although if the bleeding has been fairly slow and the clinical course correspondingly longer, some compensation may have occurred whereupon there might be a tendency for low values to be obtained. Although renal function may be impaired, in really acute cases the impairment will not have lasted long enough to produce a rise in blood urea concentration. For the same reason, the first sample of urine obtained was probably passed by the kidneys into the bladder before the onset of the bleeding, and is therefore likely to be normal in sodium and chloride concentrations and in specific gravity. In the later stages of severe shock due to haemorrhage, the secretion of urine is often completely suppressed, so later samples of urine may be nonexistent, or else small in volume and low in sodium and chloride concentrations. The renal effects of shock are considered in more detail in Chapter 15.

CONSIDER HYPOVOLAEMIA

Blood loss   **Plasma loss**   Saline loss   No evidence

Plasma loss can usually be diagnosed or strongly suspected from the clinical indications. The essential abnormality which permits the loss of plasma from the circulation is an increase of capillary permeability, sufficient to allow plasma proteins as well as the water and electrolytes of plasma to escape into the tissues. The most commonly quoted example of a condition causing this increased permeability is a *burn*, but except in wartime the other possibilities of the inflammation of large serous surfaces, such as in *peritonitis*, or the distension of the capillaries of a region whose blood supply is *strangulated*, are probably more frequent. A capillary distended by local chemicals released in inflammation, or by the back-pressure resulting from the venous obstruction in strangulation, is more permeable than a normal capillary.

In patients with plasma loss, the reduction in plasma volume compared to the unchanged red cell mass produces a marked degree of haemo-concentration, with proportionately marked rises in haemoglobin and haematocrit. Since renal excretion may have been impaired for a longer period than in acute blood loss, the blood urea is likely to be moderately raised. The urinary changes are usually much the same as in blood loss.

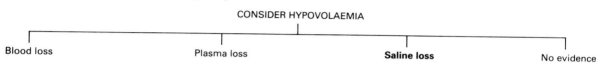

ECF depletion is due to the loss of water and sodium ions from the body. The usual route for such losses is the alimentary tract, although in hot climates sweat may be an important route, and rarely excessive loss of sodium may occur in the urine (see p. 213). Losses from the alimentary tract can be equated, in terms of their effect on the ECF as a whole, with the loss of a similar volume of 'normal' (isotonic) saline — i.e. NaCl 150 mmol/litre (9 g/litre). A combination of history and observation usually indicates that abnormal losses are occurring from the alimentary tract, as *vomiting, diarrhoea,* fluid discharge via an external fistula, or abdominal distension as may occur in intestinal obstruction (see Chapter 26).

Loss of isotonic saline results in a reduction in the size of the extracellular space and a proportionate reduction in plasma volume. Since the ECF volume in an adult is 15 litres (i.e. about five times the plasma volume), 5 litres of saline needs to be lost from the ECF before the plasma volume shrinks by as much as 1 litre. It follows that shock is slower to develop, and less severe except in the latest stages, than in blood or plasma loss. On the other hand, a typical feature of saline loss is the reduction in the pressure of the intestitial fluid, i.e. the extravascular component of the ECF. This may be gauged clinically by a reduction in skin elasticity, a reduction in the tension of the eyeballs, and, in severe cases, by the typical appearance of the face known as the *Hippocratic facies*, in which the eyeballs are sunken and the bony prominences of the face stand out as sharp ridges through the lax superficial tissues.

Haemoconcentration tends to be less severe than in plasma loss until the late stages. However, since the condition is more chronic in its development, the blood urea concentration tends to be higher. The important feature of the urine is the virtual absence of sodium and chloride ions, although oliguria and a high urine specific gravity are usually also notable.

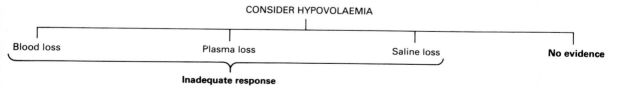

Remaining causes of shock

The two remaining causes of shock need to be considered either if the preceding varieties have been sought but not found, or if one of the preceding varieties, usually some kind of hypovolaemic shock, has been apparently adequately treated but the shock state persists.

The latter situation is often called *irreversible shock*, but the use of this term should be avoided. The usual reason why hypovolaemia fails to respond to apparently adequate treatment is that the treatment has not been adequate. If the clinician fails to grasp this point, he may waste valuable time in giving treatment for the two remaining forms of shock; especially dangerous is the fact that such treatment may produce temporary improvement in the state of shock, and result in a quite unwarranted complacency in the clinician.

Nevertheless, some cases occur in which one may be confident that none of the previous types of shock is present, or that if one is present it probably has been treated adequately. In such circumstances the possibility arises that a lack of adrenal corticosteroids or the presence of septicaemia is responsible.

Adrenocorticosteroid lack may be suspected on clinical grounds. It may be known that the patient has received corticosteroid treatment during the previous year or two, in which case his adrenal cortical response to any stress may be inadequate. Alternatively, a picture of saline depletion without any obvious route of saline loss may suggest that sodium has been lost via the kidneys. This possibility may be confirmed by finding that sodium output in the urine is high, while potassium output is low. Such patients may show associated features such as nausea and oral mucosal pigmentation, the whole syndrome being known as Addison's disease.

Septicaemia, especially with Gram-negative organisms, is a potent cause of shock. The combination of septicaemia, with its profound and widespread vasodilation in skin, muscles and viscera, with hypovolaemia is quite common and particularly resistant to treatment. The diagnosis should always be considered in shocked patients with evidence of overt or potential infection (peritonitis, respiratory tract infection, renal infection or instrumentation of the urinary tract, and operations upon or foreign bodies in the biliary passages). Suggestive clinical features are pyrexia, rigors and a warm red skin rather than a pale, sweaty, cold one, but the hypovolaemic element, if present, may mask these signs. Several venous blood samples are taken with full aseptic precautions and sent to the laboratory for the immediate examination of smears and the setting up of cultures.

The management of these forms of shock is considered in Chapter 23.

Further problems

Organ damage in shock

Paradoxically, the circulatory adjustments which maintain an adequate blood supply to the brain and keep the patient alive may themselves result in damage to important organs. The chief sensitive organs are heart, lungs, liver and kidneys. The changes produced in these organs may, if sufficiently severe, become irreversible and themselves threaten life. The possibility of such changes is a good reason for treating shock urgently, even though the condition seems to be well compensated from the cerebral point of view.

Kidneys

Renal effects are described in Chapter 15.

Lungs

The typical changes affecting the respiratory system in severely shocked patients are hyperpnoea, the respiratory movements being shallow, rapid and ineffectual, cyanosis, diminished air entry, increased dullness and added râles at the lung bases, and plain x-ray appearances suggesting pulmonary oedema — large areas of basal opacity with a tendency to circinate outlines. Arterial oxygen tension (Po_2) is low, arterial carbon dioxide tension (Pco_2) is high, and the pulmonary diffusion index reduced.

There are often many aetiological possibilities in a seriously ill patient, but it is reasonable to suppose that a reduction in tissue perfusion damages the delicate alveolar membrane and its capillary blood vessels, and allows the leakage of a protein-rich exudate into the alveoli.

Flow-chart 22.1

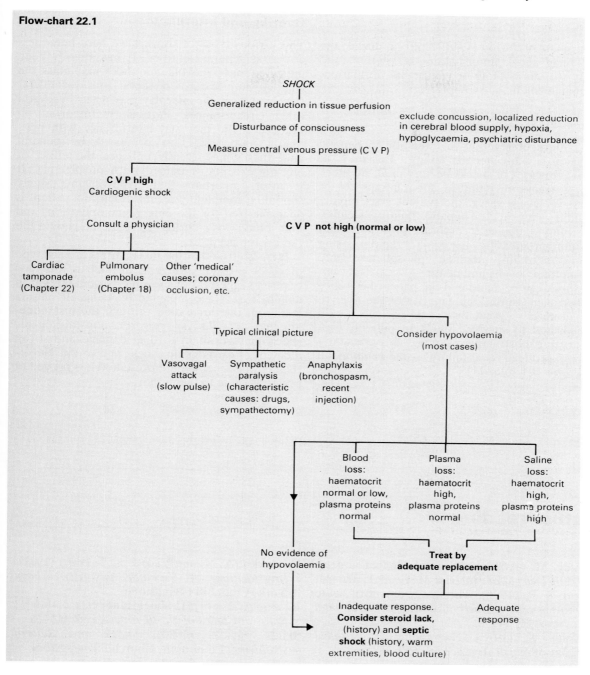

Heart

If coronary perfusion is sufficiently reduced, the heart may show abnormalities of rhythm, and finally stop in asystole or ventricular fibrillation. For management, see Chapter 21.

Liver

The pattern of reaction to reduction in hepatic perfusion is acute hepatic failure. This may, in less severe cases of shock, be very mild: no more than a transient jaundice for perhaps 24–28 hours. In severe cases, the patient goes rapidly downhill with acute hepatic failure: steadily deepening jaundice, cerebral confusion and delirium progressing to coma, rapidly rising plasma bilirubin, alkaline phosphatase and transaminase levels, and death.

If shock can be cured and the patient kept alive by special measures, the capacity of the liver to regenerate is so great that some patients would be expected to survive. Shock in patients with pre-existing obstructive jaundice is particularly likely to produce renal failure — the *hepatorenal syndrome* (Chapter 11).

Overlap and interplay

The various types of shock have here been described as separate entities. It has already been indicated that hypovolaemic shock may mask the characteristic features of septicaemic vasodilatation, and a similar interplay may occur in several other circumstances. Particularly important in practice is the fact that interference with peripheral vasoconstriction produced by general anaesthesia may greatly enhance the effect of any pre-existing or immediate hypovolaemia. It is most important that hypovolaemic shock should be completely reversed before a patient is anaesthetized for the emergency operation, and that blood loss during anaesthesia should be rapidly replaced.

It is also true that the mechanisms of each type of shock are not always as distinct as this description suggests. For example: vasodilatation in anaphylaxis is accompanied by saline or plasma loss from the circulation through the histamine-affected capillaries; severe non-cardiogenic shock may result in cardiac damage and so an element of cardiogenic shock; and so on. Nevertheless, the scheme here presented has proved of practical value to the author.

Further reading

Hobsley, M. (1968). Shock in abdominal surgery. *British Journal of Hospital Medicine* **1**, 326–34.

Joseph, S. P. (1976). The management of acute hypotension. *British Journal of Hospital Medicine* **16**, 34956.

Messmer, K. (1975). Haemodilution. *Surgical Clinics of North America* **55**, 659–78.

Moore, F. D. *et al.* (1969). *Post-traumatic Pulmonary Insufficiency*. Philadelphia, W. B. Saunders.

Nicolaides, A. N. and Yao, J. S. T. (Ed.) (1981). *Investigation of Vascular Disorders*. New York, Churchill Livingstone.

Rosen, A. J. (1975). Shock lung: fact or fancy? *Surgical Clinics of North America* **55**, 613–26.

Shires, G. T. (1984). *Shock and Related Problems*. Edinburgh, Churchill Livingstone.

Chapter 23

Acute Blood Loss

Principles of management

The principles of management of acute blood loss may be simply stated: (1) establish the diagnosis; (2) stop the bleeding; (3) restore the cardiac output to normal by replacing the lost blood with transfused blood or blood substitute.

Several difficulties may be met in applying these principles. The first is that making the diagnosis may not be easy if the blood loss is not obvious. The second is that stopping the bleeding may not be easy if the source of the blood loss is remote from the observer. The third is that in some cases of rapid bleeding it may be difficult for the clinician to decide whether principle (2) or principle (3) should take priority. In the average case, it is feasible to restore cardiac output by transfusion while arrangements are made with reasonable haste to gain access to the remote bleeding point so that it can be secured. Sometimes, however, the rate of blood loss is so great that transfusion cannot easily keep pace with it: in these circumstances, attempts at resuscitation before operation are doomed to failure and *any* operative risk must be accepted and surgery undertaken immediately if there is any hope of the patient surviving. The classical example of this unusual situation is rapid leakage from an abdominal aortic aneurysm: the only hope for the patient may lie in immediate transfer to the nearest place that will pass muster as an operating theatre and laparotomy without even cleansing the skin or undertaking other antiseptic measures. Nevertheless it must be emphasized that usually principle (3) can receive attention while arrangements are being made to approach the bleeding point at a remote site.

There are two further difficulties in applying principle (3): how does the clinician know whether his transfusion is adequate, inadequate, or excessive? And to what extent may blood substitutes be used to conserve supplies of blood? These problems are discussed immediately below. The rest of the Chapter discusses the diagnosis and special features of management of acute blood loss, in the various situations in which the clinician meets the condition.

Adequacy of transfusion

The usual mistake of the inexperienced doctor is to transfuse too little, too slowly. The danger of excessive transfusion is of course that it will overload the heart, producing an element of cardiogenic shock. In a reasonably young, previously healthy individual, the possibility that overloading will occur suddenly, and before the doctor realizes that he has restored the patient's cardiac output to normal, is remote. In the average case, the doctor simply transfuses blood at the most rapid convenient rate (i.e. without special measures such as pumps to increase the rate) until the patient is no longer shocked as judged by the usual clinical signs of conscious level, pulse rate and blood pressure, fullness of the veins, and warmth and colouring of the skin.

Problems arise with the elderly patient, or one who is known to have hypertensive, valvular or coronary heart disease. In such patients, cardiogenic shock and even cardiac arrest may be precipitated before the hypovolaemic shock has been corrected. Presumably the period of hypovolaemia has, in such patients, further damaged the heart so that it can only gradually accept again its full normal work-load. It is in these cases that the clinician should monitor central venous pressure (CVP)(see Chapter 22) by an indwelling catheter in the great veins of the superior mediastinum, so that he may get an early warning of a rise in venous pressure. An excellent way to proceed is to give blood in small, accurately measured, rapid deliveries of about 100 ml, with a pause between each delivery to measure CVP. Because of the difficulties with regard to baseline and the consequent uncertainty of the exact level of CVP, the *change* in

CVP produced by this manoeuvre is a much safer way of using CVP readings than is the actual reading obtained on any one occasion.

Inadequate transfusion is a much more common event. One reason for this is the exaggerated fear of overtransfusion; another is that a doctor often underestimates the volume of blood required. The latter may arise because the doctor underestimates the volume of blood lost (e.g. because it is internal and cannot be measured) or because an unsuspected blood loss is continuing despite measures to control haemorrhage, or because he fails to appreciate that the volume of transfusion required to restore the cardiac output to normal may be greater than the volume of blood lost because of such factors as vasodilatation due to the accumulation of lactic acid in poorly perfused areas. In cases of severe shock due to blood loss, it is advisable to catheterize the bladder and base an objective assessment of the adequacy of the transfusion upon the objective assessment of the rate of urine flow. One aims at achieving a rate of urine flow of 1 ml/min, or about 1.5 litres/24 hours, and would certainly not be satisfied with less than half that rate. Recently it has been pointed out that the direct measurement of tissue oxygen tension by placing an oxygen-sensitive needle electrode into the tissues can reveal evidence of underperfusion in many patients in whom the clinical evidence suggests that perfusion is satisfactory.

Blood substitutes

Blood is always in short supply. The available substitutes that stay in the circulation are stored dried *plasma* reconstituted with distilled water, and the range of synthetic polysaccharides known as the *dextrans*. Plasma would be ideal because it is remarkably free from all other side-effects, but carries the risk of infective hepatitis and many other communicable diseases such as AIDS (p. 30). Stored plasma is being prepared from smaller pools of donors than heretofore (thereby reducing the statistical chance of contamination), and methods for screening blood donors for the hepatitis B antigen are becoming more readily available, but the AIDS problem is still unsolved. Plasma proteins free from the fraction containing hepatitis antigen are now also available. The dextrans are available in a range of average molecular weights: thus dextran 70 has an average molecular weight of 70 000, dextran 40 of 40 000. The latter has fewer side-effects, and is the product of choice. However, dextrans cause rouleaux formation in blood and interfere with the interpretation of agglutination of red blood cells, so a sample of blood for grouping and cross-matching should be taken from the patient before dextran is transfused. Dextrans may also interfere with blood coagulation and produce a bleeding diathesis, so it is unwise to use more than 2 litres of dextran in any one transfusion.

Gelatin products (e.g. Haemaccel) do not interfere with crossmatching and seem less likely to provoke allergic reactions than do dextrans, but stay a shorter time in the circulation. Synthetic starches are becoming available and the preliminary evidence suggests that they may prove to be better than the other synthetic plasma substitutes.

Presentation

There are many ways of classifying acute blood loss. Haemorrhage may be *arterial*, *venous* or *capillary*, and this subdivision helps in the practical details of how best the bleeding may be stopped. Other classifications are into *external* (or *overt*) and *internal* (*covert*), and into *primary, reactionary* or *secondary*. Primary haemorrhage is the bleeding which results from the initial damage to one or more blood vessels, the damage being *traumatic*, or due to *disease of the blood vessels*, or *disease of neighbouring tissues* affecting blood vessels. Reactionary haemorrhage occurs in the first 24 hours, secondary haemorrhage in the second week, after operation or trauma. All these types of classification are of help in considering how patients with acute bleeding present, but the most useful is the subdivision into primary, reactionary and secondary. Primary haemorrhage presents in the field after trauma (Chapter 20), in the practitioner's consulting room or the casualty department, in the wards before elective surgery, and in the operating theatre. Reactionary and secondary haemorrhage occur later.

Primary haemorrhage

The general practitioner, on meeting primary haemorrhage due to trauma, is either able to arrest the haemorrhage immediately and definitively or must refer the patient to hospital. All patients with bleeding in the absence of trauma must also be referred to hospital, as there is no way of telling whether the bleeding will cease spontaneously.

In casualty

Here, patients present with bleeding in association with trauma, or in the absence of trauma; and the bleeding may be external or internal.

Traumatic haemorrhage may result in obvious external bleeding. The first-aid measure to control bleeding, namely the application of direct pressure to the bleeding point, should have already been undertaken in the field. In the casualty department it may be possible to apply definitive measures: a bleeding artery can be secured with artery forceps and ligatured, the bleeding edges of a scalp wound controlled with skin sutures. If more complicated procedures are necessary, or if general anaesthesia is indicated for these or other procedures, further management is deferred to the definitive operation. At that operation, the measures to control haemorrhage are no different from those used in an elective surgical operation and are considered later.

The much more difficult problem, in cases of trauma, is where shock is diagnosed but there is no external bleeding. With the proviso that in such circumstances shock could be due to the loss of plasma or saline (see Chapter 20), a patient who develops shock after being involved in trauma *must* be assumed to be losing blood internally. The site of bleeding may become manifest as epistaxis, haemoptysis, haematemesis, melaena, or haematuria, but in the absence of such clues it should be assumed that covert blood loss is occurring into the chest, the abdomen, the large muscle bulk of the posterior abdominal wall, or the swelling around the site of a major fracture, e.g. a fracture of the shaft of the femur.

Physical signs in the chest are unreliable in the diagnosis of *haemothorax*, and so a chest x-ray must be performed. The appearances of the latter depend on whether or not the lung or chest wall have been punctured, so letting air into the chest as well — *haemopneumothorax*. In either case, the initial treatment is to drain the pleura via an intercostal tube connected to an underwater seal and a suction pump. If the patient's general condition does not deteriorate, and the lung expands and drainage of air and blood slow down and cease (see Chapter 19), nothing further needs to be done. If the above conditions are not met, the chest is opened by formal thoracotomy to turn out blood clots and to find and control the bleeding vessel.

Physical signs of *intraperitoneal bleeding* are also notoriously unreliable. Usually, there is tenderness and guarding and an absence of the normal bowel sounds on auscultation. However, in many cases physical examination is entirely normal; if the patient is shocked with a normal or low CVP, and there is no evidence of blood loss elsewhere, this picture constitutes an indication for immediate laparotomy.

After trauma, the management of haematuria depends upon whether there is any possibility of a ruptured bladder or urethra. If there is no such possibility, traumatic haematuria is treated expectantly and only very rarely does it give rise to any serious degree of shock. Evidence that conservative treatment must be abandoned in favour of exploration includes increasing shock, the development of a swelling in the loin, and radiographic evidence suggesting disruption of the kidney on an intravenous pyelogram.

The problem of *intracranial bleeding* is considered in Chapter 24. The clinical features of *pericardial bleeding* with consequent cardiac tamponade are described in Chapter 22; the diagnosis of this condition depends on echocardiography or on inserting a needle into the pericardial sac through the fourth left intercostal space, 5 cm from the mid-line so as to avoid the internal mammary artery, and attempting aspiration. If the diagnosis is confirmed by obtaining blood, definitive surgery should be undertaken to open the pericardium and find and control the bleeding point.

Epistaxis, haematemesis, etc., after trauma present no particular features that will not be covered below.

Non-traumatic haemorrhage should always make the clinician think of the possibility of a bleeding diathesis, even when the cause seems obvious. If a case treated on the lines described below fails to respond, a blood sample should be sent for the determination of bleeding and clotting times and whatever other tests the local haematologist uses as a screen for coagulation defects.

Bleeding from the nose — *epistaxis* — or coughed up from the respiratory passages — *haemoptysis* — or passed in the urine — *haematuria* — only rarely produce shock. The exceptions are such irremediable lesions as leaking aneurysms of the aortic arch eroding the bronchi, carcinomas of the nasopharynx, etc. Epistaxis usually originates in Little's area, the lowermost centimetre of the mucosa of the nasal septum, where the mucosa is often thin and atrophic, and prominent blood vessels may lie close to the surface and be easily injured. Local pressure for a few minutes controls the bleeding. Occasionally, the source is posteriorly in the nostrils and packing of this region is required. The average haemoptysis needs no immediate treatment other than reassurance, but every case must be fully investigated for disease of heart, lungs or great vessels (see Chapter 18).

Non-traumatic haematuria requires special mention. If the bleeding is associated with pain or discomfort in the bladder region, or a sensation of burning in the urethra on micturition, it is probably due to acute cystitis and should be treated by sending the urine for culture and prescribing an increased fluid intake, antibiotics and rest. If the bleeding is painless, and is actually still occurring at the time the patient presents, it is wise to perform an immediate cystoscopy. Most cases of painless haematuria are due to bladder neoplasms, but occasionally one meets with a problem case where the origin of the bleeding, perhaps due to a tiny haemangioma, is obscure. In that case, immediate cystoscopy may give the best chance of determining, if the bleeding point is above the bladder, at least on which side of the renal tract it lies (see Chapter 28).

Bleeding from the gastrointestinal tract, vomited as *haematemesis* or passed via the anal canal as *melaena*, tarry black altered blood with a characteristic smell, is quite unlike the previous conditions in that, even when apparently mild, it must be treated with the greatest circumspection. Any case of haematemesis and/or melaena is potentially life-threatening. Until recently, management has been complicated by the difficulty of establishing a precise diagnosis, but the advent of the flexible gastroduodenoscope has made a tremendous improvement in the management of those cases where the bleeding arises in the stomach or duodenum.

The management of gastrointestinal haemorrhage presenting as haematemesis and/or melaena may be summarized by saying that usually there should be a preliminary period of observation combined with investigation and resuscitation, and that in most cases the bleeding stops and further decisions about management can be undertaken at leisure. Rarely the haemorrhage is so severe in the first instance that operation should be undertaken immediately. Sometimes, after the initial period of assessment it becomes manifest that the bleeding has not stopped in a reasonable period; or after an interval during which bleeding stops, it may start again during the same hospital admission. In such cases surgery is undertaken under the heading of failed conservative treatment.

The site of the bleeding has for practical purposes to lie in a fairly restricted segment of the gastrointestinal tract, starting at the lower third of the oesophagus and finishing somewhere in the small bowel. Blood in large quantities from higher regions of the digestive tract is usually expelled before it can be swallowed and vomited. Blood from lesions of the large bowel is usually evacuated so soon after being shed that the characteristic appearance of melaena, due to semi-digestion of the blood is not seen. According to level, therefore, large bowel lesions produce staining of the motions with bright or dark blood, but even the darkest stools have a tinge of red at the periphery of the dark staining.

Various rare bleeding lesions of the oesophagus, stomach, duodenum and small intestine may be encountered from time to time. Particular difficulty, for example, is occasioned by such a lesion as an angioma of the biliary passages. Nevertheless, in practice the vast bulk of the cases one encounters is due either to chronic peptic ulcer of stomach and duodenum, acute gastroduodenal erosions or haemorrhagic gastritis, malignant ulcer of stomach, or oesophagogastric varices in patients with portal hypertension.

A guess at the diagnosis may be made from the history. The easiest situation is where there is a clear-cut past history of a lesion such as a chronic peptic ulcer that might bleed, but even in this situation experience teaches that the diagnosis turns out to be the expected one in only 80 per cent of cases.

A patient with a *chronic peptic ulcer* is likely to give the typical history of epigastric pain relieved by food and alkalis, troubling him in bouts of a few days or weeks with remissions of several weeks in between bouts. Acute gastroduodenal erosions and/or haemorrhagic gastritis occur in patients who are shocked for any reason, or have otherwise been exposed to an excess of cortisol, or drugs such as acetylsalicylic acid, phenylbutazone, etc., which have similar corticosteroid-like properties. A patient with oesophageal varices is, in Europe or North America, probably suffering from chronic alcoholism or cryptogenic (i.e. cause unknown) multilobular cirrhosis; in other parts of the world (e.g. tropical and subtropical Africa) the likely diagnosis would be schistosomiasis. A patient with carcinoma of the stomach typically complains of a fairly recent loss of appetite.

On examination, clues to the diagnosis may also be found. A hard epigastric mass may represent a carcinoma of the stomach. The cirrhotic liver may be small and therefore impalpable, but it may be palpable as a hard multinodular mass moving with respiratory movements. Signs of liver failure may also be present: the typical *foetor hepaticus* of the breath, the coarse flapping tremor of the hands, spider naevi of the upper half of the body. In the author's experience, however, the much-vaunted collaterals between the portal and systemic circulations at the umbilicus (caput medusae) and the anal canal (internal haemorrhoids) are practically never seen.

Help is rarely obtained from laboratory investigations at the time when decisions need to be made urgently. The standard investigation to establish the diagnosis is an immediate examination of the appropriate parts of the gastrointestinal tract with the flexible gastroduodenoscope.

In most cases, gastroduodenoscopy gives the diagnosis, and the value of this cannot be too greatly stressed. A laparotomy for gastrointestinal haemorrhage of undetermined origin is one of the most difficult situations in general surgery, and anything that can be done to reduce the number of occasions on which the surgeon must face it is of inestimable value. Moreover there are several endoscopic techniques available for stopping the bleeding. Oesophageal varices can be injected with sclerosant, bleeding points in relation to ulcers or neoplasms can be sealed using diathermy or laser-coagulation, and tissue for biopsy can be obtained. Sometimes a lesion can be seen but it is not bleeding: it is then very important not to assume that the lesion must be the source of the haemorrhage, there may be some other source further down the alimentary

tract. In the case of peptic ulcers that are not bleeding, endoscopists describe various features – 'stigmata' – such as a sizeable artery seen end-on in the floor of the ulcer, which indicate a strong likelihood of further bleeding in the near future.

Bleeding from oesophageal varices is considered separately below. In all other cases, the decision to operate because of the presence of stigmata or the failure of conservative measures is taken sooner rather than later, in relation to the age of patient. Atherosclerotic vessels are less likely to retract adequately for effective stasis than the supple vessels of younger people. If laparotomy has to be undertaken, the exact procedure clearly depends upon what lesion is found. A chronic gastric ulcer is usually treated by partial gastrectomy, a chronic duodenal ulcer either by the same operation or by undermining the bleeding point in the floor of the ulcer with a stitch and adding a truncal vagotomy and pyloroplasty. If no cause for bleeding had been revealed by endoscopy, the alternatives lie in the first instance between angiographic techniques to demonstrate the bleeding point or laparotomy with simultaneous gastrointestinal endoscopy (if necessary, from both ends) so that the operator can manually assist the placing of the endoscope (see also p. 133).

Bleeding from oesophageal varices is another difficult problem. Two conservative lines of treatment are available: vasopressin (given by intravenous injection in a dosage of 20 units in 100 ml dextrose over 15 minutes) and local pressure. Vasopressin is a constrictor of splanchnic arterioles and therefore should reduce the pressure in the portal system. It does not, however, appear to be very reliable. Local pressure on the wall of the lower third of the oesophagus can be achieved by the apparatus known as the *Sengstaken tube*. This is a soft tube that is swallowed so that its tip lies in the stomach and can be used to aspirate the stomach contents. Near the tip is a small balloon which can be filled with air via its own channel, and when distended keeps the tip of the tube in the stomach. More proximally, in the lower third of the oesophagus, there is a larger balloon with its own channel through which this balloon, too, can be distended, thereby compressing the bleeding veins in the oesophageal wall. Gentle traction is applied to the tube so that the lower balloon compresses any varices in the stomach wall near the entrance to the oesophagus.

The Sengstaken tube is useful, but it can cause necrosis of the oesophageal wall so that the pressure in the oesophageal balloon must be relaxed every 6 hours.

If conservative measures fail, an emergency operation may be necessary. Emergency operations to shunt blood from the portal to the systemic venous systems carry a high mortality, and some form of direct attack upon the varices themselves is made. The available procedures include injection of the varices with sclerosant material via an oesophagoscope, opening the oesophagus via a thoracotomy and obliterating the varices with sutures, cutting across the stomach just below the oesophageal hiatus via an abdominothoracic approach and then reanastomosing (Tanner), and performing splenectomy and devascularizing the upper half of both curvatures of the stomach (Hassab). No controlled trial of these various procedures has been done, and every surgeon familiar with this field has his favourite operation.

In the ward before operation

If primary haemorrhage presents in the ward, its management is no different from that described above. The important consideration in the ward is that the patient is about to undergo an elective surgical operation at which primary haemorrhage is bound to occur, and certain measures must be taken to ensure that the patient is in the fittest possible position to withstand blood loss and is at no special risk from blood loss (due to blood dyscrasias, etc.). These problems are considered in Chapter 18.

At operation

A surgeon cannot cut tissues without shedding blood. There is therefore a heavy responsibility upon him in the operating theatre to minimize blood loss, and to minimize the deleterious effects of any blood loss. The subject can thus be considered under the headings of prophylaxis and replacement.

Prophylaxis of blood loss during the operation begins with the anaesthetist, who ensures that there is no build-up of carbon dioxide in the tissues due to underventilation — because a high partial pressure of CO_2 in the tissues produces arteriolar and capillary dilation — and no hint of obstruction to the airway — because that produces venous engorgement. The anaesthetist and surgeon then share the responsibility of positioning the patient so that, while the operation area is accessible to the surgeon, the posture chosen prevents any venous engorgement. For operations on the upper half of the body a head-up tilt enlists the help of gravity. Local pressure effects must also be avoided; for example, when performing adrenalectomy by the posterior approach, care is taken that the abdomen of the prone patient is not pressing against the operating table. The pressure is taken on the patient's chest and hips on built-up supports, leaving the abdomen suspended. This measure greatly reduces venous oozing in the operation field.

The question of arterial hypotension then arises. For operations in heavily vascularized regions of the human anatomy such as the head and neck, and particularly when fine structures such as the facial nerve have to be dissected and preserved, blood pressure lowered to the range 60–70 mmHg produces a much drier field and offers great advantages. The anaesthetist may use a variety of drugs such as ganglion-blocking agents (e.g. hexamethonium), or rely on the simpler combination of halothane, with its vasodilator effect, plus posture to make sure that the vasodilator effect occurs in the lower rather than the upper half of the body.

As the surgeon dissects, the important point of technique is that the larger blood vessels should be dissected free and controlled, by underrunning with aneurysm needles or clamping with artery forceps, before they are divided. For smaller vessels, diathermy is a great boon as it reduces the time needed compared with tying off vessels. Should bleeding occur despite these precautions, the ease with which it can be stopped usually depends upon whether it is arterial, venous or capillary. Arterial bleeding is the easiest, as the spurt of blood with each heart beat is easily seen and leads one to the origin. Venous is the most difficult, because the blood just wells up continuously into the field and there is no hint of where it arises. Of great assistance in this situation is a sucker: the suction clears away the pool of blood and allows the tear in the vein to be seen. A capillary ooze responds to pressure from a gauze pack soaked in either hot or cold saline. A high temperature speeds blood coagulation, while a low one stimulates capillary contraction. If rapid bleeding is produced from a large vessel, it is always worth taking time (at least 5 minutes) to exert pressure on the injured vessel with such a pack; after this the edges of the vessel have usually contracted considerably, the gush has become a stream and is easily stemmed.

Should circumstances enable the operator to foresee a situation which is bound to demand rapid transfusion, he warns the anaesthetist to transfuse 0.5 or 1 litre of blood just *before* the event. An example is in arterial surgery, where a prosthesis has been sewn between the two cut ends of an artery to replace the diseased or damaged segment: when the clamps that have prevented flow through the vessel during the suturing are relaxed, there is for a few minutes a rapid loss of blood through the prosthesis. Gradually the interstices of the woven material (e.g. Teflon) seal with formed elements laid down from the blood, and in 5 minutes the segment is watertight. During that period, however, a good deal of blood may have been lost and serious shock occur. Pretransfusion prevents the circulatory disturbance. A similar situation occurs when a *phaeochromocytoma* is removed, not because of blood loss but because of the removal of the abnormal catecholamine vasopressor effect produced by the tumour and a profound, though temporary, vasodilatation. Just before the last vein draining the affected adrenal gland is tied, therefore, a pretransfusion should be given.

After operation

Primary haemorrhage may of course occur as a coincidence from some new lesion after a surgical operation. Usually, however, bleeding during the same hospital admission is due to reactionary or secondary haemorrhage.

Reactionary haemorrhage

Reactionary haemorrhage is defined as bleeding from a wound (usually, but not necessarily, an operative wound) after the primary bleeding has been stopped, and within the first 24 hours. The responsible factors are technical faults, such as a ligature slipping off a vessel and permitting a recurrence of bleeding, and a rise in blood pressure.

A meticulous surgical technique is the only safeguard against the first factor. One special point needs emphasis with regard to the second factor: at the end of the manoeuvres within the wound, and before closing the superficial layers, the surgeon should ask the anaesthetist what the patient's blood pressure is. Whether or not formal hypotensive procedures have been invoked, the blood pressure is often low during general anaesthesia. The safe policy to adopt is to wait till the blood pressure has been over 110 mmHg for at least 5 minutes before closing the wound.

Special situations

Reactionary haemorrhage is particularly common after operations on the upper half of the body where the tissues have a particularly rich blood supply. In some areas, such as the limbs, it is convenient to reduce the risk of reactionary haemorrhage by pressure dressings that can be reduced to ordinary tightness after 24 hours. In areas where this technique is impossible or difficult to apply, suction-drainage is preferred. Efficient suction-drainage keeps the layers of the wounds apposed and is the equivalent of applying pressure from without: moreover, it gives early warning if reactionary haemorrhage occurs despite all precautions.

Suction-drainage is of particular value after mastectomy, and after operations on the face and neck. Reactionary haemorrhage after thyroidectomy is especially dangerous, because the pressure of a haematoma deep to the strap muscles can buckle the trachea and produce fatal obstruction of the airway. The correct treatment is immediate reopening of the wound, both skin and muscle, to let the blood exude; in serious bleeding there is no time for sterile precautions, let alone taking the patient to theatre, and a tray with suitable instruments kept at the bedside for 24 hours is part of the routine management of patients after thyroidectomy.

Secondary haemorrhage

Secondary haemorrhage occurs from a wound later than 24 hours after operation. In practice, the average time is about 10 days, with a spread of from 5 to 15 days. The cause of secondary haemorrhage is infection: enzymes produced by the micro-organisms or by the body's defences destroy the organizing clot which forms a weak point in the blood vessel at the area of the original injury, and bleeding ensues.

The prevention of secondary haemorrhage thus comprises all the measures designed to prevent infection of a wound as described in Chapter 20 (p. 247).

Special sites

As one would expect, wounds with heavy primary contamination and wounds in tissues with a relatively poor blood supply are particularly at risk. Prostatectomy is frequently complicated by haematuria about the tenth day, because it is difficult to keep a urethral catheter *in situ* for some days without permitting ascending infection to reach the raw surfaces of the prostatic cavity. Restorative or replacement surgery on blocked arteries is prone to this complication because the incision has been made through tissues that are relatively poorly perfused at the start of the operation. In most sites, secondary haemorrhage is usually not very dramatic and stops spontaneously, but secondary haemorrhage from a major artery is a catastrophe. It is often presaged by some minor leaks ('warning haemorrhage'), and even a few spots of blood should be taken seriously if there is a major artery in the depths of the wound.

Further problems

Massive blood transfusion

Blood for transfusion is stored at 4°C, its plasma contains a higher hydrogen and potassium ion concentration than normal, and it contains a high concentration of citrate as an anticoagulant. Quite apart from the possibility of overtransfusion and cardiogenic shock (see p. 265), blood transfused very rapidly in very large quantities carries the theoretical risks of refrigeration, metabolic acidosis, hyperkalaemia and depression of ionized calcium concentration in the plasma via the chelating effect of the citrate ion. Metabolic acidosis and hyperkalaemia do not appear to constitute practical difficulties; with regard to calcium, a reduction in ionized calcium can be demonstrated, but it reverts to normal as soon as the transfusion is completed, and although it is traditional to give 10 ml 10 per cent calcium gluconate injection intravenously with each 500 ml of blood transfused, this precaution is probably unnecessary.

The question of hypothermia, however, is of very real significance: the transfusion of large quantities of blood straight from the refrigerated store may reduce the temperature of the heart to below 25°C, and ventricular fibrillation is very likely to occur. It is mandatory, therefore, that if a really massive transfusion is necessary, the blood should be prewarmed to a temperature approaching blood heat by passing it through a long coil immersed in a water-bath at 38°C before being introduced into the patient's vein.

'Irreversible shock'

In Chapter 22, the circumstances in which the possibilities of steroid deficiency and septicaemic shock have to be taken into account have been described. The author's personal practice is that, if either of these diagnoses is suggested by clinical evidence, or by failure to reverse shock by manifestly adequate transfusion, then he treats the patient as probably having both conditions. Hydrocortisone 100 mg is given intravenously, and repeated after 30 minutes if there is no response from the blood pressure: otherwise, or afterwards, it is given in the same dosage at 4-hour intervals. Three separate samples of blood are sent for culture, and the bacteriologist is also asked to examine a smear of each immediately for micro-organisms. Any micro-organisms seen may, by their morphology and behaviour on Gram-staining, give valuable clues as to what antibiotics should be used. In the absence of any such clue, and until the results of any positive blood cultures are available, the patient is started on large doses intravenously of two antibiotics. The choice of these is determined by the advice of the bacteriologist, who bases his decision on knowledge of which organisms have been commonly isolated from infections in the hospital during the immediately preceding period.

At the same time (if it is not already in place) a superior caval line is inserted for the measurement of central venous pressure (CVP), and normal saline solution infused until the CVP is at least +10 cm above the manubriosternal angle.

If there is no response to these measures, and provided the CVP has been raised to the stated level and if the patient's cerebral circulatory state is clinically critical or visibly deteriorating, it is legitimate to try the effect of the α-blocker, phenoxybenzamine. It must be remembered, however, that this is a dangerous remedy which may produce sudden death.

No flow-diagram is given for Chapter 23, which discusses a number of separate clinical situations under the general heading of acute blood loss. The reader may wish to practise constructing for himself flow-diagrams to cover certain individual situations; e.g. haematemesis and postoperative bleeding.

Further reading

Cotton P.B. and Russell, R.C.G. (1977). Haematemesis and melaena. *British Medical Journal* **1** 37–9.

Gill, W., Champion. H.R., Long, W.B., Jamaris, J. and Cowley, R.A. (1975). Abdominal lavage in blunt trauma. *British Journal of Surgery* **62**, 121–4.

Gruber, U.F. (1969). *Blood Replacement*. Berlin, Heidelberg, New York, Springer-Verlag.

Gunning, A.J. (1976). Surgery in the haemorrhagic diathesis. In: *Current Surgical Practice*, Vol. 1, pp 34–46. Ed. by G.J. Hadfield and M. Hobsley, London, Edward Arnold.

Morgan, A.G., McAdam, W.A.F., Walmsley, G.L., Jessop, A., Horrocks, J.C. and de Dombal, F.T. (1977). Clinical findings, early endoscopy, and multivariate analysis in patients bleeding from the upper gastro-intestinal tract. *British Medical Journal* **2**, 237–40.

Schiller, K.F.R., Truelove, S.C. and Gwyn Williams, D. (1970). Haematemesis and melaena, with special reference to factors influencing the outcome. *British Medical Journal* **2**, 7–14.

Shields, R. (1976). The management of portal hypertension and bleeding oesophageal varices. *British Journal of Hospital Medicine*, **17**, 126–43.

Swain, C.P., Bown, S.G., Storey, D.W., Kirkham, J.S., Northfield, T.C., and Salmon, P.R. (1981). Controlled trial of argon laser photocoagulation in bleeding peptic ulcers. *Lancet* **11**, 1313–16.

Chapter 24

Head Injuries; Burns; Loss of Skin Cover

This chapter gives more detailed consideration to three very important aspects of trauma, two of which are closely related in that burns are a very important cause of loss of skin cover.

Head Injuries

Principles of routine management

The seriousness of a head injury is related more to the damage and disturbance of functions of the brain than to the extent of injury of the skull. The nature of concussion — the disturbance of consciousness resulting from brain damage — is not known. In the brains of those who fail to survive their injuries there is usually widespread contusion, especially on the inferior surfaces and at the poles of the cerebral hemispheres. However, histological changes can be remarkably insignificant and limited to chromatolysis, capillary haemorrhages and foci of microglial cells, even when the disturbance of consciousness has been profound and long-lasting. It does seem to be clear that the precipitating causes of concussion are acceleration/deceleration forces which cause the semi-liquid brain to undergo translational and rotational movements relative to its rigid bone case.

The causes of death in concussed patients are beginning to be better understood, and routine management is designed to neutralize these. There is no 'cure' for concussion, but if one can keep the patient alive there is always the possibility of spontaneous resolution. The fatal factors can be grouped as those acting remote from the skull and brain, and those acting within or in the skull.

Remote factors

Depending on the exact level of the depth of consciousness, the patient may have lost the benefit of his cough and gag reflexes, the control of micturition and defaecation, and the ability to feed himself. The risk that he will suffocate or develop bronchopneumonia as a result of inhaling foreign bodies, his own secretions or vomit, or even his tongue are prevented in the short term by hooking the tongue forwards and keeping him in the semi-prone position, but if the level of consciousness does not lighten within a few hours it is wise to pass an endotracheal tube. Should it be necessary to maintain this artificial airway for more than a few days, a tracheostomy is performed. The bladder may have to be catheterized, and the possibility that a full bladder is responsible for a marked increase in restlessness or agitation must always be remembered. Feeding can be a problem. During the first week, it is usually sufficient to replace water and electrolytes intravenously; later, provided that there is good control of the airway, the best technique is to pass a nasogastric tube into the stomach and to use it to deliver a homogenized blend of food and drink. Occasionally, the stomach rejects this food and it may be necessary to feed the patient by the intravenous route.

The deeply unconscious patient moves little in his bed and may not react even to painful stimuli. He is therefore at risk from the effects of pressure and other noxious agents in his immediate surroundings, such as heat and cold. A large pressure sore may develop rapidly and, in a critically ill patient, prove fatal. Nursing care must be meticulous, the patient's position must be changed every few hours, and special attention paid to the pressure points. If defaecation is not spontaneous the bowels can be controlled by an enema every 2 or 3 days.

Finally, a particular danger in the unconscious
patient is that he is unable to complain of any
symptoms, and therefore it is more difficult for
his medical attendant to make sure that there is
nothing else seriously wrong such as an intraperitoneal haemorrhage (p. 275).

Cranial and cerebral factors

While the injury to the skull is of little importance compared with the injury to the brain as a
general rule, there are circumstances in which it
can threaten life. A depressed fracture of the
skull very rarely presses on the underlying brain,
and then should be elevated as a matter of
urgency. Usually, however, depressed fractures
are compound: a fracture of the skull that brings
the subarachnoid space into communication with
the exterior renders possible the serious complication of meningitis by direct spread of micro-
organisms from the exterior. Therefore the usual
emergency management is to cut the hair away
around the fracture, remove any loose foreign
bodies or bone fragments, excise the skin edges,
apply a pressure dressing to exclude infection
and control bleeding, and give antibiotic cover.
A serosanguinous discharge from the ear or the
nose, in association with radiological evidence of
a fractured base of skull, is an urgent indication
for penicillin or ampicillin, together with a
sulphonamide. Sometimes the leak of cerebrospinal fluid is persistent and an operation has to
be performed to close the defect.

For the most part, the danger lies in the brain
damage. Occasionally this damage is, from the
outset, so severe that it is impossible for the
patient to recover. However, it is now clear that
there are a number of factors which tend to
aggravate the initial damage, and the surgeon
must guard against these. They all seem to be
concerned with raised intracranial pressure, and
consist of intracranial haematoma, swelling of
the brain inself, and hydrocephalus. The first
two of these factors usually arise acutely, during
the first few hours or days, although a chronic
form of subdural haematoma is notorious
because it is difficult to diagnose. Hydrocephalus
is a more chronic and delayed complication that
one does not seriously consider till two weeks
have passed (see below).

It can be difficult to distinguish between the
effects of a localized haematoma and those of a
generalized swelling of the brain itself. In both
cases there is a deterioration in level of consciousness and a tendency for the blood pressure
to rise and the pulse rate to fall as a result of
brain stem compression and tentorial impaction.
The respiratory centre is at first stimulated,
resulting in hyperventilation, but later there is
respiratory depression. A unilateral haematoma
tends to produce a fixed dilated pupil on the
same side, but may produce this change on both
sides, while brain swelling usually produces
bilateral pupil changes but can sometimes produce unilateral or at least asymmetric changes.

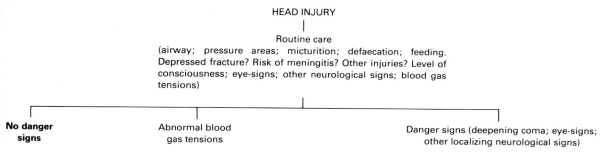

The routine care of the unconscious patient,
apart from the features described under the
heading of 'Remote factors', above, therefore
consists of frequent (quarter-hourly at first)
observations of conscious level, pulse rate, blood
pressure, respiratory rate and character, and the
size of the pupils and their reaction to light. In
the majority (perhaps 90 per cent) of patients the
period of unconsciousness is brief and indeed
may have already passed before the patient is
admitted to hospital. Because of the risk of later
deterioration due to such factors as haemorrhage
or brain swelling, the observations should be
continued for, say, 24 hours after full consciousness is regained.

The length of time that the patient should be
kept in hospital depends on the surgeon's
assessment of the severity of the injury to the

brain. Apart from the length of the period of unconsciousness, a good pointer is the duration of retrograde amnesia; i.e. for how long before the accident has the patient a blank in his memory? Anything longer than a few minutes of retrograde amnesia signifies serious brain damage, and if such a patient is allowed to return too soon to his normal activities the likelihood of chronic complaints of headache, irritability, loss of concentration and lapses of memory is high. It is fair to add that retrograde amnesia sometimes seems to be related to the progress of a claim for compensation.

Early recognition of any change in the level of consciousness is facilitated by using a numerical or alphabetical code for different levels. For example: 0 might be fully conscious and orientated; 1 = conscious but disorientated; 2 = confused but still responsive to the spoken word; 3 = responsive to touch but not the spoken word; 4 = responsive only to pain; 5 = unresponsive to all external stimuli; 6 = decerebrate rigidity.

There is one more investigation that should be performed routinely in the unconscious patient: the measurement of blood gas levels.

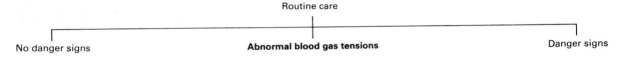

Routine care

No danger signs | Abnormal blood gas tensions | Danger signs

Indications for more active measures

One bears in mind the tendency in most cases towards spontaneous resolution, and the real possibility that any active measure might do harm rather than good. Nevertheless, evidence of deterioration, or of a failure to improve after a reasonable interval (whether or not there has been any preceding improvement), or of the presence of a factor that is likely to produce deterioration, is an indication for a more active approach.

The blood gas measurements can provide valuable evidence. Hyperventilation, with an arterial carbon dioxide tension less than 25 mmHg, indicates an early disturbance of the respiratory centre, while a raised value of 50 mmHg or more indicates hypoventilation and probably more advanced damage. Hypoxaemia, an arterial oxygen tension less than 70 mmHg, whatever its cause, is another danger signal. Both hypercapnia and hypoxaemia tend to cause swelling of the brain, and so aggravate the cerebral damage by increasing intracranial pressure. Such abnormal blood gas tensions are an indication for endotracheal intubation or tracheostomy (if not already performed) and controlled ventilation to adjust the arterial blood gas tensions to the normal range.

Even if the blood gas tensions are normal, controlled ventilation has been advocated for patients with a proved markedly raised intracranial pressure (see below) or who are subject to convulsions or decerebrate spasms.

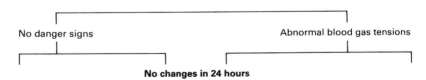

No danger signs | Abnormal blood gas tensions

No changes in 24 hours

If the above features are absent but the patient's level of consciousness does not change for some time, say 24 hours, it seems reasonable to try to reduce intracranial pressure. Logically, one should measure the pressure first, so that the condition can be accurately diagnosed and its response to treatment quantified. This can be done by making exploratory burr holes in the frontal region and via these inserting a ventricular catheter or an epidural or subdural trans-

ducer. Epidural transducers are used more often than subdural and carry less risk of infection than an intraventricular catheter. This procedure is therefore in some centres performed routinely in all patients with severe head injuries, while others reserve the technique for patients whose conscious level is deteriorating, or in whom the burr holes are in any case indicated because of the clinical suspicion of an intracranial haematoma.

Methods for the reduction of intracranial pressure include hyperosomotic agents, corticosteroids and controlled ventilation.

Hyperosmotic agents

The two drugs most commonly used are urea and mannitol, each given intravenously to produce a diuresis and consequent dehydration of all tissues, including the brain. Each drug has its protagonists: urea is reliable in its effect and lasts for 8 hours, but has more complications than mannitol, the effect of which lasts only 5 hours.

Corticosteroids

The rationale for these drugs is that they have anti-inflammatory properties, and they do seem to have a good effect in reducing cerebral oedema around abscesses or tumours in the brain. However, their value in patients with head injury is more controversial.

Controlled ventilation

If the intracranial pressure is above 30 mmHg and the use of drugs has failed to reduce this pressure, it is reasonable to try the effect of controlled ventilation. In expert hands the technique has often proved valuable.

In some centres thiopentone is given hourly to deeply unconscious patients who are being therapeutically ventilated. It is said that thiopentone reduces the metabolic requirements of injured neurones, particularly in the presence of cerebral oedema, and thereby reduces the level of permanent brain damage.

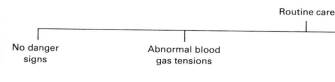

Routine care

No danger signs   Abnormal blood gas tensions   **Danger signs** (deepening coma; eye-signs; other localizing neurological signs)

The problem of intracranial haematoma

The clear-cut case of a patient with lateralizing eye-signs and deteriorating conscious level requires urgent exploration for an intracranial haematoma that has probably arisen in the extradural space. However, in such cases the lesion has probably produced a great deal of brain damage already that might have been avoided had the diagnosis been made earlier. The possibility of an intracranial haematoma also has to be considered if a patient fails to respond to measures designed to lower intracranial pressure, or does respond and then relapses.

In the last resort, burr holes must be made, but if there is no indication for urgency (the patient's condition is static or only slowly deteriorating) there is a case for lesser investigations first. These include plain x-rays (the shift of a calcified pineal from the mid-line may indicate a haematoma), and ultrasonography and carotid angiography, but undoubtedly the big advance in this field is transaxial computerized tomography (the CT-scan). In this technique the resistance of individual zones of the field under examination to the passage of x-rays arriving in different directions is built up by computer-performed calculations into a composite picture of the

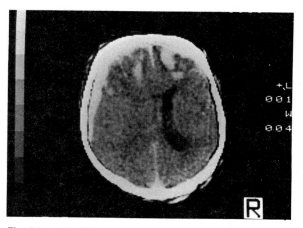

Fig. 24.1 The CT-scan is an axial section from a man aged 60 taken 24-hours after head injury. Skull x-ray showed a linear fracture at the vertex and the scan was performed because of deterioration in the level of consciousness.

There is a high density extracerebral, apparently subdural haematoma over the left frontal and anterior parietal convexity. There are multiple haemorrhages into contused frontal lobes, which are more extensive on the left side. There is compression of the left lateral ventricle, with shift of the mid-line towards the right, and some dilatation of the right lateral ventricle.

Recent blood clots are of high density and appear white on CT. Note the large amount of information that this technique can provide. (Provided by Dr Brian Kendall.)

densities of the tissues. In this way the relatively small difference in density between one soft tissue and another (for example, brain and haematoma) is emphasized sufficiently to produce an image in which the boundary between the one and the other can be seen. In any centre in which this machine is available, it is routine for this investigation to be used in any patient who has sustained a head injury but is not obviously improving. Being non-invasive and relatively simple to perform it can be used repeatedly to assess changes, as well as for initial assessment (Fig. 24.1 see p. 285).

Burr holes

In patients where burr holes are deemed necessary because of failure to improve with measures to reduce intracranial pressure, or because it is felt necessary to measure intracranial pressure or to exclude an intracranial haematoma without direct evidence of its presence or because of evidence from CT-scanning, it should be a neurosurgeon who makes this difficult decision and takes the necessary action. The placing of such burr holes will depend upon the neurosurgeon's judgement of the best sites in relation to his own experience, the nature of the patient's injury and the details of the clinical picture.

By contrast, every surgical resident who is responsible for the first-line management of emergency admissions must be prepared to deal with the extreme emergency of an extradural haematoma. The patient's deterioration may well be so rapid as to leave no time for seeking a neurosurgical opinion. The burr hole should be made on the side of the dilated pupil, or (if there is no help from the eye-signs) on the side of a fracture of the temporal bone in the region of the middle meningeal artery. The surface marking for the burr hole is a point 5 cm above the mid-point of a line joining the front of the external auditory meatus to the lateral angle of the orbit. Enough bone is nibbled away from the circumference of the burr hole to enable clot to be evacuated and the bleeding arrested. There should be no hesitation about repeating the process on the other side if no clot has been found on the first side, and to make burr holes at the site of maximal bruising of the scalp which is likely to be the site of the fracture which has caused the extradural haemorrhage.

Prolonged unconsciousness

Naturally, the longer the period of unconsciousness, the more remote the chance of complete recovery. Youth is a favourable prognostic feature, while fixity of the pupils for more than 48 hours, decerebrate rigidity with paralysis of all four limbs for 1 month, or the absence of any improvement in the first month, are all unfavourable. As time passes, and the hopes of relatives and medical attendants ebb, it becomes even more difficult to spot factors which might be inhibiting recovery. Even at a late stage, one must remember the possibility of a chronic subdural haematoma in particular as a cause of failure to recover. Recently, another possible factor has become manifest — hydrocephalus. There is no doubt that some patients do develop this complication after a severe head injury, sometimes not till months or years have passed. Signs of rising intracranial pressure may indicate the need for computer-assisted tomography and thus lead to the demonstration of ventricular dilatation. In such patients the treatment of the hydrocephalus by inserting an artificial shunt between the ventricle and the peritoneum can lead to useful improvement. However, in patients in whom hydrocephalus can be demonstrated although there is no demonstrable increase in intracranial pressure, shunting is less likely to result in any improvement. Single readings of CSF pressures may be normal, but continuous recording over 2 or 3 days may demonstrate spikes or plateaux of raised intracranial pressure.

Of all patients who have been unconscious more than a month, about half ultimately die of their head injury. Of the remainder, about one quarter end up with a complete recovery or only minimal disability, one-half have a definite residual disability but can live a useful life, and the remaining quarter are more or less completely dependent. The care of these last is a burden to their relatives or the appropriate institution, but this is a price that society must willingly pay for the reclamation of the other three-quarters, since there is usually no way of deciding at the beginning into which group an individual will ultimately fall.

Flow-chart 24.1

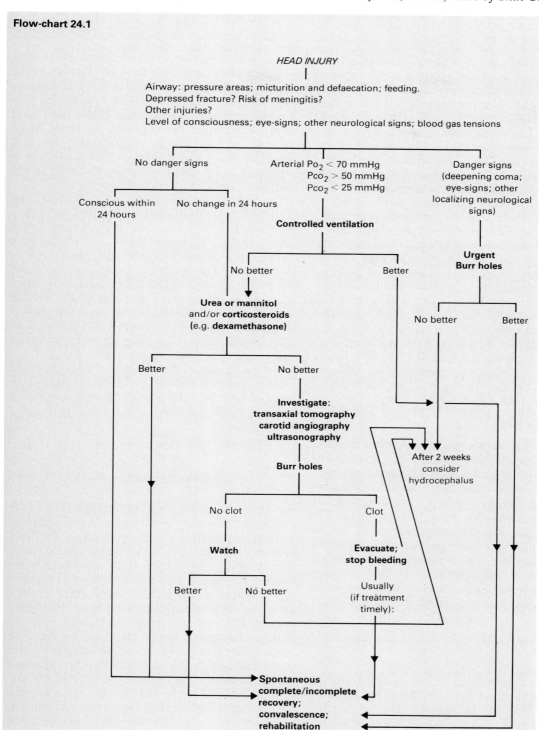

Burns

A burn is usually thought about as an injury due to exposure to heat, but several other types of physical agent produce very similar lesions: cold, light and other electromagnetic radiations such as x-rays, and chemicals such as caustic alkalis and acids. The distinguishing characteristic of a burn is the rapid destruction of an area of the superficial tissues (skin or mucous membrane) which, at least at first, is large compared to the depth to which the agent penetrates. Since the prognosis is strongly influenced by the depth of the injury, urgent steps to limit the action of the agent are required. In the common burn due to heat, if the part involved is small enough for this to be feasible, it should be immersed in cold water or otherwise cooled as quickly as possible. Chemicals should be washed off the burned surface in chemical burns, and this mechanical action is probably much more effective than a chemical antidote such as a weak alkali for acid burns, especially if one has to wait for the antidote. The exposure to radiation, if still continuing, must be stopped immediately. Unfortunately, by the time the patient reaches a doctor the time for such action is often past.

Threats to life

The burns may be combined with other forms of injury and these may constitute their own threat to life. From the viewpoint of the burns themselves, the most immediate threat comes from burns from flaming vapours such as petroleum, since the patient may have inhaled these. The resulting acute inflammatory oedema of the respiratory passages may produce acute anoxia, and an immediate tracheostomy may be needed. If the burns extend right down to the pulmonary alveoli, the resulting pulmonary oedema may be so severe as to be irremediable and rapidly fatal.

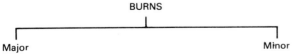

The other urgent threat to life results from the acute disturbance of the body fluids produced by the burn. One of the normal functions of the integument is to limit the loss of water by evaporation from the surface: when the effect of the destruction of an area of the body surface is added to the effect of damage to capillaries in the less severely affected subjacent and adjacent zones, with resultant exudation into the neighbouring tissues, it is clear that the primary effect of a burn is to cause a loss of water and electrolytes and plasma proteins. The rate of this loss depends primarily on the area of the burn, and hardly at all upon the depth of the burn. Since the rate of loss can be considerable, so that oligaemic shock can develop within 1 hour, it is important to be able to estimate the area of the burn with speed and reasonable accuracy.

The 'rule of nines' is useful in this context. The head and neck, each upper limb, and separately the front half and the back half of each lower limb, severally represent 9 per cent of the total surface area, while the trunk represents 4 x 9 = 36 per cent. This estimate leaves 1 per cent for the perineum and external genitalia. Any burn affecting as much as 20 per cent of the surface area of an adult, or 10 per cent of the surface area of an infant, will almost certainly need an intravenous infusion to keep up with the losses and allow for normal requirements.

For minor burns, it is usually sufficient to make certain that the patient increases his intake of fluids above the normal and takes a nourishing diet.

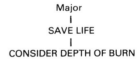

For major burns, the nature and quantity of replacement by the intravenous route can be worked out from first principles along the lines indicated in Chapter 22. However, the disturbance produced by a burn is so reproducibly related to its surface area that a number of regimes are available which yield a fairly accurate estimate of the requirements in any individual patient. For example, Muir and Barclay estimate that in the first 4 hours after the burning, an adult patient requires a volume of plasma (in millilitres) given by multiplying the patient's weight in kilograms by half the percentage surface area of the burn, and that the same volume will be needed in each of the second and third 4-hour periods. After this the rate of exudation of plasma protein into the wound usually lessens, but it proceeds at about half the initial rate for a further 24 hours at least, i.e. until 36 hours after the injury. The basal intake of normal saline and

5 per cent dextrose (p. 222) must be continued throughout this period, and experience shows that deep burns (see later) require some blood as well.

Notwithstanding such calculations, the patient's clinical condition, especially the central venous pressure and the urine output via a catheter in the bladder, must be taken into consideration and the scheme modified appropriately. The serial measurement of haematocrit is particularly useful in assessing the loss of plasma. For comments on the possible value of diuretics in preventing renal damage in shocked patients, see p. 181.

The problem of infection

The dead burned tissue is an excellent medium for the growth of micro-organisms, and once these have become established the patient lives with the ever-present threat of septicaemia. Moreover, some organisms have a particularly deleterious effect locally by deepening the burn: the β-haemolytic Streptococcus is the worst offender in this respect, and skin grafts will not take in its presence. The common organisms are *Pseudomonas aeruginosa* and the coagulase-positive Staphylococcus. Since infection is inevitable until the wound has become covered by living skin, the achievement of skin cover at the earliest possible moment is the aim of the local treatment of the burn.

It is with respect to the healing process that the depth of the burn is of crucial importance. The presence of only erythema and blistering defines a superficial burn: healing is spontaneous and rapid. If all sources of epithelium have been destroyed, the burn is said to be deep. Spontaneous regeneration of skin can occur only from the edges of the burn, and in anything like a sizeable burn the restoration of skin cover will take a long time. Some form of skin grafting is therefore essential. On the other hand, if islands of epithelium are still viable in the form of the linings of sweat and sebaceous glands, hair follicles, etc., regeneration takes place from these islands and the process of healing is greatly accelerated. Such burns are said to be partial-thickness burns, and grafting is not necessary.

CONSIDER DEPTH OF BURN

Deep burn, small area   Deep burn, large area; mixed burns   Superficial burns

The principle of local management may thus be said to be: encourage the spontaneous healing of partial-thickness burns, especially by limiting infection; but excise slough from full-thickness burns as soon as possible and replace their cover with a suitable skin graft. The snag is that it may be difficult or impossible to distinguish between partial- and full-thickness burns in the early stages. Theoretically, a pin-prick should elicit pain in an area of partial-thickness burn, but no pain from an area of full-thickness loss. Since the patient may be shocked and in severe pain from his injuries at first, even great care and patience on the part of the examiner may fail to yield the distinction in the early stages. It may, of course, be obvious that certain areas of the burn are deep, but nearly always there are also some areas of doubtful depth. It is unusual, therefore, that a burn can immediately be totally excised and grafted, although the occasional deep electrical burn, often sharply demarcated and localized to the region of contact with the electrical apparatus that caused the injury, can be treated in this ideal way.

In most cases, one waits: prophylactic oral or systemic antibiotics are given to reduce the chance of septicaemia. The nature of this antibiotic cover should be decided in consultation with the bacteriologist, in the light of information about prevalent organisms. The burns themselves are treated by one of two methods: exposure or dressings.

Exposure of the burn rapidly leads to coagulation and the formation of a solid crust of dead tissue and exudate. This crust is inevitably infected, but its dryness prevents too free a penetration of organisms into the living tissues beneath. Dressings, on the other hand, are moist, but seek to lower bacterial contamination by their content of antiseptic or antibiotic agents. The consensus of opinion favours dressings for most patients, but there are factors which demand the use of exposure. For example, the very young and the very old may be restless and unco-operative, and it may be difficult to keep the dressings in place. Certain regions are also more suited to exposure; for example, the face and the perineum. The most popular antibacterial agent to use in the dressings at the moment is silver sulphadiazine.

Whichever method is used, a solid eschar or slough forms in the area of full-thickness burns, while spontaneous re-epithelialization occurs in the area of partial-thickness burn. In the case of full-thickness circumferential burns of a limb or digit, the tendency for this eschar to contract may produce a strangulating effect on the tissues distal to the eschar, and it is necessary to slit the eschar longitudinally in such cases – a painless procedure.

Opinions differ as to whether the eschar should be excised as soon as there is a clear demarcation from the area of partial-thickness burn, or whether it should be left to separate sponta-neously or with the help of a desloughing agent such as eusol in paraffin. The modern tendency seems to be towards more aggressive treatment, because of the continuing threat of septicaemia until healing has been achieved. Even before the demarcation of the slough is obvious, some sur-geons use a technique called tangential grafting to assist in distinguishing the area that needs grafting. Larger and larger tangential slices are cut from the region of the centre of the burn until the presence of bleeding points at the peri-phery indicates that the zone of partial-thickness burn has been reached.

Once the slough has been removed, provided that the bacteriology of the wound is favourable (*Ps. aeruginosa* in particular produces a large purulent exudate that floats the graft off), a skin graft is applied.

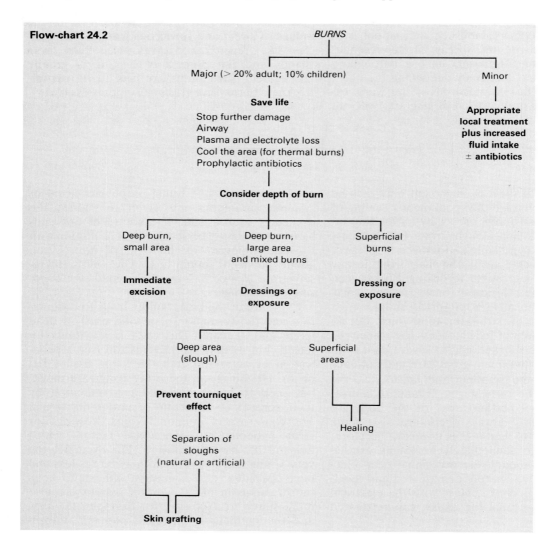

Flow-chart 24.2

BURNS

Major (> 20% adult; 10% children) — Minor

Save life
Stop further damage
Airway
Plasma and electrolyte loss
Cool the area (for thermal burns)
Prophylactic antibiotics

Minor: **Appropriate local treatment plus increased fluid intake ± antibiotics**

Consider depth of burn

Deep burn, small area — Deep burn, large area and mixed burns — Superficial burns

Deep burn, small area: **Immediate excision**

Deep burn, large area and mixed burns: **Dressings or exposure**

Superficial burns: **Dressing or exposure**

Deep area (slough) — Superficial areas

Deep area (slough): **Prevent tourniquet effect** → Separation of sloughs (natural or artificial)

Superficial areas: Healing

Skin grafting

Loss of skin cover

Skin grafts are partial thickness or full thickness; another form of full-thickness cover is provided by pedicled skin flaps. Defects of muscle together with the overlying skin can be repaired with myocutaneous flaps. Finally, free transfer of a variety of tissues from remote areas can be achieved using microvascular techniques for anastomosing small vessels.

Partial-thickness (Thiersch) grafts

These are cut to such a thickness that islands of epithelium are left intact in the deeper layers of the epidermis, in sweat and sebaceous glands and hair follicles, so that the lesion produced by cutting the graft is comparable to a partial-thickness burn (p. 289). In consequence, the area from which the graft has been taken (the donor area) heals spontaneously by regeneration from these islands.

Partial-thickness grafts survive by diffusion of nutrients from the recipient area into the graft, until new blood vessels grow into the graft. It is the thinness of the graft which makes survival likely. The thinner the graft, the more likely it is to survive but the less good the cosmetic result.

Normally, partial-thickness grafts are used where the cosmetic result is not important (in non-exposed areas of the body), and where the grafted area is unlikely to be subjected to much wear and tear. They are not suitable for areas bearing weight or exposed to friction. Because of their high incidence of taking, they are also used in the first instance to provide early cover in emergency situations such as burns, where factors such as infection might militate against the survival of a thicker graft, even though subsequently a full-thickness graft may need to be substituted as a definitive procedure.

In cases where large areas of skin have been lost (e.g. major burns) the patient's convenient donor areas may not suffice to give complete skin cover. In such situations, Thiersch grafts are cut very thinly from the available areas so that they will heal rapidly and shortly provide a second crop of skin grafts, and the grafts are cut into small pieces ('postage stamp grafts') and laid on the donor area with spaces between them, thus eking out the grafts to the required area. Other techniques include the use of skin from related donors (i.e. relatives who volunteer) or

from animals such as the pig. Such grafts are ultimately rejected by immunological mechanisms, but by that time the second crop may be ready.

Full-thickness grafts

Free skin grafts are only likely to succeed if they are fairly small: since they have been completely cut off from their normal blood supply and have to survive by diffusion till a new blood supply grows into them, their greater thickness compared with Thiersch grafts greatly limits their area. For practical purposes, their use is restricted to recipient areas that enjoy an excellent blood supply, such as the face. Ovals of skin, of full thickness but carefully cleansed of all fatty tissue because the latter has a very poor blood supply, may be obtained from the loose skin behind the pinna, or immediately below the clavicle. The resulting defect in the skin is easily closed by primary suture. The upper limit in size for a full-thickness free graft (Wolfe graft) is about 6 x 2.5 cm.

Pedicled skin flaps

Pedicled skin flaps retain a portion of their normal blood supply at one end, while their free portion is rotated or otherwise rearranged into the position of the defect. Unless the base of the pedicle has been constructed so as to include a generous blood supply from a neighbouring artery, it is a safe rule that the length of the flap should not exceed two and a half times the width of the base. However, in particularly vascular areas such as the scalp this ratio can safely be exceeded. The area left denuded by raising the flap can sometimes be closed by primary suture, or else a Thiersch graft is used. In the latter case it follows that the flap should be so designed that the donor area is suitable for covering by a partial-thickness graft, on cosmetic and mechanical grounds.

In cases where a full-thickness flap is needed of rather larger dimensions than can safely be raised in one step, the surgeon may use the technique of the delayed flap. A quadrilateral pedicle is raised along its length, but left attached at both ends, and the resulting defect is closed suitably. Only after several days have passed and the pedicle has recovered from the trauma of the operation and developed an enhanced blood supply from its two ends is it detached from one end and swung into its new position on the donor site.

Moving the pedicled flap from the nearest suitable donor site, where the skin has the requisite qualities, to the recipient area may require ingenuity or staged operations. Sometimes use can be made of the mobility of one portion of the body relative to another. For example, the patient can be confined to bed and a pedicle from one calf can be applied to the opposite shin, or a denuded finger can be buried in a tube raised from the anterior abdominal wall. Sometimes, however, it is necessary to swing a pedicled flap and attach its free end to a new site intermediate between the donor and recipient areas, and after a new blood supply has developed through this new site of attachment the latter is used as the base of a new rotation to or towards the donor site.

Partial-thickness and free full-thickness grafts are techniques that the general surgeon should be prepared to tackle, but the pedicled flap requires special expertise if acceptable results are to be obtained: if possible, the help of a plastic surgeon should be sought when a pedicled skin flap appears to be indicated. There is no question but that such help is mandatory if the more complex procedures described below are under consideration.

Myocutaneous flaps

It has recently become recognized that skin derives most of its blood supply from the same blood vessels that nourish the subjacent muscle. In some areas the arterial supply and venous drainage of a large muscle mass is conveniently concentrated in a pedicle of a single artery and vein. It is then feasible to mobilize a large block of the muscle and its overlying skin, leaving the nutrient artery and vein attached, and displace the mobilized tissues to repair the defect. An example is the use of the latissimus dorsi to construct a new breast after mastectomy.

Vascularized free-transfer grafts

The principle of myocutaneous flaps can be extended by modern techniques for anastomosing small vessels, using the improved vision provided by the operating microscope. The feeding artery and vein of the mobilized tissue can be anastomosed to any suitable artery and vein in the neighbourhood of the defect. This makes the method independent of the necessity for keeping intact the vascular pedicle of the graft, and tissue (including even nervous tissue – for example, a portion of the anterior tibial nerve to repair a defect in the facial nerve) can be moved with its blood supply from any available donor site to virtually any site of the body where there is a deficiency of tissue.

These last two paragraphs cover very exciting recent advances, and to the author's mind constitute in a very real sense the major growth area of the subject.

Further reading

Head injury

Harrison, M. J. G. (1976). The diagnosis of brain death. *British Journal of Hospital Medicine* 16, 320–23.

Lewin, W. (1976). Changing attitudes to the management of head injuries. *British Medical Journal* 2, 1234–9.

Potter, J. M. (1974). *The Practical Management of Head Injuries*, 3rd edn. London, Lloyd-Luke.

Burns

Lawrence, J. C. (1974). The healing of tangentially excised and grafted burns. *Burns* 1, 75–82.

Lynch, J. B. (1973). Thermal burns. In: *Plastic Surgery. A concise guide to clinical practice*, 2nd edn., Chapter 24. Ed. by W. C. Grabb and J. W. Smith. Boston, Little, Brown.

Muir, I. F. K. and Barclay, R. L. (1974). *Burns and their Treatment*, 2nd edn. London, Lloyd-Luke.

Chapter 25

An Approach to the 'Acute Abdomen'

Every doctor knows what he means by an 'acute abdomen', but a formal definition is rarely attempted. This is a pity, because to be able to define a phenomenon is at least to begin to understand it.

The most important point about the 'acute abdomen' is that every case is potentially lethal. Starting from this basic fact, one may attempt the definition that *'the acute abdomen' is any situation in which the patient complains of acute abdominal symptoms that suggest a disease which definitely, or possibly, threatens life.*

This definition begs the question of what one means by *acute*: there is no really satisfactory answer, but on the basis that a patient with an untreated acute abdomen is either dead or better in a week, one might say that *acute* means that the history, or the recent exacerbation of symptoms, has lasted less than 8 days.

The advantage of the definition of acute abdomen given above is that it focuses attention on the acute abdomen as a threat to life.

The menaces

Death from acute intra-abdominal disease results basically from sepsis or from *acute disturbances of the body fluids*, i.e. losses of blood, plasma or saline. Bleeding may result from trauma to the abdominal wall or to the intra-abdominal viscera, or it may result from the erosion of blood vessels by disease. Plasma and saline losses result from peritonitis, which may be due to infection entering the peritoneum from the exterior, to rupture of a hollow viscus, or to liberation of inflammatory agents into the peritoneal cavity from some other source (e.g. the pancreas). Rupture of a hollow viscus, in turn, may be due to trauma, to localized disease, or to a raised intraluminal pressure consequent upon obstruction of the lumen with accumulation of the secretions of the viscus proximal to the block. Intestinal obstruction alone can produce disturbances of the body fluids other than blood. Even when peritonitis is primarily non-infective, secondary infection may occur. All these factors are heavily interrelated, but consideration of this in this way provides clues for the general practitioner who has to decide whether to send a patient up to hospital as an emergency admission.

General practice

For every one patient with a 'real' acute abdomen, the general practitioner probably sees ten with acute abdominal symptoms which turn out to be self-limiting. Unless he is to bombard the hospital with a mass of unnecessary work, he must develop criteria for recognizing the 'real' case, or at least for recognizing that the chance of real trouble is too high to be accepted in the patient's home. Certain criteria arise from our consideration of the menaces. There are three situations in which it is essential that the patient should be transferred to hospital, and three further which suggest that referral be carefully considered.

Trauma

A patient with any abdominal symptom following trauma must be immediately referred to hospital. Trauma that has destroyed the integrity of the abdominal wall, thereby opening the way into the peritoneum for external infection, is an obvious example, but blunt trauma is notorious for producing delayed rupture of solid viscera (such as the spleen) with bleeding, or of hollow viscera (such as the duodenum) with perforation and peritonitis. Even the mildest nausea, diarrhoea or abdominal pain after trauma therefore makes it essential that the patient be transferred to hospital. There should be no exception to this rule, no matter how trivial the trauma may appear to have been. In any patient with unexplained abdominal symptoms and signs, inquire carefully about a history of trauma, perhaps mild and forgotten, during the previous week.

Shock (see Chapter 22)

This feature, too, makes referral to hospital mandatory. The statement applies just as much to patients without as to patients with abdominal symptoms. Every case of shock except the vasovagal attack needs a hospital admission, even if the curative measure (as, for example, the adrenaline in anaphylactic shock) has been taken immediately by the general practitioner. The importance of stipulating shock, however, is that in the presence of abdominal symptoms the practitioner will look very closely for minor degrees of peripheral circulatory failure which might otherwise escape notice. For example, after superficial veins have been emptied by external pressure they might be slow to refill.

Disturbance of body fluids

Whether or not the features of shock are sufficiently pronounced to be recognizable, any evidence of extracellular depletion constitutes grounds for referral. Minor degrees of loss of skin elasticity, or clear-cut evidence of oliguria, require assessment in hospital.

The preceding three factors have had all-or-none significance. The remaining three are more difficult to interpret, and require modification in the light of other considerations.

Obstruction

If a reasonable suspicion of obstruction of the bowel arises, the patient should be referred to hospital. The clinical features of intestinal obstruction are colicky abdominal pain, nausea, vomiting, abdominal distension and constipation (see p. 308). Many patients, particularly children, with gastroenteritis have all these features except that constipation is replaced by diarrhoea. The presence of diarrhoea should therefore distinguish between these two diagnoses. Unfortunately, diarrhoea may occur in intestinal obstruction (spurious diarrhoea, p. 138) so that the distinction is not clear-cut.

Obstruction of other hollow viscera usually gives fairly characteristic clinical pictures (e.g. gall bladder pain, renal colic, uterine colic), and also constitute grounds for admission except in the case of labour pains where the delivery has been arranged to take place at home. Details of these patterns are given in Chapters 26, 27, 28.

Peritonitis

The advanced case of generalized peritonitis is obvious, but the early case, or the case of localized peritonitis, may give much more difficulty. The cardinal features are constant abdominal pain, tenderness and guarding; other features are described below (p. 302). In equivocal cases of peritonitis, or of obstruction, the final principle of *time* may make up the practitioner's mind for him.

Time

Any acute abdominal symptom that goes on long enough should result in referral to hospital as an emergency. Obviously it can be difficult to describe how long is enough. The doctor has to gauge the severity of the symptoms on a sliding scale against time. A patient with really severe abdominal pain will need to be admitted at once, whereas milder obscure symptoms can be watched. A safe rule is that unexplained abdominal symptoms which are no better at a second consultation 24 hours after the first constitute grounds for admission.

Hospital: basic evaluation

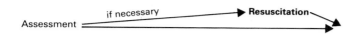

Resuscitation

The three principles of management of patients following physical trauma apply no less to examples of the acute abdomen. Any threat to life naturally takes precedence over all other considerations, including even the question of the diagnosis of the underlying condition.

In patients with acute abdominal symptoms, any immediate threat to life usually comes from haemorrhage or from plasma or saline depletion. The recognition and differential diagnosis of these conditions are discussed in Chapter 22. In most patients, however, the hypovolaemia is less severe and its correction can be undertaken more gradually, and concurrently with the working out of as exact a diagnosis as possible. Further observations on the management of shock in abdominal cases are given in subsequent sections of this Chapter.

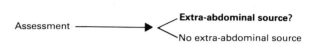

Extra-abdominal sources

It is a good rule that the surgeon presented with an acute abdominal problem should always consider, at an early stage, the possibility that the signs and symptoms are derived from a source outside the abdomen, or are manifestations of a systemic disease that does not require an abdominal operation. Failure to apply this rule is bound to result in a mistake one day, even though most patients with acute abdominal symptoms and signs have an intra-abdominal cause.

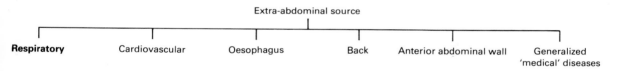

Respiratory system

The anterior abdominal wall is innervated by the lower six intercostal nerves as well as the first lumbar nerve, and in consequence a disturbance in the chest can produce referred pain and tenderness related to the abdomen. Careful clinical examination of the chest, and a plain radiograph whenever possible, should precede a definitive diagnosis and, particularly, a laparotomy. An important source of confusion is a lobar pneumo-nia affecting the right base in a child, with consequent pain and tenderness in the right lower quadrant of the abdomen. Acute appendicitis is inevitably suspected, especially as physical signs in the chest may be very slight in an early basal pneumonia. However, the true diagnosis may be suggested by a tinge of cyanosis, or by activity of the accessory muscles of respiration producing, for example, working of the *alae nasi*. The reverse situation may also arise: acute cholecystitis may mimic a right lower lobar pneumonia.

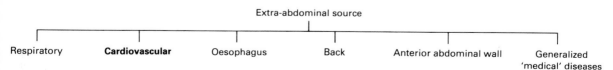

Cardiovascular system

Pain due to ischaemia of cardiac muscle is typically felt behind the sternum, and radiates as a constricting band around both sides of the chest, upwards to the jaw, and along both arms, particularly the left. Occasionally, the pattern of distribution of the pain is atypical: it concentrates on the lower retrosternal and the subjacent epigastric region and may lack its typical upward radiation. In such circumstances it is easily confused with upper abdominal pain (see p. 95 and Chapter 27) and may give rise to the possibly calamitous decision of inflicting an unnecessary laparotomy, with all its increased strain on cardiac and peripheral circulatory performance, on a patient who is already suffering from a myocardial infarction.

There is no easy way of avoiding this mischance. Certainly any suggestion of cardiogenic shock should result in a request for the opinion of a physician. Beyond that, any symptom or sign that might originate in the cardiovascular system must be carefully assessed, and any patient with the picture of upper abdominal pain who does not fit into a clearly defined surgical pigeon-hole should be considered as a possible example of this problem.

In practical terms, before summoning a physician it will save time to get a plain chest radiograph and an electrocardiogram performed, and to send a sample of blood for subsequent enzyme studies. The choice of enzymes measured depends on those used by the local laboratory for identifying the products of degeneration of cardiac muscle; e.g. aspartate aminotransferase (AST).

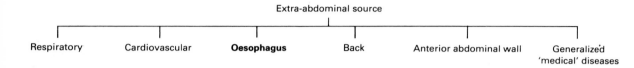

Oesophagus

The oesophagus, mostly an extra-abdominal structure, may on rare occasions cause confusion because oesophageal pain tends to have a similar distribution to cardiac pain, and like cardiac pain may be preponderantly epigastric. The causes of acute oesophageal pain include oesophageal spasm, acute peptic oesophagitis and peptic ulceration of the oesophagus.

Oesophageal spasm usually has an antecedent history: an immediate bout of gastronomic excess, truncal vagotomy, or pregnancy. The radiological appearance on swallowing an opaque meal, taken in conjunction with the very acute history, should be diagnostic. The peptic lesions may be much more difficult to diagnose from the clinical picture, and may result in an exploratory laparotomy that fails to identify the cause. Characteristically, however, these lesions are accompanied by dysphagia, which should lead to oesophago-gastroscopy.

Bleeding from the lower oesophagus may be the source of haematemesis or melaena, and is considered on p. 276.

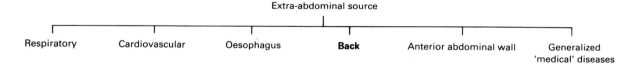

The back

The lower thoracic and first lumbar nerves can be directly irritated by pressure, direct trauma, or inflammatory changes in the spinal structures (cord, canal, and column) or paraspinal muscle masses. Possible lesions are legion and include, for example, haematomas, fractures of osseous borders of the intervertebral foramina, and vertebral metastases. The safe rule here is to examine the back and the nervous system thoroughly in all cases of trauma and whenever there is objective evidence of damage to a nerve or nerves supplying the abdominal wall. Such evidence of damage is usually hypoaesthesia or hyperaesthesia in the area of skin innervated by the nerve. The fact that these findings are usually in fact referred phenomena from intra-abdominal disease should not detract from the application of this rule.

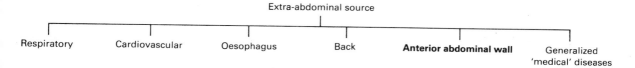

The anterior abdominal wall

Apart from the fact that a wound of the anterior abdominal wall needs treatment in its own right, as well as if it has breached the whole depth of the wall with a consequent risk of peritonitis or intra-abdominal bleeding, the anterior abdominal wall is more likely to cause chronic, rather than acute, symptoms that simulate intra-abdominal disease (see p. 98). However, spontaneous haematomas occasionally occur; for example, in the rectus sheath. The important diagnostic manoeuvre is palpation of the affected area with, and without, voluntary contraction of the muscles of the abdominal wall; if the trouble is in the abdominal wall, pain and tenderness will be greater when the muscles are contracted; if the trouble is intra-abdominal, the tenderness at least will be less.

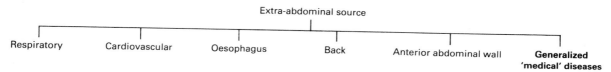

Generalized ('medical') diseases

If the surgeon suspects a cause in this group, the advice of a physician should be urgently sought.

A comprehensive list of these diseases cannot possibly be given, since many generalized disorders may on occasion manifest themselves with symptoms and signs which are strictly, or emphatically, abdominal. They are best grouped according to which type of acute abdomen they simulate — shock, obstruction or peritonitis.

Shock due to blood loss may result from any generalized disorder of coagulation and haemostasis. The bleeding may occur into the lumen of the alimentary tract, producing obvious haematemesis or melaena, but it is important to remember that bleeding may simulate other abdominal pictures. It may occur into the wall of the bowel, producing a disturbance of mobility and colicky abdominal pain, as in Henoch–Schönlein purpura, or into the peritoneum or parietes, as in the pseudo-tumour that is characteristic of haemophilia. The pseudo-tumour is a large haematoma between the iliacus muscle and its covering fascia: the mass expands till it becomes palpable in the lower quadrant of the abdomen. A careful history of any bleeding tendency must be taken if mistakes with this group of conditions are to be avoided.

Intestinal obstruction may be mimicked by the colicky abdominal pain produced by poisoning with lead or with strychnine, or by acute porphyria, or by the lightning pains of abdominal tabes.

An apparent generalized peritonitis may in fact be due to the combination of fluid and electrolyte disturbance with paralytic ileus, nausea and vomiting, and some (usually fairly mild) abdominal discomfort in patients with adrenal failure (see p. 214) or diabetic coma. The latter should be diagnosed by the examination of the urine that should be routine for every patient admitted to hospital, but it is surprising how often a nurse's report that the urine contains sugar is overlooked by the medical attendant.

Basic symptoms

The following sections analyse the significance of the common symptoms of acute surgical abdominal disease. The most important symptom is abdominal pain. Other symptoms are important primarily in determining whether the source of the trouble is the gastrointestinal, urinary or genital tract, but the nature of the actual pain sheds important light on the mechanism producing it, and the likely prognosis in the absence of effective treatment.

Abdominal pain

Basically there are two types of abdominal pain: intermittent and continuous.

Intermittent pain is a term that should be re-

served for pain which occurs for a short period
(of the order of a few minutes), and is interspersed with periods of complete remission, when
there is no pain at all, lasting for a few minutes
up to perhaps half an hour. The specific and detailed definition of intermittent pain must be
stressed, because only if it is defined in this way
is it a useful surgical concept. Truly intermittent
pain is characteristic of the pain produced by obstruction of a hollow viscus, and is probably related to the vigorous peristaltic activity in the
muscular wall of the viscus proximal to the
block. It often has other characteristic features:
that it is felt deeply in the abdomen but is poorly
localized, and that it makes the patient writhe
and press his abdominal wall. However, lack of
such features should not be permitted to obscure
the decision that the pain is intermittent. It is
obvious that intermittent pain corresponds with
the frequently used term *colicky* pain. There is,
however, a snag in using the words colic and *colicky:* they were originally used by doctors to describe any severe abdominal pain. As a result,
many typical pains are called 'colicky' that are
not intermittent. The pain of an obstructed gall
bladder or common bile duct is usually called a
gall-bladder colic, but it is nearly always a constant pain.

Constant pain is a term used for a pain that is
present for hours or even days without any
period of complete relief. It is important to recognize that the constancy implied is one of the
presence of the pain in time, not necessarily one
of its *intensity*. A better word would be *continuous*, but *constant* is usually used. A constant
pain may be steady in its intensity, or alternatively it may be combined with an intermittent
pain and may therefore appear to vary in time,
even to the extent that the unwary clinician is
ready to accept it as a purely intermittent pain
because the background of continuous pain between the colicky exacerbations is so mild.

Continuous pain raises the possibility of peritonitis or strangulation, or the impending rupture of a distended structure, and for this reason
may require more urgent interference than simple mechanical obstruction. This difference in
significance is the main reason for insisting on a
very strict definition of intermittent, or colicky,
as distinct from continuous, or constant, abdominal pain.

The *site* of abdominal pain is of crucial importance: this statement is expanded in Chapters 26,
27, and 28.

Gastrointestinal symptoms

The presence of these symptoms suggest, but
certainly do not fix, the gastrointestinal tract as
the source of the trouble. They may be grouped
according to whether they direct attention primarily to the gastroduodenal regions, the small
intestine, or the large intestine. On the whole,
the presence of an individual symptom is by no
means as important to diagnosis as is the presence of two or more in combination in a characteristic pattern.

Gastroduodenal symptoms include anorexia,
nausea, vomiting, regurgitation, water-brash,
retrosternal burning ('heartburn') and haematemesis. *Small intestine symptoms* other than pain
are confined to borborygmi (vigorous peristalsis,
obvious to the patient by sensations of movement and sounds of gurgling), abdominal distension and steatorrhoea − the passage of bulky,
pale-coloured motions that tend to float rather
than sink, may actually look greasy, and are produced by an excess of fat in the faeces.

Large bowel symptoms comprise a change in
bowel habit (towards either constipation or diarrhoea, or alternating bouts of each), melaena,
passage of blood per anum, and passage of
mucus per anum.

There is, of course, considerable overlap in
the significance of the digestive tract symptoms
of these three groups.

Urinary tract symptoms

These are mentioned here for completeness, but
are considered in more detail in Chapter 28.
They comprise renal and ureteric pain, haematuria, suprapubic pain and burning, and the
various symptoms that may be grouped as
dysuria — discomfort associated with the act of
micturition. Rigors suggest acute renal tract
infection (or cholangitis, p. 325).

Genital tract symptoms

In the female, the onset of normal parturition
ushers in the most typical of all the intermittent
pains; uterine colic or labour pains. Similar intermittent pain occurs in abnormal labour states
such as premature labour, abortion and the closing phases of a tubal pregnancy. Any pain in the
pelvis may be gynaecological in origin, and complaints of disturbances of the periods may streng-
then the evidence.

In the male, testicular pain may be referred to high in the abdomen, a diagnostic trap if the scrotum and its contents are not properly examined.

Basic signs

The following sections analyse the significance of the basic signs that may be of value in the diagnosis of the acute abdomen: extra-abdominal; parietal; suggestive of peritonitis; suggestive of intestinal obstruction; abdominal masses; and signs elicited on rectal examination.

Extra-abdominal signs

These include the signs of shock (Chapter 22), finger-clubbing, any oral abnormality such as a coated tongue or foetor, abnormal enlargement of lymph nodes especially the supraclavicular nodes on the left side, and signs of liver failure (Chapter 11).

Parietal signs

Evidence of trauma affecting the abdominal wall is noted. The external hernial orifices are inspected and palpated as described in Chapter 13, for evidence of a hernia, and the femoral pulses are palpated to obtain evidence of possible occlusive or aneurysmal disease of the major abdominal vessels.

Signs suggestive of peritonitis

These are very important. On inspection, the abdominal wall does not move with the ventilatory movements of the chest.

Tenderness on palpation of the abdominal wall can be difficult to assess. Every patient finds it uncomfortable to have his abdominal wall palpated, and some are more sensitive than others. It is essential that the examiner's forearm is horizontal and the hand flat: pressure is then exerted with the pulps — not the tips — of the fingers by flexing the wrist and the metacarpophalangeal joints. Differential tenderness between one area and another helps in the assessment: a localized area of maximal tenderness is more likely to be meaningful than a diffuse tenderness to an equal degree all over the abdomen.

Guarding is an involuntary contraction of the abdominal muscles subjacent to a palpating hand when the pressure of the fingers is increased: it is usually accompanied by tenderness, but tenderness is not always accompanied by guarding. The important feature of this definition is the phrase *involuntary contraction*: the examiner has to decide whether the contraction that he feels is reflex, or made at the will of the patient. *Rigidity* is an exaggeration of guarding: the abdominal muscles concerned are contracted all the time, so that the abdomen feels hard — board-like rigidity — from the instant the examiner's hand lightly touches it rather than from the moment a light touch becomes firm pressure. Small, rapid, gentle excursions of the hand and fingers are often more accurate in eliciting tenderness, guarding and rigidity than are larger, stronger, slower movements. Localized tenderness, involuntary guarding and rigidity must be diagnosed as due to peritoneal irritation unless there are very strong indications to the contrary.

A number of other signs that are supposed to indicate peritonitis are described, but the author finds them much less reliable. *Rebound* or *release tenderness* describes a *sudden* increase in pain when the examiner suddenly removes his hand from a sore spot. This sign is certainly present in most cases of peritonitis, but its value is reduced by the fact that it is also often present in gastroenteritis, simple intestinal obstruction, or indeed any condition where bowel is distended. *Crossed tenderness* refers to pain in the right iliac fossa when pressure is exerted on the left iliac fossa: it is supposed to indicate acute appendicitis, but is rarely present in that condition and may be present in the absence of any serious intra-abdominal disease. *Psoas spasm* is elicited by passively moving the right hip in the direction of extension and external rotation; resistance due to the spasm is said to indicate an inflamed appendix lying against the psoas muscle, but the author has never found this sign useful. Finally, *hyper-* or *hypoaesthesia* of the skin overlying the area of peritoneal irritation may occasionally be present, but the real importance of this sign is that it should direct attention to the possibility that the nerve involved is being directly stimulated (see p. 296). In *generalized* peritonitis, *bowel sounds* are nearly always absent.

Signs suggestive of intestinal obstruction

These include distension and abnormalities of the bowel sounds.

Abdominal distension can be a very difficult sign to assess, since the shape (i.e. the protuberance) of the abdomen is not much help if the examiner has not seen the patient when his abdomen was normal. Increasing distension can be measured with a tape-measure, passed round the abdomen at a level marked in terms of fixed (i.e. bony) landmarks, but the only clear-cut demonstration that a patient must be distended when he is first seen is that the umbilicus is everted. Otherwise the decision is basically subjective, and based upon the patient's history that the abdomen is swollen, and upon the examiner's impression that the resistance of the abdominal wall to deformation by light pressure is greater than average. This latter point can, of course, be impossible to assess in a very sensitive or truly tender patient.

Assuming that distension is present, the surgeon must decide on the cause. *Flatus* results in hyperresonance to percussion. *Ascites* produces: shifting dullness — i.e. the flank, dull to percussion with the patient supine, becomes resonant when he lies on the opposite side and the air-filled intestines float upwards to the now-uppermost flank region; and fluid thrill — the propagation of a pressure wave, created by tapping or flicking the abdominal wall, through the liquid filled abdomen to be felt by a hand resting on the opposite flank. The passage of this wave through the tissues of the abdominal wall itself should be prevented by an assistant who presses the ulnar border of his forearm on to the abdominal wall along the mid-line. *Faeces* are indentable. A large *tumour*, practically filling the abdomen, can be difficult to distinguish from ascites, particularly if it is a soft ovarian cyst. A pregnant uterus or large fibroids are easier to diagnose. The management of abdominal masses is considered in Chapter 10.

The *bowel sounds* may be absent or increased. Their presence constitutes strong, but not overwhelming, evidence against the possibility of peritonitis or intraperitoneal bleeding, or some other cause of intestinal paralytic ileus. Increased bowel sounds are typically met in mechanical intestinal obstruction, and are more easily recognized than described; they may be tinkling, or amphoric (echoing as in a large cavern), or loud gurgles in a long sequence (peristaltic rush).

Abdominal masses

The diagnosis of abdominal masses is discussed in Chapter 10.

Signs on rectal examination

Melaena, and blood in the stool, can be diagnosed by inspecting the gloved finger after digital examination. A tumour palpable in the rectum — either the apex of an intussesception or a neoplasm in the sigmoid palpable through the wall of the rectum — may explain intestinal obstruction. Tenderness and masses in relation to the uterus and adnexae may require vaginal examination to sort out a gynaecological cause for the acute abdomen. Tenderness high on the right side suggests the acute inflammation of an appendix lying in the pelvic position. Rectal tenderness is even more difficult to gauge than abdominal: it is worth while always starting the assessment by pressing gently, directly backwards on to the sacrum. The reaction of the patient to this manoeuvre gives a baseline from which any excess of tenderness can be gauged. It is also most important to compare the one side with the other.

The sign of emptiness ('ballooning') of the rectum in intestinal obstruction is, in the author's opinion, valueless.

Basic special investigations

The following investigations, taken in conjunction with the history and the physical signs, permit a confident working diagnosis in most patients. Not all these investigations are needed in every patient, and a few patients need other special investigations, some of which (like the transaminases) have already been mentioned.

Blood should be sent for an immediate haemoglobin or haematocrit estimation, preferably also for immediate urea determination, and for the measurement next day of electrolytes to yield a baseline. The first sample of urine is all-important (p. 268), and its volume and specific gravity should be measured in addition to performing the usual tests for sugar, reaction, albumin and bile; should facilities be available for an immediate estimation of urinary sodium or chloride, this may be most valuable. These tests are important for the assessment of any disturbance of the body fluids. A chest radiograph and plain films of the abdomen in the erect and supine positions are vital in the diagnosis and management of mechanical and paralytic intestinal obstruction or suspected perforation. Serum amylase determinations are requested if there is any reason to suspect acute pancreatitis, and in any patient with acute upper abdominal pain whose cause cannot be definitely diagnosed. Ultrasound examination of the abdomen is often very helpful to chart swellings of organs (e.g. acute pancreatitis), abnormal masses (stones and tumours) and collections of liquid (cysts and abscesses). CT-scanning is in the author's experience less helpful, and even if available in a centre may not be accessible in an emergency.

No extra-abdominal source
|
LOOK FOR 'PATTERNS'

Pattern sorting

The stage is now set to discuss the strategy of the management of a patient with acute abdominal symptoms. The basis of this strategy is to recognize certain patterns which demand definite lines of approach, leaving a residuum which requires a further period of observation or special investigations. In particular, the strategic emphasis is not so much upon deciding the nature of the disease causing the symptoms as upon the threat to life. Thus the points at issue are: is the patient bleeding, has he got peritonitis, has he an acute disturbance of the body fluids that is producing , or may go on to produce, shock?

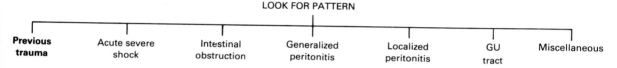

The importance of trauma

Every patient with acute abdominal symptoms, not matter how mild, that are not clearly located to the immediate vicinity of the antecedent trauma, should have his abdomen explored. Experience teaches that damage to intra-abdominal structures may result in very little in the way of symptoms and signs at first, but may progress to a sudden collapse with a high fatality rate. The fact is that, when patients who have suffered blunt trauma to the abdomen and have localized abdominal pain or tenderness elsewhere than the site of impact are subjected to laparotomy, a very high proportion are found to have serious intra-abdominal damage such as tears of mesentery with bleeding vessels, contusions of the large bowel that will probably perforate in a few days, and ruptures of the splenic capsule that will probably lead to catastrophic haemorrhage later. A four-quadrant tap and peritoneal lavage can help in demonstrating intraperitoneal bleeding, although a negative result is not conclusive.

Although it has been standard teaching that a penetrating wound of the abdominal wall always demands a laparotomy, recent evidence from centres with a large experience of the problem suggests that as long as the patient does not show signs of shock it is usually safe to try to avoid laparotomy. Surgeons not exposed to a high incidence of patients with stab wounds usually prefer to explore the abdomen as a routine. There is no doubt that all gunshot wounds of the abdominal wall should lead to a laparotomy, even in the absence of shock.

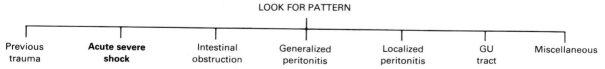

The importance of very acute shock

Reference has been made to many aspects of this subject. Sudden, severe shock that is not cardiogenic or due to vasodilatation can only be caused by loss of blood or plasma. Burns, peritonitis and strangulation, the usual causes of plasma loss, usually present with characteristic clinical features, so if they are absent it can be presumed that blood is being lost. If there is a history of trauma, and a chest radiograph excludes substantial bleeding into the thorax and there are no large haematomas at fracture sites, etc., to account for the blood loss, then intra-abdominal bleeding must be assumed and laparotomy performed.

The management of bleeding from the gastrointestinal tract presenting as haematemesis or melaena has already been discussed.

Intraperitoneal bleeding that does not follow obvious preceding trauma is the remaining consideration in this section. Sudden severe shock without an identifiable site of blood loss elsewhere means either septicaemia or else intra-abdominal haemorrhage; in the absence of septicaemia, the diagnosis must be intra-abdominal haemorrhage, even if there is no clear-cut history of trauma. For one thing, the trauma may have been very mild and thus hardly noticed; for another, the causative lesion (for example, an ectopic pregnancy) may have caused

no symptoms or signs as it developed. It is often taught that blood in the peritoneal cavity is very irritant and produces severe peritoneal symptoms and signs, but this cannot be true, at least in every case. The intraperitoneal route for blood transfusion is well recognised in infants and does not seem to produce any local tenderness or guarding, and haemorrhage from a ruptured spleen may have to be diagnosed, in an unconscious patient, simply from the shock and in the absence of any guarding (p. 275).

Help concerning the *site* of the bleeding may be obtained from various features of the history (e.g. gynaecological, such as a missed period in a ruptured ectopic pregnancy), or the examination (e.g. particularly a mass; a shocked patient with a palpable aneurysm of the abdominal aorta is bleeding from the aneurysm unless proved otherwise at laparotomy). However, the site is of much less importance than the decision that haemorrhage is occurring and that laparotomy must be undertaken.

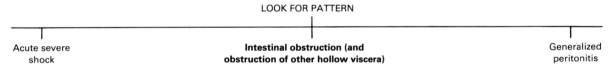

LOOK FOR PATTERN

| Acute severe shock | Intestinal obstruction (and obstruction of other hollow viscera) | Generalized peritonitis |

Intestinal obstruction

The decision that intestinal obstruction is present is very important since the condition is incompatible with life. The way in which the decision is

reached, and the further management of the various types, is considered in Chapter 26.

Obstruction of other hollow viscera is considered in Chapter 27 (bile duct) and Chapter 28 (ureter).

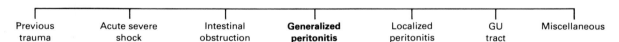

LOOK FOR PATTERN

| Previous trauma | Acute severe shock | Intestinal obstruction | Generalized peritonitis | Localized peritonitis | GU tract | Miscellaneous |

Generalized peritonitis

Sudden onset

This condition is diagnosed by the presence all over the abdomen of the signs of peritoneal irritation — tenderness, guarding, and maybe rigidity — together usually with the absence of bowel sounds. If it has started *suddenly*, it must be assumed that perforation of a hollow viscus has occurred and laparotomy must be undertaken so that the leak can be sealed. As in the case of

intraperitoneal haemorrhage, the diagnosis of the site of the leak is of secondary importance. Most such leaks arise in the gastrointestinal tract, particularly from the stomach or duodenum, the appendix, the caecum or the sigmoid colon. This picture can be produced by acute pancreatitis, but it is safer to perform a laparotomy on a patient with acute pancreatitis than not to perform laparotomy on a patient with peritonitis because of a mistaken diagnosis of acute pancreatitis.

The management of sudden generalized peritonitis is based on the twin principles of restoring the circulating volume and then performing a laparotomy and stopping the leak. The fluid lost from the circulation is basically plasma (p. 268), and so plasma or a plasma substitute should constitute the bulk of the replacement although some saline may be required to replace loss by vomiting. Stopping the leak depends upon the site and the cause. A perforated appendix is removed; a perforated peptic ulcer of the stomach or duodenum is repaired with a plug of neighbouring omentum. A perforation due to a carcinoma of stomach or colon demands resection, with immediate restoration of the continuity of the gastrointestinal tract in the case of the stomach, but delayed restoration in the case of the large bowel (see p. 145). Generalized peritonitis in association with diverticular disease of the sigmoid colon is a particularly difficult and controversial problem (p. 235). Rupture of a solitary diverticulum of the caecum can usually be treated by exteriorizing the affected bowel as a temporary caecostomy.

Less often, the leak arises in the urinary or the genital tract. Appropriate symptoms and signs may have led to an accurate diagnosis beforehand, but in any event the principles of the operative treatment remain the same. An intraperitoneal or extraperitoneal rupture of the bladder is repaired and the suture line protected by indwelling urethral continuous drainage. The ureter may leak into the peritoneum as the result of blunt trauma, and very rarely a large hydronephrosis may rupture.

Very rarely, laparotomy reveals no leak. This may be because a tiny leak (e.g. from diverticular or peptic ulcer disease) has already healed spontaneously. Bacterial infection also occasionally reaches the peritoneum via the blood, or via the genital tract in females (i.e. the fallopian tubes). The author has no personal experience of this condition, which used to be common but now seems to be very rare; however, if there is no leak there is clearly nothing the operator can do but take specimens of the peritoneal exudate for culture, clean the peritoneal cavity with saline, and close the abdomen, treating the infection in general with a broad-spectrum antibiotic till the bacteriologist can give specific information about the nature of the organism and its sensitivity.

Two further points need to be made about generalized peritonitis. The first is that the peritoneum and the patient recover very well from soiling of the peritoneum with faeces and the secretions of the normal gastrointestinal tract, provided that the circulation is maintained and the leak is sealed: it is a *continuing* leak that is tolerated very badly. As a rider to this remark, it must be emphasized that soiling with faeces from an *obstructed* alimentary tract is quite a different matter: presumably because of a change in flora, the incidence of septicaemia is greater and the mortality is correspondingly high. The second point concerns after-care; the role of drainage of the peritoneal cavity and of antibiotics. Both measures are traditional, and the author uses the second but not the first. It has been shown experimentally that a few hours after the abdomen has been closed, any drain that has been left in the peritoneal cavity is draining only a tiny area in its immediate vicinity and is therefore valueless. Unless there is some other indication for a drain (e.g. a suture line) the author therefore relies on a thorough cleansing of the peritoneal cavity with normal saline at the conclusion of the operation, paying special attention to those areas — the subphrenic spaces, the pelvis, the lesser sac and the paracolic gutters — where localized collections of pus are known to be prone to form.

Less sudden onset

If the pain and other symptoms (e.g. nausea, vomiting, prostration) take an hour or more to develop fully, the possibility arises that the generalized peritonitis is due to acute pancreatitis, a condition for which laparotomy is not indicated. The problem of acute pancreatitis is further considered in Chapter 27. However, a gradual onset is perfectly compatible with a perforation which has developed following some acute symptoms, and in any case of doubt laparotomy should be performed (p. 324).

Flow-chart 25.1

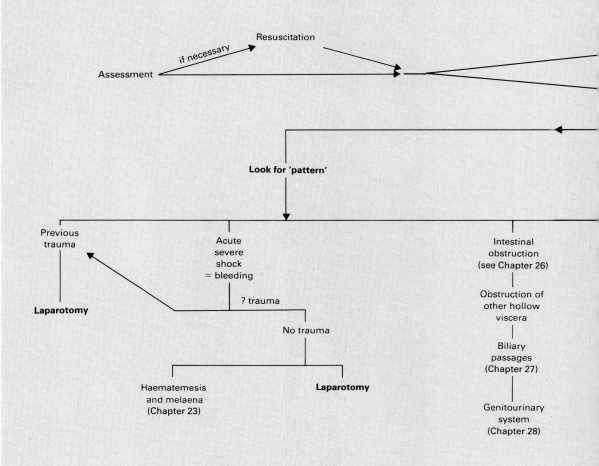

AN APPROACH TO THE ACUTE ABDOMEN

Assessment —— if necessary —→ Resuscitation

Look for 'pattern'

Previous trauma

Laparotomy

Acute severe shock = bleeding

? trauma

No trauma

Haematemesis and melaena (Chapter 23)

Laparotomy

Intestinal obstruction (see Chapter 26)

Obstruction of other hollow viscera

Biliary passages (Chapter 27)

Genitourinary system (Chapter 28)

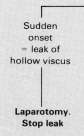

Sudden onset = leak of hollow viscus

Laparotomy. Stop leak

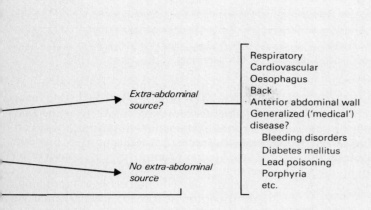

Respiratory
Cardiovascular
Oesophagus
Back
Anterior abdominal wall
Generalized ('medical')
disease?
    Bleeding disorders
    Diabetes mellitus
    Lead poisoning
    Porphyria
    etc.

*Extra-abdominal
source?*

*No extra-abdominal
source*

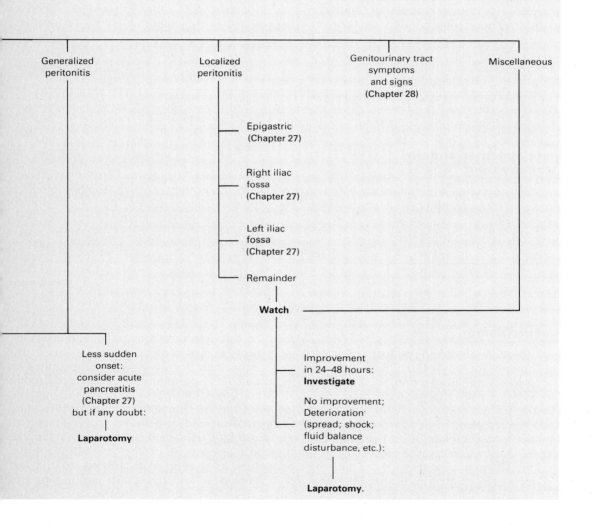

Generalized
peritonitis

Localized
peritonitis

Genitourinary tract
symptoms
and signs
(Chapter 28)

Miscellaneous

Epigastric
(Chapter 27)

Right iliac
fossa
(Chapter 27)

Left iliac
fossa
(Chapter 27)

Remainder

Watch

Less sudden
onset:
consider acute
pancreatitis
(Chapter 27)
but if any doubt:

Laparotomy

Improvement
in 24–48 hours:
Investigate

No improvement;
Deterioration
(spread; shock;
fluid balance
disturbance, etc.):

Laparotomy.

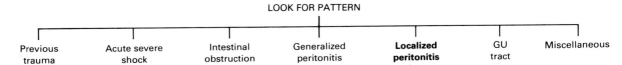

Localized peritonitis

If the signs of peritonitis are elicited in a localized area only of the abdomen, and bowel sounds are still present, a diagnosis of localized peritonitis should be made. This situation can be classified into subgroups: epigastric, right iliac fossa, left iliac fossa, and others. They are discussed in Chapter 27.

The residuum consists of those conditions that are difficult to place in any of the previous categories. In the absence of any evidence of trauma, shock, depletion of the extracellular fluid, or intestinal obstruction, conservative management is indicated in the first instance — i.e. wait and

see. Further evidence of the nature of the underlying cause may be provided by a palpable mass, a fistula, skin discoloration (p. 325), or the findings on rectal examination. If despite these considerations no more exact diagnosis is possible, and if the patient improves on conservative management, the cause will probably never be discovered. If the patient becomes more ill, if the signs of peritonitis spread, and particularly if circulatory changes develop or the haematocrit rises, laparotomy is advised. Failure to improve on conservative management for 48 hours, maybe even for 24 hours, should also lead to laparotomy. In the immortal words of Moynihan, 'it is safer to look and see than to wait and see'.

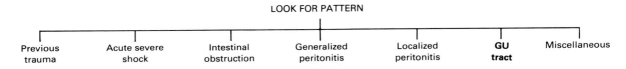

The acute abdomen and the genitourinary tract

When a patient presents with an acute abdomen plus some signs and symptoms suggestive that

the source is in the genital or urinary tract, special considerations arise; the problem is considered in Chapter 27.

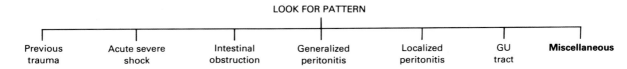

Residual problems

In a sense, there should be no residual problems, since the absence of any of the features considered previously in this section should mean that there is no threat to life, and the patient by our definition is not an example of the acute abdomen. Nevertheless, a few awkward cases always remain who complain of acute abdominal pain of persistent type and yet show no sign of a threat to life. The management of these patients should be identical with that of localized peritonitis not definitely situated in the epigastrium or

right or left lower abdominal quadrants. One must stress that abdominal pain persisting without improvement for 24—48 hours constitutes an indication for laparotomy even if there are no abnormal signs on physical examination. The length of time the surgeon waits before deciding to operate depends on the severity of pain, on the possibility of a medical cause, and on the surgeon's assessment of the reliability of the patient as a witness. With respect to the last point the opinion of a paediatrician or a psychiatrist can be invaluable in appropriate cases.

Further reading

Boey, J.H. and Dunphy, J.E. (1985). The acute abdomen. In: *Current Surgical Diagnosis and Treatment*. Ed. by L. W. Way. Los Altos, California, Lange.

Cope, Z. (1983). *The Early Diagnosis of the Acute Abdomen*, 16th edn. Oxford, Oxford University Press.

Chapter 26

The Acute Abdomen; Intestinal Obstruction

The management of this condition really depends upon the answers to five questions that the clinician must ask himself. They are:
1. Is intestinal obstruction present?
2. If it is present; is it mechanical or paralytic?
3. If it is mechanical; is it simple or strangulation-obstruction?
4. Is it affecting small or large bowel?
5. Finally, whether mechanical or paralytic; is there any disturbance of the body fluid compartments?

It will be noted that not one of the five questions is concerned with the *cause* of the obstruction. The exact nature of the obstruction may certainly influence what is done at any laparotomy, or even in certain cases whether a laparotomy is advised; the philosophy of the surgeon's approach to a case of intestinal obstruction is, however, far more dependent on the answers to the five questions than on the cause.

Is obstruction present?

Most cases are clear-cut and the answer straightforward, at least in mechanical obstruction. The characteristic features are anorexia, nausea and vomiting; abdominal distension; increased bowel sounds; intermittent (colicky) abdominal pain; and absolute constipation, i.e. constipation for flatus, the complaint that no flatus has been passed per anum for longer than the subject and the doctor would consider normal.

A snag already arises that the typical colicky abdominal pain is absent in cases of paralytic intestinal obstruction. Again, anorexia, nausea and vomiting may be inconspicuous in low (distal) obstruction, and distension may be non-existent in very high (proximal) obstruction. Finally, constipation may be difficult to assess if the obstruction is very acute, so that there has been no time for the absolute constipation to declare itself, or if the obstruction is partial, in which case some flatus may still be being passed.

The final and clinching evidence, in most of the difficult presentations, is given by plain radiographs of the abdomen, and these are discussed in a later section.

Some explanation of the genesis of the symptoms and signs in intestinal obstruction is helpful in approaching the variations described. The aqueous exocrine secretions of the upper reaches of the alimentary tract into its lumen amount to 8–12 litres each 24 hours. The loss of water in the faeces is normally less than 0.5 litre daily. The vast proportion of the secreted water is reabsorbed by the lower reaches of the bowel, to some extent by the large bowel, but mostly by the distal 1 m or so of the ileum. If the obstruction is placed distally in the large bowel, there is little disturbance of the water reabsorption and so vomiting is not a prominent feature; however, swallowed air is still prevented from reaching the anal canal and builds up in gut, so absolute constipation and abdominal distension are accentuated features. By contrast, if the obstruction is very high in the alimentary tract, in the region, say, of the stomach and duodenum, the salivary, oesophageal and gastric secretions collect in and distend the stomach until copious vomiting rapidly occurs, and no swallowed gas or alimentary secretion passes on into the intestine to produce abdominal distension.

The safe rule on the difficult case is that if the abdomen is distended with gas, or if vomiting is intractable, then whether or not absolute constipation or intermittent abdominal pain are present, x-ray studies of the abdomen are essential.

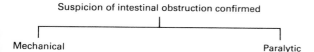

Suspicion of intestinal obstruction confirmed

Mechanical   Paralytic

Mechanic or paralytic?

If vomiting and/or abdominal distension are associated with intermittent abdominal pain and increased bowel sounds that sound 'obstructive' (p. 300), the obstruction is mechanical; if there is no pain and the bowel sounds are absent, the obstruction is paralytic. An important variant is vomiting and/or abdominal distension with pain but no bowel sounds. This combination suggests that strangulation (see below) is complicating mechanical obstruction. These decisions must always be checked by plain abdominal radiographs (see later).

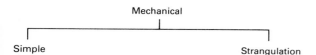

Mechanical

Simple   Strangulation

Simple or strangulation?

This question applies only to mechanical obstruction. Simple obstruction defines a mechanical obstruction to the lumen of the bowel without any primary interference with tissue perfusion. Strangulation as a term on its own is an entirely different concept from intestinal obstruction: it defines an interference with the relatively narrow vascular pedicle servicing a particular part of a tissue or organ, or the whole organ, by a mechanical constricting factor. The nature of the constricting factor is irrelevant to the definition; it may be the presence of tight surrounding structures, or the twisting of the pedicle itself. The essential pathophysiology of the disturbance which ensues is that, because venous pressure is much lower than arterial pressure, the veins are constricted first, and strangulation is basically a venous engorgement. In consequence, the capillaries of the affected part become distended by the mounting venous pressure, and since a distended capillary is a damaged and therefore leaky capillary, protein-rich material exudes into the interstitial space of the tissues. There is a mounting stasis on the arterial side of the circulation also, until finally no more blood can enter the part and tissue death becomes inevitable.

It is instructive to compare this sequence with the events in ischaemia, i.e. a primary reduction of the arterial inflow below an extent compatible with the health of the tissues or organ being perfused. In ischaemia the tissues are pale and desiccated, instead of plum-coloured and dripping with oedema fluid. Ischaemia which occurs gradually causes a gradual withering away of the tissues — *mummification* — because the dry field inhibits the growth of micro-organisms; by contrast, strangulation results in an early infective gangrene because of the moistness of the tissues.

The student often speaks of strangulation as though it were a variety of intestinal obstruction. Clearly there is a confusion of ideas here. Strangulation of tissue that is not bowel may occur: a common example is strangulation of a portion of greater omentum in an external hernia. Moreover, even if the tissue strangulated is bowel, it does not necessarily follow that intestinal obstruction is present: it is possible for a portion only of the complete circumference of the bowel to be trapped in the sac and strangulated (*Richter's hernia*), and in this case the continuity of the bowel lumen is maintained.

The distinction between simple mechanical obstruction and mechanical obstruction with strangulation is made on the basis of symptoms, signs and special investigation.

Symptoms

The cardinal feature is the pain. Assuming that the obstruction starts as the simple type, the pain begins as the typical intermittent (colicky) pain of mechanical obstruction. When strangulation supervenes, the mounting concentration of the products of metabolism such as pain factor and kinins, which are normally washed away by the circulation, produce a constant pain or dull ache which persists between the episodes. The nature of the pain also changes. Colicky pain is poorly localized by the patient, and when bowel is the origin the pain is felt approximately in the midline and diffusely about it: the patient says that he feels he wants to press his abdominal wall in the region where he feels the pain so as to get relief. The pain of strangulation is localized to the region of the affected bowel, and is sharper, for reasons explained in the next paragraph. This cardinal feature of continuous abdominal pain outweighs any lack of confirmatory evidence of strangulation from physical signs or special investigations.

Signs

The exudate on the peritoneal surface of the bowel — rich in enzymes and other biologically active substances, and later in micro-organisms as the bowel loses its integrity and becomes permeable to these — results in, at first, a localized,

and, in due course, a generalized, peritonitis. Thus the local sharp pain is associated with local tenderness and guarding, and in due course, if untreated, these symptoms and signs spread, the bowel sounds disappear, the abdominal wall becomes rigid, and generalized peritonitis has set in. The patient looks correspondingly more ill.

Special investigations

The most useful special investigation, if the volume of tissue strangulated is large, is the haematocrit (or haemoglobin). Loss of a large volume of protein-rich liquid into the strangulated part directly depletes the plasma, and thus the blood, volume; serial haematocrit estimations therefore show a sharper rise than in the case of plasma loss resulting from a contraction of the whole extracellular space in saline depletion. By the same token, the patient looks more ill, his circulation more depleted, than one would have expected from the amount of vomiting and distension displayed, and this combination of a patient more ill than expected with a haemoconcentration greater than expected is highly suggestive of strangulation. These qualitative considerations are given a more quantitative treatment on p. 316.

It is also said that a marked elevation of the white cell count supports a diagnosis of strangulation in addition to the obstruction, but the author has found this investigation much less helpful.

Small or large bowel?

Obviously, this question refers only to mechanical obstruction, since paralytic ileus as a clinical problem usually affects both the small and the large bowel.

The main features that indicate high (proximal) rather than low (distal) bowel (p. 308) correspond roughly to the distinction between small and large bowel obstruction, and the site of the colicky pain in the abdomen is also a rough guide: high for small bowel and low for large. However, the intermediate territory of distal small bowel and proximal large bowel gives rise to a mixed clinical picture with regard to these features. Clear-cut colicky abdominal pain is more common in small bowel than in large bowel obstruction: in the latter the pain and tenderness

of a distended caecum in the right iliac fossa, in cases where the iliocaecal valve is still competent, is more prominent than symmetrically placed griping pain. If distension is clearly delimited to the central part of the abdomen, the obstruction is likely to be in the small bowel, whereas large bowel obstruction usually produces more distension in the flanks than centrally.

The most important means of distinguishing small from large bowel obstruction (and, incidentally, both of these from paralytic ileus) is plain radiology of the abdomen in the erect and supine positions (Figs. 26.1 and 26.2). The diagnostic features are the gas shadows in the intestinal lumen, best seen in the supine film, and horizontal levels between gas and liquid contents in the erect film.

Gas in the gastrointestinal tract is mainly swallowed air, although a small portion is derived from fermentation. There is normally a gas bubble in the fundus of the stomach, separated by the horizontal level from the liquid of the resting gastric contents. The quantities of gas in the normal small intestine are too small, and too broken up by the churning movements of the small bowel, to show on a plain x-ray, but as the water is absorbed and the faecal content of the bowel becomes solid and discrete, so does the likelihood of seeing distinct shadows of gas in the lumen increase. It is normal to see large gas shadows throughout the large bowel, including the rectum and sigmoid colon.

In small bowel mechanical obstruction, the small bowel proximal to the block becomes distended with intestinal secretions and swallowed gas, and the typical appearances of loops of small bowel distended with gas in the supine film, and of multiple gas/fluid levels in the erect film, result. The gas shadows in small bowel obstruction (Fig. 26.1) tend to be centrally placed in the abdomen, disposed in a stepladder pattern, and the valvulae conniventes are represented by straight lines that tend to cross the whole lumen of the bowel, and meet the bowel wall on each side at a right angle without indenting the bowel wall at the junction. Distal to the block, any gas originally present is quite soon expelled per anum, any fluid is absorbed in the normal way, and the large bowel significantly contains no gas shadows.

In large bowel obstruction, once the ileocaecal valve becomes incompetent, the raised pressure of the large bowel proximal to the block is transmitted to the small bowel, and the radiological evidence of small bowel distension with gas and liquid appears. The important distinction, however, is that distended large bowel as shadows and gas/fluid levels are also present in the large bowel proximal to the obstruction. The gas shadows in the large bowel (Fig. 26.2) tend to lie peripherally (though any redundancy of the transverse colon or of the sigmoid obscures this feature), and the segmentation effect of haustration draws in the line of the wall but does not extend across the whole bowel lumen to the opposite wall. Distension of the caecum is a particularly helpful feature. Beyond the obstructions, there is no gas in the large bowel including the rectum.

In paralytic ileus, all regions of the bowel are distended and contain gas and gas/fluid levels: this applies in the large bowel right down to the rectum, thereby distinguishing paralytic ileus from mechanical large bowel obstruction with an incompetent ileocaecal valve.

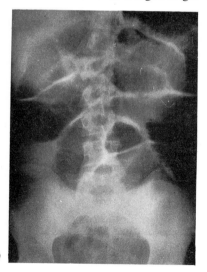 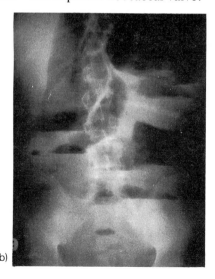

(a) (b)

Fig. 26.1 Plain x-rays of the abdomen in small bowel intestinal obstruction. (a) Supine. The gas shadows lie on the whole centrally in the abdomen, the loops are distended, and the valvulae conniventes are well seen as lines crossing the whole width of the bowel. (b) Erect. This view shows more clearly the distension of the loops and the multiple gas/liquid levels.

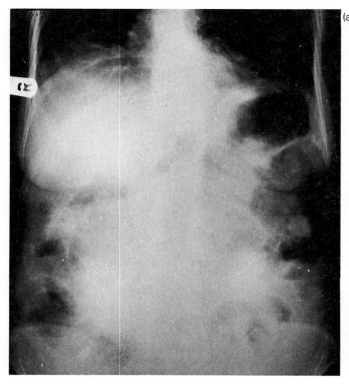

(a)

Fig. 26.2 Plain x-rays of the abdomen in large bowel intestinal obstruction. (a) Supine. The gas shadows in the distended loops of bowel are disposed peripherally rather than centrally in the abdomen, and the haustrations indent the margins of, but do not cross the whole of, the bowel (though there is an exception to this rule in the left upper quadrant).

Circulatory disturbance?

Enough has been written on the subject of recognizing shock (Chapter 22) and diagnosing blood, plasma and saline losses to make further comment here superfluous. However, in the following sections on the management of the various types of intestinal obstruction, it is important to appreciate that the correction of any disturbance of the body fluid compartments has a very high priority among the other aspects of management described, and must be well advanced before general anaesthesia can be contemplated.

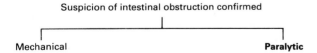

Suspicion of intestinal obstruction confirmed

Mechanical   **Paralytic**

Management

Paralytic ileus

Paralytic ileus is not in itself a diagnosis, but merely a description of a pattern of reaction of the intestines to some insult. The insult itself must be sought and, where possible, eliminated, whereupon the ileus can confidently be expected to settle down spontaneously. The parts of the gastrointestinal tract whose mobility is most affected are the stomach and the colon; despite

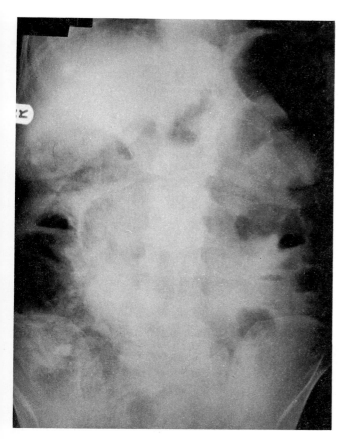

(b)

Fig. 26.2 Contd. (b) Erect. This shows the multiple fluid levels in the dilated loops. Note particularly in this view the distended caecum, containing much solid faeces as well as gas: this is a characteristic feature in large bowel obstruction when the ileocaecal valve remains continent.

the name 'ileus', the small bowel is relatively unaffected by this condition. Common causes are generalized or localized peritonitis, haematomas of the posterior abdominal wall, and a recent laparotomy which is said to act via mechanical handling of the bowel. Although pain is not a feature of paralytic ileus itself, many of the predisposing insults are painful. The diagnosis can be particularly difficult after laparotomy: a leak in an intestinal suture line may produce local peritonitis and paralytic ileus, and the pain of the peritonitis can be difficult to distinguish from the pain of the incision in the abdominal wall.

Views differ as to whether potassium deficiency can produce paralytic ileus: the author feels that such a deficiency certainly aggravates any disturbance of the motility of the bowel, but probably does not initiate ileus. Opiates certainly inhibit gastric emptying, and slow gastric emptying is an important feature of paralytic ileus. Any correctable cause is corrected; otherwise, the management of paralytic ileus is to give intravenous fluids and electrolytes and to try to

keep the gastrointestinal tract as empty as possible by nasogastric suction. If gas and liquid accumulate in the bowel and cause distension, this factor can itself cause a reduction in normal bowel movements and prolong the period of paralytic ileus.

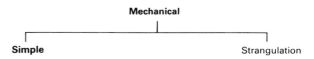

Simple small bowel obstruction

The strategy of management is to aim at a surgical operation to remove the obstructing agent. However, in the absence of any evidence of strangulation there is no great urgency, and preparation of the patient for operation by nasogastric aspiration and intravenous fluids can be reasonably leisurely.

Nasogastric aspiration is designed to reduce the distension of the digestive tract proximal to the block so as to minimize the risk of perforation.

Depending on the nature of the obstruction, deflation of the bowel sometimes has a positive therapeutic value. If the obstruction is due to kinking of a loop of bowel by an adhesion to some fixed point (e.g. the anterior abdominal wall), then increasing distension of the proximal loop tends to increase the kinking and perpetuate the obstruction; deflation of the proximal loop gives the bowel a chance to straighten itself, thereby relieving the obstruction.

After a suitable period on this conservative regime, the patient is reassessed: if the abdomen is less distended and there is still no evidence of strangulation, the conservative management may be pursued, but if there is an increase in distension or any other evidence of deterioration, laparotomy is undertaken. Emptying the stomach through the nasogastric tube is particularly important in preventing inhalation of vomitus during induction of anaesthesia. The decision between continuing the conservative approach and laparotomy can be a fine one, and demands experience. In general, the safe rule is to err on the side of an unnecessary laparotomy, particularly if the patient has not had a previous abdominal operation. In the much commoner event that there is a scar from a previous laparotomy, adhesion obstruction is overwhelmingly the most likely cause and experience teaches that the conservative approach often succeeds. The author's practice in cases with an abdominal scar is to review the patient at 24-hour intervals (with plain radiographs of the abdomen as well as the clinical signs), and if the situation has deteriorated at one assessment from the previous one, or has remained static for two consecutive assessment periods, he advises laparotomy.

The use of a very long tube (Miller–Abbott) for aspiration, suitably weighted to assist it in passing the pylorus, and with an inflatable balloon at its tip, has been advocated for cases of adhesive obstruction. The idea is that, once radiological screening shows that the tube has negotiated the pylorus, the balloon is blown up and is gripped by the gut wall and carried onwards to the site of the obstruction by peristalsis. This should result in very efficient deflation of the intestine and a greater chance of relieving the obstruction. In the author's experience, such tubes pass very well along the normal gastrointestinal tract, but very poorly along an obstructed tract.

The laparotomy

A collapsed loop of small bowel is found, and traced proximally to the site of obstruction, which may be outside the wall, in the wall, or within the lumen of the bowel.

Lesions outside the wall include kinking by adhesions or bands — inflammatory or congenital — or trapping in an internal hernia through a congenital or acquired (postoperative) hole in the mesentery, or into one of the congenital peritoneum-lined recesses of the posterior abdominal wall in the neighbourhood of the fourth part of the duodenum or the ileocaecal junction. Volvulus around an adhesion to a fixed point may also be placed in this group. The obstructing agent is removed; bands and adhesions are divided, hernias reduced and their necks obliterated to prevent recurrrence, and any volvulus untwisted. The bowel at the site of the recent obstruction is carefully inspected for direct or vascular damage (see p. 155); assuming it is intact and viable, it is left in place. Finally, the proximal bowel, if markedly distended despite nasogastric aspiration, is deflated; this measure facilitates closing the abdomen and probably reduces any tendency to postoperative ileus. Deflation is best achieved by gently milking the gas and liquid in the intestine proximally into the stomach, whence the anaesthetist removes it by aspiration via the nasogastric tube.

Lesions in the wall causing obstruction are rare; they may be congenital, inflammatory or neoplastic, but usually demand resection of the affected segment of bowel and immediate restitution of the continuity of the digestive tract by end-to-end anastomosis. Immediate reanastomosis can be performed with reasonable safety in small bowel despite the presence of severe obstruction, presumably because the blood supply of small bowel is so rich that the junction heals very well and leakage is uncommon. The situation in large bowel is quite different. The rest of the management is as for lesions outside the wall.

Lesions in the lumen, such as a gallstone, should if possible be broken up by the operator's fingers from outside the wall of the bowel and milked distally into the large intestine. If this manipulation is not possible, the bowel is deflated via the stomach as described previously, and the obstruction is milked proximally to an area of bowel whose wall has not been subjected to the pressure of the stone, etc., and removed via a small incision in the wall.

Simple large bowel obstruction

The wall of large bowel is less well supplied with blood than is small bowel, and therefore is more susceptible to damage and more likely to perforate. Perforation is a calamity because faecal peritonitis when the bowel has been obstructed carries a high fatality rate. Moreover, the ileocaecal valve may remain competent till a late stage, and this may result in a disproportionately rapid build-up in pressure in the closed loop between the valve and the obstruction. For these reasons, large bowel obstruction is an emergency situation which demands early decompression of the bowel. Nevertheless, the capacious nature of the large bowel means that there is plenty of slack to be taken up, and there is usually time to repair any circulatory deficit without undue haste, and to administer one, or even two, enemas.

The reason for the enemas is twofold. First, particularly in the case of lesions of the left side of the colon, where the bowel contents are solid, the final obstructing agent at any area of narrowing of the bowel may be a mass of hard faeces, and the enema may dislodge this and relieve the obstruction, thus removing the urgency from the case. Secondly, particularly in elderly patients, *pseudo-obstruction* is not very uncommon: the patient presents with an apparently typical large bowel obstruction due to a constricting lesion of the sigmoid colon, and the clinical diagnosis is even supported by typical x-ray appearances. However, if laparotomy is undertaken no cause of obstruction is found, the bowel just tapering down to normal dimensions at a point corresponding to the x-ray level of the apparent obstruction. An enema usually relieves pseudo-obstruction and prevents an unnecessary laparotomy.

The nurse giving the enema is instructed to report on the result obtained on evacuation; faeces is not as important as flatus in diagnosing relief of the obstruction since the faeces may have been present in the rectum since before the obstruction occurred. If one enema gives a moderate result, it may be worth trying the effect of a second, 2 hours later. If an enema fails to relieve the obstruction, a limited barium enema helps in excluding pseudo-obstruction.

If the obstruction is relieved by the enema, the situation is no longer urgent and investigation of the nature of the obstruction by sigmoidoscopy and barium enema or colonoscopy can be undertaken. Such investigations are, of course, nega-

tive if the case was one of pseudo-obstruction. However, if the obstruction is not relieved, operative decompression of the bowel is mandatory. The principle of the operation is to relieve the distension; removal of the obstructing lesion and restoring continuity of the bowel are often not feasible at the first operation, for reasons discussed in Chapter 12.

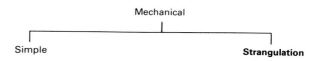

Strangulation

Any evidence suggesting strangulation increases the urgency of the case. Resuscitation must be carried out within 1 hour, and large volumes of fluid may be needed so it is often wise to have a central venous pressure manometer in the great veins (p. 265). In patients with large bowel obstruction strangulation is uncommon, but gross dilation of large bowel, and pain and tenderness in the region of the caecum are indications of a similar urgency.

Circulatory disturbance

No patient should be submitted to a general anaesthetic and surgical operation in a state of shock, unless the shock is due to bleeding at such a rapid rate that transfusion cannot keep pace with it. This principle cannot be too strongly re-emphasized, and repletion of the body fluids accordingly precedes the operative management described above, in all patients with intestinal obstruction.

The problem of the early recognition of strangulation is sometimes simplified by careful consideration of the circulatory state. In a patient with haemoconcentration due to loss of plasma or saline from the circulation, the proportionate reduction in plasma volume can be assessed from the change of haematocrit value or haemoglobin concentration by assuming that the red cell mass stays constant. In terms of haematocrit values, suppose H_1 is the haematocrit (percentage) in normal circumstances and H_2 the observed haematocrit in the shocked state, then simple algebra leads to the conclusion that

Flow-chart 26.1

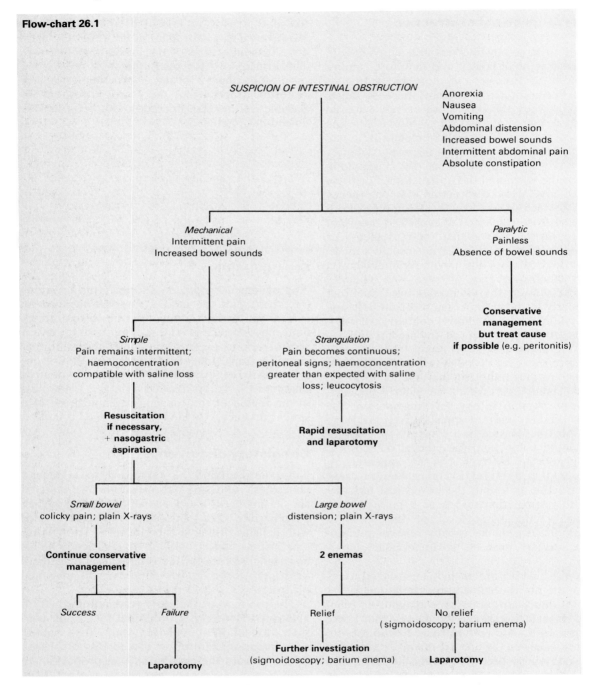

SUSPICION OF INTESTINAL OBSTRUCTION

Anorexia
Nausea
Vomiting
Abdominal distension
Increased bowel sounds
Intermittent abdominal pain
Absolute constipation

Mechanical
Intermittent pain
Increased bowel sounds

Paralytic
Painless
Absence of bowel sounds

**Conservative
management
but treat cause
if possible** (e.g. peritonitis)

Simple
Pain remains intermittent;
haemoconcentration
compatible with saline loss

Strangulation
Pain becomes continuous;
peritoneal signs; haemoconcentration
greater than expected with saline
loss; leucocytosis

**Resuscitation
if necessary,
+ nasogastric
aspiration**

**Rapid resuscitation
and laparotomy**

Small bowel
colicky pain; plain X-rays

Large bowel
distension; plain X-rays

**Continue conservative
management**

2 enemas

Success

Failure

Relief

No relief
(sigmoidoscopy; barium enema)

Laparotomy

Further investigation
(sigmoidoscopy; barium enema)

Laparotomy

Fall in plasma volume
(expressed as percentage of original)

$$= 100 \left[1 - \left(\frac{H_1}{100 - H_1} \times \frac{100 - H_2}{H_2} \right) \right]$$

For example, if $H_1 = 45$ and $H_2 = 52$, then the percentage fall in plasma volume is

$$100 \left[1 - \left(\frac{45}{55} \times \frac{48}{52} \right) \right] \text{ or 24 per cent}$$

Within the values of haematocrit that one usually encounters, a simple form of this expression is that for each 1 per cent rise of the haematocrit reading, the fall in plasma volume is approximately 4 per cent.

If the patient is an adult of approximately average size, his plasma volume when normal can be assumed to be 3 litres. The fall in plasma volume in the shocked patient is therefore about 750 ml. This might be due to a loss of 750 ml of plasma directly from the vascular compartment. On the other hand, the loss might be saline, and to produce this fall in plasma volume, a pure loss of saline shrinking the whole extracellular compartment would need to be five times this figure

(since the extracellular compartment is normally about 15 litres, i.e. five times the plasma volume). Thus, this argument indicates a pure saline deficit approaching 4 litres. The surgeon then asks himself whether the history and physical findings are compatible with a loss of saline or of plasma. If the patient had a case of intestinal obstruction that, on ordinary criteria, appeared to be simple, yet there had been no vomiting and the abdomen was only slightly distended, a change in haematocrit of this order would indicate that the loss must have been closer to 750 ml plasma than to 4 litres normal saline, and it would be far safer to diagnose obstruction *with strangulation* and to proceed accordingly.

One difficulty in applying this technique is that one rarely knows the patient's haematocrit in normal circumstances, since he is usually admitted as an emergency in the shocked state. In most patients it is reasonable to assume a normal value of 45 per cent. Pre-existing polycythaemia is rare, while pre-existing anaemia simply minimizes one's calculation of requirements of saline or plasma, and it becomes obvious when the calculated requirements have been infused that the patient is not cured of his shock and more is needed.

Particular problems

Small bowel obstruction without previous laparotomy

The commonest cause of small bowel obstruction is a strangulated external hernia, and such a hernia should be carefully sought in every case. A small strangulated femoral hernia in particular may be easily overlooked, especially if the patient is fat and the abdominal symptoms and signs of associated intestinal obstruction are gross and overshadow a small tender lump in the groin. The next commonest cause is adhesions due to a previous laparotomy, and as already stated the accent can be placed on conservative management unless there is clear evidence of accompanying strangulation.

If neither of these two causes is present — i.e. the hernial orifices are empty and the abdomen bears no scars (the 'virgin' abdomen, as it is often called) — the clinician should weight his

management towards laparotomy. There is always a place for conservative measures in the first instance, but if definite improvement is not apparent at each reassessment there should be no hesitation in advising laparotomy.

Subacute small bowel obstruction

This is another serious situation that should incline the surgeon towards laparotomy. Unlike large bowel obstruction, which is usually gradual in its onset, small bowel obstruction generally starts suddenly. Should the onset in fact be gradual, perhaps with short periods of colicky pain and nausea interspersed with symptomless intervals, the unwary clinician may persist with conservative measures for too long. The fact is that a subacute picture like this is given by many serious conditions such as gallstone ileus and mesenteric vascular occlusion, so that early recurrence of small bowel obstruction or an insidious course should be considered strong indications for exploration.

Mesenteric vascular occlusion

Occlusion of mesenteric arteries or veins results in gangrene of variable lengths of bowel, depending upon the precise site of the obstruction. For example, the whole of the midgut can be involved or the damage may be localized to a short segment. This is one of the most difficult situations encountered by the surgeon performing a laparotomy for intestinal obstruction or for generalized peritonitis. A length of bowel, usually small intestine, looks plum-coloured, oedematous, or even frankly gangrenous and perforated, as though it had been strangulated, but no mechanical cause of strangulation is apparent.

Whether it is the vein or the artery that has been occluded makes no difference to the morbid anatomical changes in the affected loop as seen by the naked eye. The ischaemic damage to the intestinal mucosa resulting from arterial obstruction seems to produce predominantly a paralytic effect on the capillaries and small venules so that they become distended and leak protein-rich fluid, just as they would if the mesenteric vein had been affected. This strangulation-like lesion results in a marked haemoconcentration and a correspondingly severe peripheral circulatory failure, features which may have given rise to a preoperative suspicion of the diagnosis. The passage of dark blood per rectum is another pointer, but this is likely to be seen only in the rarer colonic form of the disease rather than in the small intestinal form. Arterial obstruction may be due to thrombosis supervening on an atheromatous plaque, and an antecedent history of abdominal pain after meals (the so-called 'mesenteric angina'), resulting from the increased circulatory demands of digestion acting on a bowel with a relative impairment of its blood supply, may lead to a suspicion of this diagnosis. The other form of arterial obstruction is an embolus, and the presence of a potential cause of embolus formation (e.g. atrial fibrillation) in a patient with intestinal obstruction should alert one to the possibility of this diagnosis. If there has been a preoperative suspicion, arteriography can confirm the diagnosis. However, it is most unusual for the diagnosis to be suspected, let alone made, before the operation.

The vessels usually affected are the superior mesenteric artery or vein, and consequently the lesion is usually in small bowel. A similar disturbance can occur in the colon, usually in the region of the splenic flexure where the blood supply is poor relative to the rest of the large bowel; however, such patients present with rectal bleeding, generalized peritonitis due to perforation, or later large bowel obstruction due to healing with scarring and stricture formation. The length of the lesion in the small bowel depends upon the exact site of the block in the main vessel, whether proximal or distal, and presumably upon the efficiency of the collateral circulation from neighbouring segments of bowel in the individual case.

The operator must distinguish between an arterial and a venous block. In the former, arterial pulsations are absent in the mesentery near the affected bowel, and the zone of oedema and colour change extends from the bowel only a short distance into the mesentery. In venous occlusion, arterial pulsations are present in the mesentery, and the zone of oedema extends a long way towards the root of the mesentery.

The principles of management are first to excise dead bowel but as little as possible if the lesion is extensive, to attempt to relieve an arterial obstruction (but not a venous one), to make a primary anastomosis if bowel has been resected and, finally, to repeat the laparotomy 24–48 hours later (the 'second-look policy') so that one can see whether the bowel of doubtful integrity that has been left in the patient has survived or whether further excision is necessary. The technique of relieving an arterial obstruction is to open the ileocolic artery at a convenient site and pass a Fogarty catheter (p. 351) towards the site of the block. If the tip of the catheter can be negotiated past the block, the balloon is distended and the catheter withdrawn, whereupon the balloon drags out the clot. Naturally, this can work only if the obstruction is an embolus rather than thrombosis. In the event of failure to restore pulsations to the arteries distal to the block, an attempt is made to achieve a retrograde perfusion of the mesenteric vessels by anastomosing the ileocolic artery to a suitable systemic artery such as the right iliac artery. Attempts to disobliterate the superior mesenteric vein, on the other hand, have met with little success, and most authorities advise that the abdomen should be closed, after any necessary resection of small bowel, without such an attempt, and anticoagulation with heparin used in an attempt to limit the extent of the mesenteric venous thrombosis.

If the patient survives (and the mortality of these conditions is variously quoted at 60—80 per cent), his further prognosis depends upon how much small bowel he has left. Patients with less than 1.5 m of small intestine beyond the duodenojejunal flexure rarely survive for as long as 1 year, due to the problems of intestinal hurry and consequent malabsorption. Patients with very small amounts of functioning bowel can be kept alive for long periods by intravenous feeding, but no adaptation of the gut to increase absorption takes place unless some food is also given by the oral route.

Intestinal obstruction in infants

Obstruction of the digestive tract in infants falls into two clearly defined groups from the viewpoint of management: those that are present at birth and therefore present within the first week of postnatal life, and those that present later, usually not till 4 weeks have passed. The importance of this distinction is that surgery of the neonate is a highly skilled and specialized field so that the emphasis must lie in very early diagnosis and rapid transfer of the infant to the appropriate specialized unit, whereas babies in the latter group are tougher and the likely conditions producing the obstruction are more readily amenable to surgical correction by the nonspecialist surgeon. Even in the latter group, the best results are likely to be obtained by the specialist units.

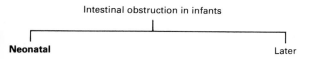

Neonatal intestinal obstruction

The cardinal feature is persistent vomiting. All infants, particularly premature ones, are likely to vomit or regurgitate from time to time, but it is the persistence of the vomiting, its recurrence with every attempt to feed, that should alert the clinician to the possibility of a congenital form of obstruction. Should the baby have attacks of coughing and cyanosis during the feeding, the likelihood of a very high obstruction, with involvement of the respiratory tract as in a tracheo—oesophageal fistula, is high. Should the vomiting

be bile-stained, the obstruction must be distal to the ampulla of Vater. Should the vomiting start only after the first few days, and abdominal distension be prominent, the site of obstruction is likely to be low in the alimentary tract, i.e. in the large bowel as in Hirschsprung's disease.

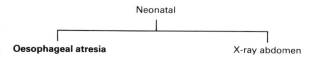

As soon as the possibility of intestinal obstruction is seriously entertained, the baby should be transferred to a paediatric surgical unit in an incubator to prevent heat loss. A nasogastric tube should be passed into the stomach if possible (failure to reach the stomach may suggest a diagnosis of oesophageal atresia) and the stomach should be kept empty by frequent aspirations. A further precaution against the aspiration into the lungs of vomit should be the maintenance of the semiprone coma position.

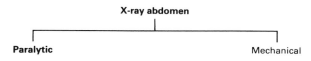

The initial steps at the paediatric surgical centre are to assess fluid and electrolyte balance and to confirm the diagnosis of intestinal obstruction. Plain x-rays of the abdomen in the erect and supine, and sometimes in the lateral positions, are most important, and if the stomach has been kept empty it is helpful to inject 50 ml of air down the nasogastric tube. Gas present throughout the small and large bowel is diagnostic of paralytic ileus, and the common causes of paralytic ileus at this age are septicaemia, birth trauma and peritonitis. The former two conditions are diagnosed by accompanying evidence such as behavioural and neurological manifestations of birth trauma or evidence of a septic focus or of positive blood culture in septicaemia, and they are treated conservatively. In peritonitis there may be calcification in the peritoneal exudate visible in the plain films and the gas shadows in the plain films are separated from each other by the peritoneal fluid, while if the cause of the peritonitis is the perforation of a hollow viscus there is probably gas under the diaphragm. Laparotomy is clearly necessary for cases of neonatal peritonitis.

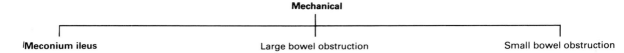

If the small bowel is seen to be distended in the x-ray but contains the typical mottled shadows of meconium and does not contain the gas/liquid levels that one would normally expect in small bowel obstruction, the diagnosis is probably meconium ileus, i.e. mechanical obstruction produced by masses of abnormally viscid meconium. This condition occurs in a minority of patients suffering from mucoviscidosis, a disease in which many mucous secretions are abnormally viscous. Provided there are no complications — such as perforation of the bowel and peritonitis, volvulus of a distended loop or a concident atresia — the obstruction is usually relieved by the use of sodium diatrizoate (Gastrografin) enema. Laparotomy is necessary for such complications, or in cases where the enema has been unsuccessful.

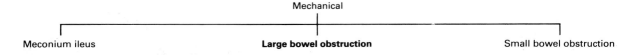

In babies with large bowel obstruction (early and pronounced abdominal distension and apppropriate radiological appearances), management depends primarily on the results of the rectal examination. This may disclose an atresia of the anorectum requiring operative correction, or it may release a long plug of inspissated meconium followed by a gush of liquid stool, or it may be essentially normal. In either of the two latter situations, the presence of Hirschsprung's disease should be suspected. This is a condition in which a variable length of the distal colon stretching proximally from the anorectal junction lacks intramural nervous plexuses and (presumably in consequence) propulsive power. It is diagnosed by barium enema which shows the typical cone-shaped narrowing from dilated normal bowel above to aganglionic bowel of normal calibre below, and by histological examination of specimens of mucosa and submucosa obtained by suction biopsy via a sigmoidoscope. In severe cases of this condition, the aganglionic segment has to be excised and an end-to-end anastomosis performed, usually after a preliminary colostomy. If the diagnosis is not substantiated, conservative measures (rectal washouts) or no treatment at all may be necessary.

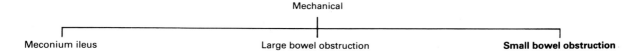

Small bowel mechanical obstruction at this age always requires a laparotomy and correction of the lesion, which may be an atresia, a stenosis, or a malrotation. Details of the management of these conditions, and of babies with oesophageal atresia, are outside the scope of this book.

Obstruction in later infancy

Many of the conditions causing obstruction of the digestive tract after the first 4 weeks of the first year are similar to situations that have already been described for the adult, e.g. strangulated external hernia. However, there are two diseases peculiar to this age which require special mention.

Congenital hypertrophic pyloric stenosis Persistent, forceful ('projectile') vomiting after every meal develops during the second or third month. Once suspected, the diagnosis can be confirmed

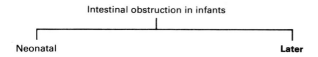

Flow-chart 26.2

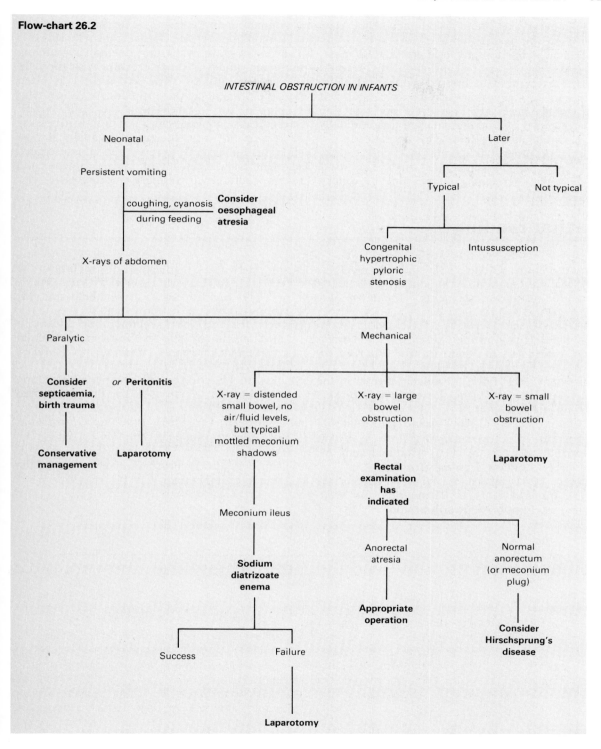

by examining the infant's abdomen while it is being fed: the hypertrophied pyloric muscle can be felt as a horizontally orientated oval mass, above and to the right of the umbilicus. In mild cases, treatment with antispasmodics (atropine methonitrate; Eumydrin) may be successful, but it is usually necessary to operate and split the hypertrophied pyloric musculature longitudinally down to the mucosa (Ramstedt's operation).

Intussusception This condition occurs usually between 6 and 12 months after birth. The infact presents with screaming attacks due to colicky abdominal pain, vomiting and the passage of dark blood per rectum ('redcurrant jelly stools'). The diagnosis is by barium enema; by running the enema fluid in under pressure with the help of visual control by x-ray screening, it is often possible to reduce the intussusception or telescoping of the proximal into the distal bowel. Should this technique fail, operation is necessary to reduce the intussusception manually if possible, or, failing that, to resect the intussuscepted segment and its sheath of intussuscipiens, and restore continuity by primary anastomosis.

Further reading

Barnett, W.O., Oliver, R.I. and Elliott, R.L. (1968). Elimination of the lethal properties of gangrenous bowel segments. *Annals of Surgery* **167**, 912−19.

Fraser, G.C. and Berry, C. (1967). Mortality in neonatal Hirschsprung's disease with particular reference to enterocolitis. *Journal of Pediatric Surgery* **2**, 205−11.

Gourevitch, A., (1971). Duodenal atresia in the newborn. *Annals of the Royal College of Surgeons of England* **48**, 141−58.

Le Quesne, L.P. (1976). Acute intestinal obstruction. In: *Current Surgical Practice*, Vol 1, pp. 168−84. Ed. by G.J. Hadfield and M. Hobsley. London, Edward Arnold.

Marston, A.M. (1986). *Vascular Disease of the Gut: Pathophysiology, Recognition and Management.* London, Edward Arnold.

Nixon, H.H. (1976). Intestinal obstruction in the newborn. In: *Current Surgical Practice* Vol 1. pp. 149−67. Ed. by G.J. Hadfield and M. Hobsley, London, Edward Arnold.

Noblett, H.R. (1969) Treatment of uncomplicated meconium ileus by Gastrografin enema: a preliminary report. *Journal of Pediatric Surgery* **4**, 190−97.

Shields, R. (1965). The absorption and secretion of fluid and electroytes by the obstructed bowel. *British Journal of Surgery* **52**, 774−9.

Wangensteen, O. (1955). *Intestinal Obstruction*, 3rd edn. Springfield, Illinois, Charles C. Thomas.

Wilson, J.P. (1975). Postoperative motility of the large intestine in man. *Gut* **16**, 689−92.

Chapter 27

Epigastric pain; Pain in the Right Iliac Fossa; Pain in the Left Iliac Fossa

Acute epigastric pain

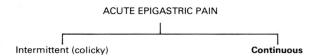

Some comments on this topic have already been made (Chapter 25). Acute upper abdominal pain may be intermittent, or else continuous, typical or atypical. Intermittent pain is due to simple intestinal obstruction or to gastroenteritis, continuous pain with intermittent exacerbations is due to strangulation obstruction, and the management of these conditions has been considered. The problems arise with continuous pain.

The subdivision of continuous pain into typical and atypical requires comment. In this context, typical means that the whole clinical picture is recognizable as being due to a specific intra-abdominal condition. The picture of generalized peritonitis, whatever its cause, demands laparotomy. The important specific conditions within the upper abdomen that give rise to acute abdominal pain are perforation of the stomach or duodenum, acute cholecystitis and acute pancreatitis.

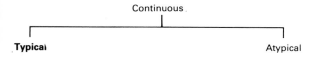

Typical continuous epigstric pain

The only way the clinician can decide whether the patient's problem falls into this category is by comparison of the clinical features present with the standard or classical descriptions of the three chief diseases within this category. Detailed descriptions follow.

Perforation of an ulcer of stomach or duodenum

The speed of *onset* of the pain is most important; a sudden onset, i.e. the patient who is normal at one instant but has severe epigastric pain the next, is practically pathognomonic of perforation of a peptic ulcer or gastric carcinoma.

A *history* of chronic dyspepsia or of recent anorexia may suggest the basic underlying condition, but is certainly not always present.

The *pain* tends to be mid-line, but may radiate to one or other shoulder-tip or elsewhere in the abdomen; tenderness and guarding are epigastric and symmetrical, and there is little movement of the upper abdominal wall during the ventilatory cycle. It is important to realize, however, that the localized form of peritonitis being considered in this chapter, due to a small perforation with only local soiling of the peritoneal cavity, may not stay localized: symptoms and signs may progress, often downwards towards the right iliac fossa in the first instance, until the peritonitis is general.

The important *radiological* evidence is gas under the diaphragm (Fig. 27.1). The best views to ask for are posteroanterior and lateral views of the chest in the erect position. The presence of gas under the diaphragm in general confirms that a hollow viscus has perforated, but it must be stressed that absence of this sign does not exclude perforation, since the sign is present in

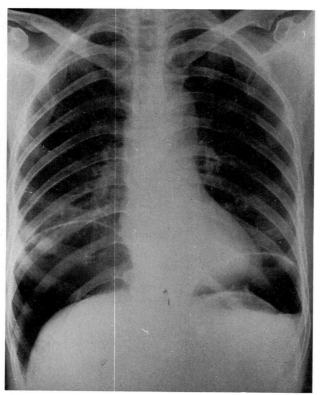

Fig. 27.1 The radiological appearances of gas under the diaphragm. There is a large quantity of gas in the peritoneal cavity, and the diaphragms are seen as thin curved white lines demarcating the gas in the lungs from the gas in the abdomen. A chest x-ray like this is more likely to show gas under the diaphragm than is an erect plain x-ray of the abdomen. The separate air bubble in the stomach can be easily distinguished from the gas in the peritoneum in this x-ray, but usually patients with perforation of a hollow viscus have much less free peritoneal gas than this patient had and the distinction may be very difficult. In such cases a lateral erect view of the diaphragm may help.

only about half the cases of perforation. The presence of gas in the peritoneal cavity can, albeit rarely, be normal in the female because of the anatomy of the female genital tract. It is also a normal finding after recent laparotomy or laparoscopy.

Acute cholecystitis

The speed of *onset* of the pain is never instantaneous, and may be very gradual.

A *history* of known gallstones, or of chronic dyspepsia suggestive of gallstones, strongly favours the diagnosis of acute cholecystitis, but certainly such a history is often lacking.

The *pain* tends to be mid-line, although it is sometimes maximal in the right upper quadrant of the abdomen rather than in the mid-line, and radiation round the ribs to the back, round the right side more than the left, or straight through to the back is also a common feature.

Tenderness is maximal in the right upper quadrant also, in the region of the gall bladder; even if there is no tenderness when the subject is at rest, there may be tenderness during deep inspiration (Murphy's sign). Guarding, if present, is maximal here too.

Jaundice is a strong pointer towards gallbladder disease, while of course the presence of a palpable *gall bladder mass* (see Chapter 10) leaves no room for doubt (but beware the mass of a carcinoma of the hepatic flexure of the colon).

Acute pancreatitis

This disease is rarely as acute in its onset as perforation, but otherwise it may simulate practically all the signs and symptoms of perforation and of acute cholecystitis, including jaundice. The diagnosis is suggested by a history of previous attacks of biliary pain, of chronic alcoholism, or rarely by present or recent mumps.

The typical biochemical features of a raised serum amylase (greater than 1000 international units/ml) and urinary amylase concentration may occur also in perforation, acute cholecystitis and high intestinal obstruction, but strongly suggest the possibility of pancreatitis. The plasma calcium concentration may in severe cases fall below 2.25 mmol/litre (9 mg/100 ml). The timing of these biochemical changes is important: serum amylase is usually raised only during the first 24–48 hours, urinary amylase during the third and fourth days.

Rarely, bruising in the flanks (Grey Turner's sign) or around the umbilicus (Cullen's sign) may help to clinch the diagnosis.

Natural history

The handling of a patient who may have one of these three conditions is decided by a consideration of the natural course and eventual outcome of the three diseases.

Perforation

A small perforation in the stomach or duodenum due to peptic ulceration may leak a small quantity of gas and liquid from the digestive tract into the peritoneum, and may then be spontaneously sealed by a plug of omentum. In these circumstances, there may be no serious complications. However, the patient is always at risk of developing localized infection and abscess formation, and, far worse, of the contamination spreading to the general peritoneal cavity and producing generalized peritonitis. Moreover, the perforation may have been due to a carcinoma of the stomach, or even of a colonic diverticulum or carcinoma (see later), and therefore be most unlikely to heal spontaneously. For these reasons, clinicians usually operate upon patients in whom a diagnosis of perforation has been made, although conservative management is occasionally acceptable, for example in a ship at sea.

Acute cholecystitis

The natural history of acute cholecystitis is that it usually settles down in 1–4 days when treated expectantly. Complications can occur, but perforation of the distended gall bladder is unlikely. These factors suggest that conservative management is suitable, but it should be pointed out that some clinicians prefer to operate: the matter is discussed later (p. 328). The presence of jaundice is an important factor whose effect is considered in Chapter 11.

Acute Pancreatitis

In no other acute abdominal condition is the eventual outcome more difficult to predict at first assessment. Three out of every four patients have *oedematous pancreatitis* and recover without requiring any treatment other than simple support. The fourth patient has the haemorrhagic type of the disease and develops serious complications that require intensive care and special intervention; the chance of death in this group is about one-third. There is no safe way of predicting which the fourth patient is! Indeed many patients are not even diagnosed as having acute pancreatitis until post-mortem: when these cases are included in the analysis, the apparent overall mortality of 10 per cent rises to 20 per cent.

The majority with the mild form certainly do not require a laparotomy. On the other hand, if the patient were developing the haemorrhagic form there would be good reason to undertake any measure that might cut short the attack (see below).

Scheme of action

The following constitutes the writer's personal approach to the problem. Alternatives are considered in the next section.

Evidence of generalized peritonitis requires laparotomy. Next, the radiological demonstration of gas under the diaphragm constitutes an indication for immediate laparotomy. Even to this statement one very occasionally meets exceptions, such as when the patient is getting better and there are strong medical, social or geographical contraindications to surgery. However, the rule remains a good one. If there is no gas demonstrable under the diaphragm but the balance of clinical evidence favours perforation and the serum amylase is less than 1000 international units, immediate laparotomy is performed.

In the absence of generalized peritonitis, an ultrasound examination of the upper abdomen is urgently requested.

Ultrasound is efficient for demonstrating gallstones, but the presence of gallstones does not itself confirm a diagnosis of acute cholecystitis: however, the ultrasound can demonstrate oedema of the wall of the gallbladder and this feature is diagnostic. If an adequately experienced surgeon is available, then the best management is early cholecystectomy – i.e., not immediately if it is the middle of the night, but on a routine list the next day. Such an operation should not be undertaken unless facilities for peroperative cholangiography are available,

Flow-chart 27.1

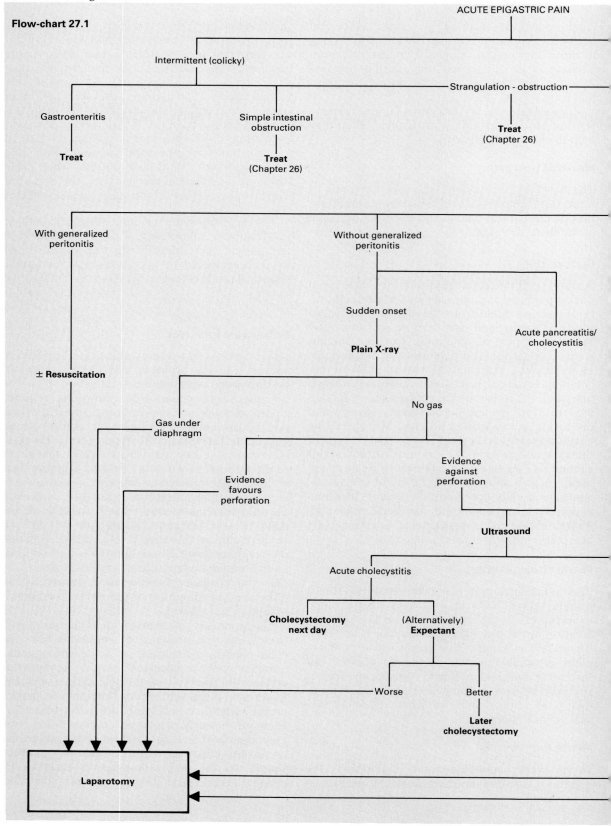

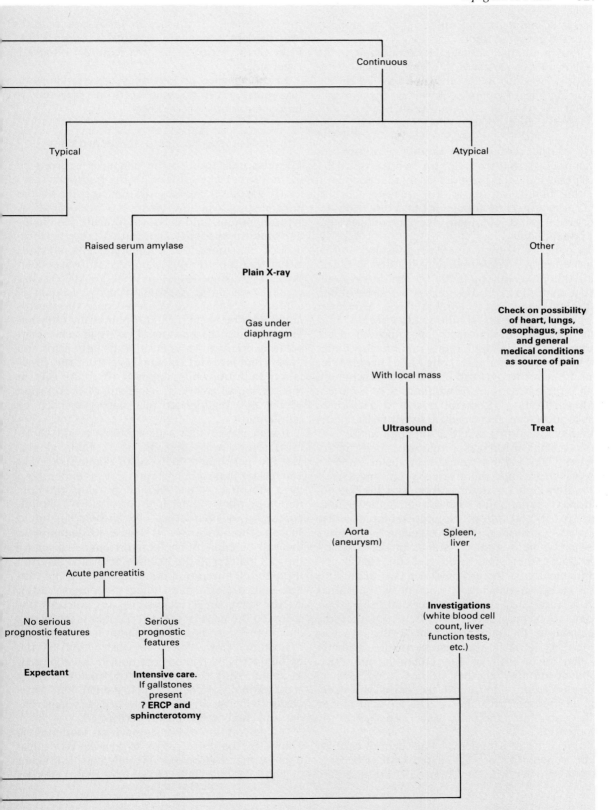

since it is mandatory to ensure that no stone is left in the common duct.

Ultrasound also efficiently demonstrates the swelling of the pancreas in a case of acute pancreatitis. This has made surgeons less dependent on biochemical evidence. However, *hyperamylasaemia* (> 1000 international units/litre) is present in four-fifths of patients. The level of the serum amylase is not useful in predicting the severity of the disease, but among a number of other factors that do help are hypoxaemia (P_{O_2} < 60 mm Hg), the presence of methaemalbumin in the blood, an early low plasma calcium (< 2 mmol/litre on admission) and bloodstained peritoneal fluid obtained by paracentesis and peritoneal lavage.

In patients without sever prognostic features, the treatment is conservative in the first instance, with the provision of fluids by the intravenous rather than the oral route. Large volumes of colloid may be needed to combat shock. However, should the patient's condition deteriorate, particularly in the direction of generalization of the peritonitis, and should there remain any doubt about the true diagnosis, one should remember that it is safer to perform laparotomy in a patient with pancreatitis than to withhold it in a patient with perforation. Remember that a perforated peptic ulcer can also produce hyperamylasaemia and may not show gas under the diaphragm.

And what if serious prognostic features are present? The patient should be transferred to an intensive care unit and given oxygen, and a careful watch kept for deterioration and for complications of pancreatitis such as pancreatic pseudocyst (p. 107). If the ultrasound examination also showed gallstones (and especially if there seemed to be a stone or stones in the common bile duct), there is a good case for ERCP and sphincterotomy. Recent evidence that in patients with gallstone-associated pancreatitis, gallstones can be recovered from the faeces after an attack seems to have proved the old theory that the mechanism of gallstone pancreatitis involves temporary impaction of a stone in the sphincter at the lower end of the common bile duct. Sphincterotomy, whether or not it releases an impacted stone, may relieve the spasm and oedema of the sphincter that might have produced reflux up the pancreatic duct and hence the pancreatitis.

In the United Kingdom, 60 per cent of cases of acute pancreatitis are associated with gallstones, 20 per cent with alcohol abuse. There is a case for ERCP even if no serious prognostic features are present. In many countries (e.g. USA, France) the ratio of the two main aetiologies is reversed.

In the absence of gallstones, severe deterioration may lead, in the hands of some surgeons, to heroic measures (see below).

The laparotomy for acute epigastric pain

The first indication of the diagnosis is given by the nature of any effusion in the peritoneal cavity. If gas is released by the first incision in the peritoneum, a hollow viscus has perforated. A serosanguinous fluid is typical of acute pancreatitis, while food particles indicate a large perforation of the stomach or duodenum. Pus indicates either that a peritonitis from any cause has been present for some time, or that an abscess has ruptured into the peritoneal cavity. Islands of white chalky material scattered over the peritoneum are due to fat necrosis: pancreatic enzymes liberated into the peritoneal cavity in acute pancreatitis break down neutral fat to fatty acids and these combine with calcium ions from the circulation to form white deposits of soap. Bile in the peritoneal cavity is diagnostic of perforation of the gall bladder or bile ducts, stomach or duodenum.

If acute cholecystitis is unexpectedly found, cholecystectomy and per-operative cholangiography are performed. It is again emphasized that emergency laparotomy should not be undertaken in a hospital which cannot provide on-table radiology when required, as per-operative cholangiography is mandatory. Nevertheless, should such a situation arise, it is wise to decompress the gall bladder by cholecystostomy — draining the gall bladder to the exterior by a tube inserted through the anterior abdominal wall and the fundus — or to perform a cholecystectomy (p. 101). At the same time, if possible, any calculus obstructing the neck of the gall bladder is mobilized and removed by digital manipulation via the cholecystostomy hole. Such an obstruction to the cystic duct is by far the commonest cause of acute cholecystitis, but the non-obstructive variety is occasionally encountered. If the gall bladder is perforated, usually the whole organ is gangrenous and cholecystectomy is performed.

If a perforation of the stomach or duodenum is found, the operator needs to answer two questions: is the ulcer benign or malignant; is it acute or chronic? Duodenal ulcers may reasonably be assumed always to be benign, but there is greater difficulty in assessing gastric ulcers. Clearly, if there are secondary deposits on serosal surfaces nearby, or in other organs such as the liver, or if the ulcer in the stomach is associated with a large region of induration that stiffens the greater portion of the stomach walls, a diagnosis of malignancy must be made. In less clear-cut cases, however, it is safer to err on the side of diagnosing a benign ulcer rather than a carcinoma. The standard operation for perforated benign ulcer of stomach or duodenum is to repair the hole with a plug of omentum applied as a pedicled graft. However, in specially selected cases (a chronic ulcer as attested by much surrounding fibrosis, recent perforation, little soiling of the peritoneal cavity, a fit fairly young patient and no medical contraindications to prolonging the operation), it is reasonable to consider whether the patient should receive definitive ulcer surgery rather than just having the leak repaired. The important criterion is, would the patient have merited definitive surgery to cure his ulcer if he had presented at that moment with all the other clinical features present but without the perforation? If the answer to this questions is 'Yes', then in the selected group the writer does truncal vagotomy and anterior gastroenterostomy (or pyloroplasty) for duodenal ulcer, and Billroth I partial gastrectomy for a gastric ulcer. For perforated carcinoma of the stomach one must assume that any form of treatment is only palliative since there must be intraperitoneal spread of tumour, and some form of excision and anastomosis is performed, depending upon the exact circumstances of obvious spread of the lesion. If possible, one aims at a Billroth II partial gastrectomy here also (not a Billroth I because of the risk of malignant recurrence and obstruction at the relatively narrow anastomosis), or, failing that, a total gastrectomy.

Acute pancreatitis may be oedematous, or haemorrhagic/necrotic, and the appearance presented by the pancreas corresponds with these adjectives. Apart from removing gallstones by cholecystectomy, and if necessary by choledocholithotomy, there is no surgical procedure that can rationally be applied. However, some experts advocate debridement and drainage, and even removal of all or most of the pancreas, for necrotizing haemorrhagic pancreatitis.

Alternative action for acute cholecystitis

Some surgeons still advise expectant treatment for acute cholecystitis — rest in bed, a liquid diet by mouth and careful observations. If there is much vomiting the liquid should be given intravenously and the stomach kept empty by nasogastric aspiration. The observations comprise pulse rate hourly, temperature every four hours, an enquiry about pain at the same intervals, and a mapping out of the size of any gallbladder mass that is palpable. Should there be marked signs of systemic infection (fever, malaise, rigors), broad spectrum antibiotics are added. Expectant treatment is continued until all symptoms or signs have subsided, or until it has to be abandoned in favour of laparotomy. Grounds for intervention include septicaemia, a rising pulse rate, signs of spreading peritonitis, and increase in the size, tenderness and associated pain of any mass.

```
                          Continuous
              ┌──────────────┴──────────────┐
Typical                                  Atypical
```

Atypical continuous epigastric pain

This is a large problem, since the possible diagnoses cover a very wide field, including such difficult situations as appendicitis in a high-lying appendix. A few guiding principles may be stated, however. If an aortic aneurysm is palpable, it must be assumed to be leaking and immediate laparotomy performed. If some other mass is present — spleen or liver — it usually becomes necessary to explore the abdomen, but preferably only after appropriate investigations have been peformed. Two special investigations are of paramount importance; radiographs to demonstrate gas under the diaphragm, and the serum amylase concentration. It is surprising how often obscure upper abdominal pain turns out to be due to a perforation or to acute pancreatitis. Upper gastrointestinal endoscopy is also necessary. Finally the possibility must be carefully considered that the symptoms may be arising from extra-abdominal structures, especially the heart or the oesophagus (p. 295).

If all these considerations fail to solve the problem, the surgeon must have recourse to ex-pectant management with careful observation, until either the patient improves or a definite indication for laparotomy arises − deterioration in general condition, increasing pain, shock, or peritonitis.

Pain in the right ilac fossa

This presentation is dominated by the question has the patient got acute appendicitis? The conventional approach is to describe the typical features of an 'average' case of acute appendicitis.

Typical acute appendicitis

Pain is almost invariably the first symptom, although occasionally there may be a prodromal period of anorexia, change in bowel habit and malaise. Pain gradually begins, of an intermittent (colicky) nature, in the central region of the abdomen. After some hours the pain moves downwards and to the right, until it is concentrated in the right iliac fossa; at the same time, its character alters and it becomes continuous and worse on movement. Localized tenderness and guarding are present in the right iliac fossa from an early stage. Rebound tenderness, crossed tenderness and psoas spasm are also described but are of less value (see p. 299). The anorexia persists and there may be vomiting, the tongue is furred and the breath foetid. There is a mild pyrexia, usually of the order of 38−39° C (100−101° F). Should the appendix perforate, the signs and symptoms of generalized peritonitis appear.

Strategy

The snag with the typical picture is that obviously one cannot expect to see every feature in every case. If the clinician works, then, from the typical picture, nearly every case of pain in the right iliac fossa that he meets will pose the question, are *sufficient* of the features of the typical picture present so that I must diagnose acute appendicitis? In many instances, only a few features of the typical picture are missing, and the decision is easy; but sometimes the problem is far more difficult. What, for instance, is the clinician to decide if the pain started in the right iliac fossa instead of centrally, and was continuous from its onset, and the patient has a clean tongue and a temperature of 40° C?

The writer's suggestion for dealing with this problem is to start from the opposite end by asking, what is the least evidence that will lead one to make a diagnosis of acute appendicitis in the absence of any contrary evidence? The justification for this approach is that acute appendicitis is by far the commonest of the conditions presenting with acute pain in the right iliac fossa, that the penalties for missing the diagnosis — generalized peritonitis, septicaemia, later sterility in the female — may be very severe, and that appendicectomy does not have a very deleterious effect upon most of the conditions that may mimic acute appendicitis.

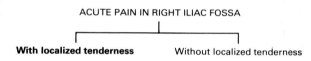

Localized tenderness

The minimal criteria suggested are acute pain and *localized* tenderness in the right iliac fossa; the addition of localized guarding represents a tremendous strengthening of the indication for operation, even if some contrary evidence is available (see below). The fact that tenderness must be localized is stressed, and indeed the sign of tenderness itself can be difficult to assess in some patients. Children provide some of the most difficult problems: a long time may be needed, talking to the child, while the clinician's hand rests on the child's abdominal wall, and gentle palpation is only started after the child's confidence has been won. Even in the absence of abdominal tenderness, the finding of tenderness on digital examination of the rectum constitutes an adequate criterion for diagnosing appendicitis. This clinical picture results from acute inflammation of an appendix that is lying in a pelvic position. The tenderness associated with a retrocaecal appendicitis may be located to the right flank, while — most difficult of all — there may be no tenderness or guarding if the appendix lies behind the loops of the small bowel in the retroileal position.

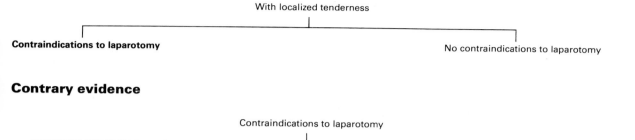

With localized tenderness

Contraindications to laparotomy   No contraindications to laparotomy

Contrary evidence

Contraindications to laparotomy

| Appendix mass | GU symptoms and signs | Referred pain from other systems | Referred pain from abdominal wall | Generalized diseases | Other GI diseases |

'Appendix mass'

This is by far the best contraindication to appendicectomy; a mass palpable in the right lower quadrant of the abdomen. Usually only the upper and medial border of the mass can be felt distinctly. The inverted commas placed around the words 'appendix mass' are stressed: the conclusion that the mass is a zone of omentum and coils of small intestine wrapped around an inflamed appendix is natural, and probably correct, but occasionally the diagnosis turns out to be some quite different condition such as carcinoma of the caecum or ileocaecal tuberculosis.

Operation is contraindicated because the adhesions make approach to the appendix difficult: adherent structures are likely to be damaged, and the tissues at the base of the appendix are probably friable so that it is difficult to invaginate the stump of the appendix neatly into the caecum. Management is therefore expectant, and similar to the expectant treatment for acute cholecystitis. The patient rests in bed, takes an oral liquid diet, and has his pulse rate charted hourly, his temperature every 4 hours; the outline of the mass is marked out, and the white cell count is measured each day; broad-spectrum antibiotics may be added if malaise, fever and headache are prominent; and, most important of all, opiates are forbidden. Usually within a few days pain and fever subside and the mass shrinks. Occasionally, the patient does not improve on the expectant regime. Indications for operation include evidence of abscess formation, septicaemia, or a threatened failure in the mechanisms localizing the infection, with consequent spreading peritonitis. Features suggesting the development of an abscess are localized pain, bogginess and increasing tenderness of the tissues superficial to the mass (these tissues may be the anterior abdominal wall, rectum or vagina), an increase in fever with an emphasis on a swinging temperature, a rising pulse rate and an increase in the leucocyte count. A pelvic abscess may be felt as a bulging mass per rectum or vagina, and causes the passage of mucus per rectum. Septicaemia, which may or may not be associated with local evidence of an abscess, is suggested by increased constitutional disturbance such as malaise, pyrexia and headache. The threat of generalized peritonitis is heralded by a spreading of the pain, tenderness and guarding from the right lower quadrant of the abdomen, an increase in the size of the mass, an increase in the pulse rate, or the disappearance of bowel sounds. In cases of abscess formation, the surgical intervention is limited to drainage of the abscess through the surface at which it points. If there is no abscess, but septicaemia or spreading peritonitis, the appendix must be removed. The decision to perform a laparotomy is very serious, since it is bound to cause a spread of infection throughout the peritoneal cavity with a consequent risk of generalized peritonitis. Such a decision should therefore not be taken without excellent evidence that it is necessary. The aim of the operator is to prevent continuing infection of the peritoneal cavity, and this can only be done by removing the appendix. To perform the necessary appendicectomy and close the defect in the caecum without damage to adherent structures can test the skill of the most experienced operator. After all, it was in the hope of avoiding this situation that conservative management was initially adopted, and it is fortunate that the vast majority of patients with appendicitis presenting with a mass do settle with the conservative approach.

In patients who respond satisfactorily to the conservative management it is important that they should be warned from the beginning that appendicectomy will be necessary in the near future even if the present symptoms subside. Once a patient has had appendicitis with a mass, the risk of a subsequent recurrence of acute appendicitis is high and should be obviated by a prophylactic routine appendicectomy 8–12 weeks later ('interval appendicectomy'). By this time, inflammatory adhesions should have resolved sufficiently for the operation to prove technically straightforward.

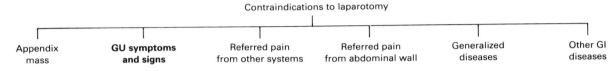

Genitourinary symptoms or signs

Clinical features suggestive of disorders of the genitourinary tract may coexist with pain in the right iliac fossa, and the combination forms an important clinical problem. Many cases of genitourinary disease presenting with pain in the right lower abdominal quadrant do not require an immediate surgical operation, so that the decision to operate is difficult. Moreover, gynaecological conditions requiring operation often demand specialized expertise by the operator and therefore referral to a gynaecological surgeon, or best of all, seeing the patient together and if necessary operating together, is the best line of management. These important problems are considered in Chapter 28.

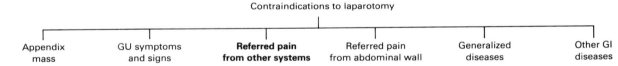

Diseases of other systems

Pain may be referred to the right lower quadrant of the abdomen from the chest, spine or nervous system. A right basal pneumonia, especially in a child, can closely mimic acute appendicitis, and one must look out for evidence of respiratory embarrassment; a slight tinge of cyanosis, or the fact that the accessory muscles of respiration such as the alae nasi are working, may indicate the true diagnosis and lead to x-raying the chest. A psoas abscess, whether tuberculous or pyogenic, is a rare disease today in the Western world, but the signs of irritation produced in the psoas muscle are identical with those produced by the inflammation of a neighbouring appendix. Careful examination of the spine and, if necessary, the taking of spinal x-rays, are indicated if any clinical feature suggests the possibility of this diagnosis. Much the same considerations apply to neurological disease. The right lower quadrant of the abdomen is innervated by the tenth, eleventh and twelfth thoracic and the first lumbar nerves; any disease affecting these nerves, from herpes to the pressure of local tumours, may be misinterpreted as arising within the abdominal cavity. Rarely, an acutely inflamed appendix produces hyperaesthesia of the skin overlying the right lower quadrant. The mechanism is said to be a reflex irritation of the sensory nerves to the abdominal wall via nerve endings in the parietal peritoneum, against which the appendix is lying. Whatever the mechanism, this phenomenon certainly occurs.; yet it cannot be too strongly stressed that both hyperaesthesia and hypoaesthesia may be due to disease directly affecting the nerves, and the presence of these signs demands a careful neurological examination and scrutiny of the back.

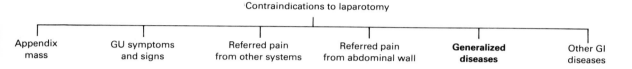

Pain from the abdominal wall

An important characteristic of tenderness arising from an intra-abdominal organ is that it is reduced when the patient is asked to tense his muscles of the anterior abdominal wall. By contrast, tenderness arising in the abdominal wall itself is unchanged, or often worse, when the muscles are contracted. This important sign enables the surgeon to distinguish such conditions as a haematoma of the rectus muscle (this can occur after surprisingly mild trauma, so that the patient may not volunteer the appropriate history, deeming it irrelevant) from acute appendicitis.

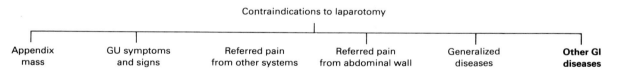

Generalized diseases

This heading includes any condition which, while not specifically producing pain in the right iliac fossa, may on occasion be associated with such pain. Any condition with generalized abdominal pain, and particularly if vomiting be associated, may sometimes produce pain that is worst in one region. Important examples are lead colic and diabetes mellitus. Obviously it is not possible to give a complete list of such conditions; the only way in which one can hope to avoid mistakes is to insist an unceasing clinical vigilance. The two examples quoted might be recognized respectively by noting a blue line on the gums, and by finding glycosuria on routine examination of the urine. Infective hepatitis (look for bile pigments in the urine) and Addison's disease (adrenal failure; note hypotension and a low plasma sodium concentration) are other uncommon examples that the author has met. Sickle cell crisis has become an important differential diagnosis in much of the UK. Only in extreme urgency should a black patient have an anaesthetic without a sickling test — and then the anaesthetist must assume that the patient has the disease.

Contraindications to laparotomy

| Appendix mass | GU symptoms and signs | Referred pain from other systems | Referred pain from abdominal wall | Generalized diseases | **Other GI diseases** |

Other gastrointestinal diseases

These form the most difficult group to distinguish. Acute gastroenteritis usually produces a generalized colicky abdominal pain that never becomes localized or continuous, but the associated vigorous vomiting or diarrhoea may result in muscle tenderness that may happen to be worse one side than the other. The lack of true guarding is a warning to be conservative in one's approach. Large bowel obstruction is an important diagnosis to eliminate in the elderly patient. Mistakes may occur through the build-up of back-pressure in a colon obstructed in its distal half: the resulting accumulation of gas and faeces produces, if the ileocaecal valve remains competent, a distension of the whole of the proximal bowel, but the caecum seems to be particularly susceptible. The distended caecum is painful and tender, and these features together with other features of large bowel obstruction that also occur in appendicitis (e.g. change in bowel habit, nausea and vomiting) may result in the wrong diagnosis. The elderly patient should not undergo appendicectomy without preceding erect and supine abdominal x-rays.

Another important condition that may be difficult to distinguish from acute appendicitis is a 'leaking' duodenal ulcer. The initial epigastric pain of the ulcer perforating may be interpreted as the early central pain of acute appendicitis. If only a small leak occurs, followed by sealing of the perforation, the irritant duodenal juices gravitate to the right iliac fossa and there produce local pain and tenderness, thereby simulating acute appendicitis to a nicety.

Finally, there are a host of other diseases of the digestive tract that can produce localized pain and tenderness in the right iliac fossa. They include regional ileitis (Crohn's disease), ileo-caecal tuberculosis, carcinoma of the caecum, diverticular disease, actinomycosis, and many other diseases that produce inflammation or perforation of the terminal ileum and caecum. When these diseases present with acute pain and tenderness in the right iliac fossa, it is unlikely that they will be diagnosed correctly. Usually the surgeon diagnoses acute appendicitis and operates with the intention of performing appendicectomy. During the operation, or often only after the operation, does it become clear that one of these diseases has been the true cause of the clinical presentation.

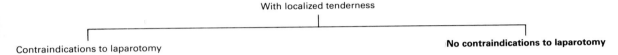

Operation for acute appendicitis

The surgeon will be faced with three possible situations.

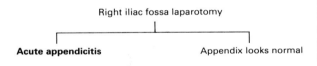

First acute appendicitis is confirmed. The appendix is then removed and its ligated stump usually invaginated into the caecum with a purse-string suture. If generalized peritonitis is present as a result of rupture of the appendix, all exudate or pus is aspirated from the peritoneal cavity and the latter washed out with normal saline solution. A localised abscess cavity with rigid walls, produced by a localised perforation of the appendix with good walling off by the adjacent structures, may need an indwelling drain via a separate stab incision, but these circumstances are not often met. Do not dissect more widely than is needed to perform the operation. General laparotomy will only spread infection.

free fluid in the peritoneal cavity. In these circumstances it is essential to check the other structures which may give rise to the clinical picture with any frequency. The terminal ileum for at least 90 cm (3 ft) and its mesentery are inspected for regional ileitis, mesenteric adenitis, and an inflamed Meckel's diverticulum. Other possibilities are diseases of the female pelvic organs or acute diverticulitis of the sigmoid colon. If no abnormality is demonstrated, the surgeon concludes that there is no serious intra-abdominal cause for the patient's symptoms, removes the appendix and closes the abdomen. It is not culpable to find oneself in this position. If the surgeon maintains a sufficiently high index of suspicion to avoid missing obscure cases of acute appendicitis, he will inevitably find a 'lily-white' appendix and a normal abdomen in a high percentage — perhaps one-third — of his operations for 'acute appendicitis'. This is right and proper: the danger to the patient of an unnecessary appendicectomy is much smaller than that of conservative management of acute appendicitis, though this statement may need modification in special circumstances, such as that of a small ship at sea.

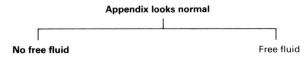

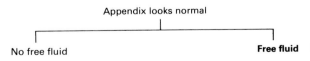

The *second* situation the surgeon might meet is that the appendix looks normal and there is no

The *third* possible situation is that the appendix looks normal but that there is free fluid in the peritoneal cavity. It is clear that some patho-logical process is occurring and its nature must be elucidated. The appearance of the fluid may help in tracking its source — the serosanguinous effusion of pancreatitis for example, or food particles in a case of perforated peptic ulcer. If no lesion can be found in the right lower quad-rant, the gridiron incision is closed and general laparotomy performed through a mid-line or paramedian incision.

Management of other diseases found

Diseases of the female pelvic organs are con-sidered in Chapter 28. Perforated peptic ulcer is treated as described on p. 328. Acute pancrea-titis does not usually require any specific oper-ative measures. Acute cholecystitis is probably best treated by cholecystectomy. (See p. 328 for further details). An intestinal mass in the region of the caecum is presumed to be a carcinoma (although less often the true diagnosis is even-tually demonstrated by the pathologist to be Crohn's disease or tuberculosis of the caecum) and a right hemicolectomy is performed. In the case of acute terminal ileitis, the surgeon usually

removes the appendix and a mesenteric lymph node for histology. If the base of the appendix is itself inflamed a fistula may result, but the risk is not increased by appendicectomy over that following laparotomy alone. Serological testing for *Yersinia enterocolitica* is carried out immedi-ately and again four weeks later: if positive (60 per cent of one series) there are no problems and no risk of further trouble. However, if the serology is negative, there is a greater than 50 per cent chance that the lesion will prove to be Crohn's disease. This by no means exhausts the list of conditions which may be revealed, but the vast majority of cases are covered by those that have been mentioned.

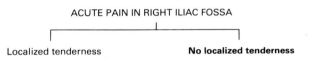

Without localized tenderness

These patients are treated conservatively: either they become worse and an operation becomes necessary or they improve and are cured.

Pain in the left iliac fossa

Pain localized in the left iliac fossa is unusual in the absence of tenderness, guarding, etc. In other words, the common problem in this region is localized peritonitis.

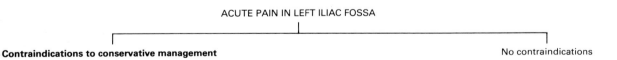

The usual considerations apply that peripheral circulatory failure, evidence of associated intes-tinal obstruction, or an intensification for or spread of the symptoms and signs, are indica-tions for laparotomy; however, in the absence of such indications, experience teaches that a con-servative policy is justified in the first instance because most cases turn out to be due to sig-moid diverticular disease which tends to resolve spontaneously. The details of the conservative regime are the same as for an inflammatory mass in the right iliac fossa (p. 331).

ACUTE PAIN IN LEFT ILIAC FOSSA

Contraindications | No contraindications to conservative management

Flow-chart 27.2

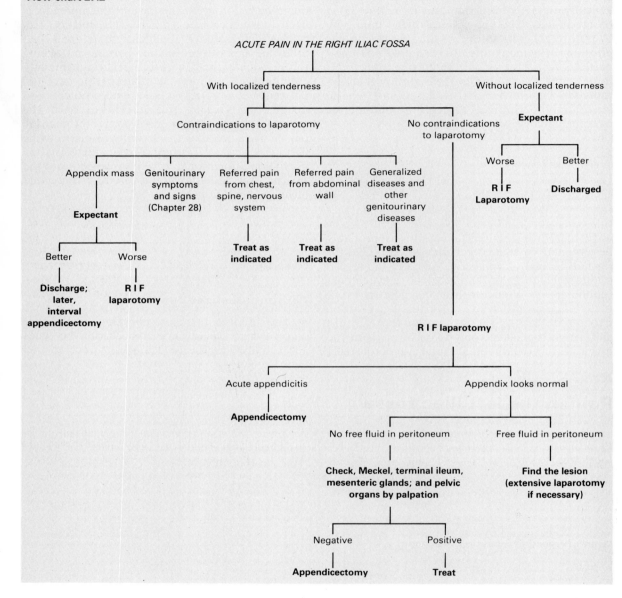

The usual outcome is that symptoms and signs gradually subside, and a few days later the patient is investigated by sigmoidoscopy and barium enema or colonoscopy. If these investigations yield negative results, the patient is discharged from hospital and reviewed once more, about a month later, in the out-patient clinic. In these circumstances, the true diagnosis is never determined, but it is probable that some relatively unimportant condition such as spontaneous torsion of an appendix epiploicae was responsible. However, the investigations usually reveal abnormal radiographic appearances in the region of the rectosigmoid, either carcinoma or diverticular disease. It is most important to remember that these are both common conditions, and therefore often coexist: the undoubted presence of diverticula does not itself rule out the possibility of carcinoma. Further observations on how this problem should be tackled are presented in Chapter 12.

Contraindications to conservative management
|
GENERAL LAPAROTOMY

Occasionally it becomes necessary to perform a laparotomy. This should be conducted through a vertical mid-line or paramedian incision because the chances of requiring access to a large part of the abdominal cavity are far higher in this situation compared to the corresponding one of localized peritonitis in the right iliac fossa. Once again the mischief is usually to be found in the large bowel, in the region of the rectosigmoid. The pathological basis of the lesion is usually carcinoma or diverticular disease, and the distinction between these can often not be reliably made on the naked-eye findings unless there is obvious evidence of malignancy such as peritoneal seedling deposits or hepatic metastases. The primary event that produced the localized peritonitis is local perforation, with the formation of a pericolic abscess as a result of adhesions of omentum, loops of small bowel, etc. If this process of localizing the inflammation succeeds, conservative management succeeds. If the inflammatory mass extends, or the abscess bursts to produce generalized peritonitis, or if small bowel obstruction is produced by the kinking of an adherent loop of intestine or large bowel obstruction results from the cicatrizing effect of the primary lesion, the resultant change

in the clinical picture provides the indication for laparotomy.

The exact operative procedure depends on the findings. Bowel obstruction must be relieved, the peritoneal cavity cleaned out if generalized peritonitis has occurred, and the possibility of any continuing leak of large bowel contents into the peritoneal cavity prevented. Small bowel obstruction is readily relieved by the division of adhesions to free the kinked loop, but large bowel obstruction requires the fashioning of a colostomy at some site proximal to the obstruction. The best procedure for preventing a continued leak is to excise the segment of diseased colon and restore continuity with an end-to-end anastomosis, with a proximal colostomy to ensure freedom from distension of the bowel at the suture line. However, colonic anastomoses do not heal as reliably as those in small bowel, and many think it unwise to attempt a primary anastomosis in the presence of the added disadvantage of acute inflammatory change. Moreover, if any question of carcinoma arises, the dissection to remove a generous portion of the mesentery of the colon with its contained lymph nodes that may harbour metastases is likely to favour the spread of infection by opening fresh tissue planes and may be fraught with danger to neighbouring anatomical structures such as the ureter that might be difficult to identify within the inflammatory mass. It is true that high-dose, short-term antibiotic treatment is very effective if there is no continuing source of contamination; this makes it generally preferable to do the standard type of sigmoid resection with lymph node clearance (p. 144). The standard view therefore is that sigmoid colectomy should be performed, the colon proximal to the resection brought out as a colostomy, and the proximal cut end of the distal colon brought up to the surface as a mucous fistula, or (if it will not reach) oversewn and left in the pelvis (Hartman's operation). The subsequent operation to restore continuity can be very difficult.

If one is sure that one is not dealing with carcinoma there is another possibility — the Paul-Mikulicz operation (Fig. 27.2). The sigmoid colon is mobilized so that the bowel containing the lesion can be exteriorized, and the loop resected leaving the proximal and distal ends of the bowel issuing from a separate incision in the bowel wall as a double-barrelled colostomy. Thus the proximal colostomy is combined into the anatomy of the resection and there is no primary anastomosis. However, the spur that has been formed by stitching together the neighbouring aspects of the proximal and distal ends of bowel can, in the period of about 2 weeks after the operation, gradually be crushed by the application and gradual tightening of a special clamp called an enterotome, and this greatly facilitates the subsequent closure of the colostomy. The snag about this operation is that in most instances one is not achieving a radical clearance of the lymph drainage, so that it should usually be reserved for those patients in whom one is certain that the possibility of carcinoma of the colon does not arise. In practice this usually means free perforation of a diverticulum (rather than of a diverticular abscess) and sigmoid volvulus.

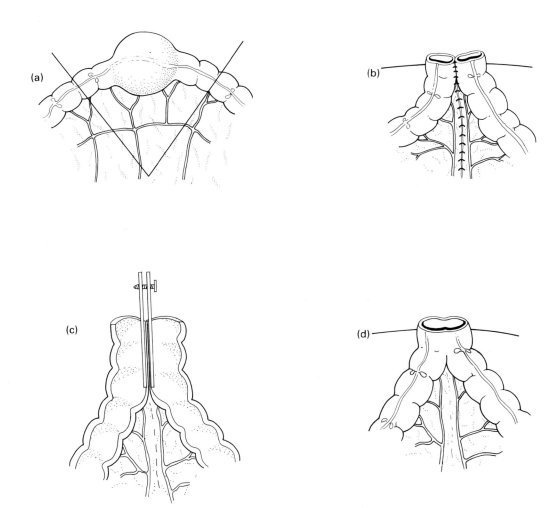

Fig. 27.2   (a) The straight lines indicate the limits of conservative excision of the sigmoid colon, including the mass representing the lesion, together with the associated wedge of mesentery. (b) After the excision the proximal and distal cut ends of colon remaining are sewn together over a distance of about 8 cm to form a spur. Note the row of sutures uniting the cut edges of the mesentery so that there is no hole through which internal herniation can occur. Note also the rotation of the bowel to ensure that the mesentery does not become crushed by the clamp. (c) On a larger scale, the position of the enterotome is indicated: its two limbs straddle the spur. A turn of the screw each day tightens the enterotome until it destroys the spur by pressure necrosis. The completion of this process is signalled by the enterotome working free. (d) The appearance of the loop after the spur has been crushed. Closure of the colostomy and completion of the anastomosis can now be readily achieved by mobilizing the loop from the abdominal wall and suturing together the edges of the stoma.

Flow-chart 27.3

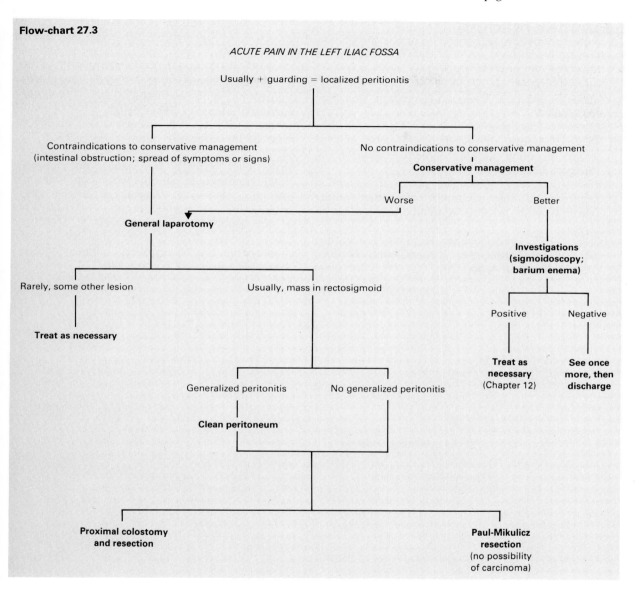

ACUTE PAIN IN THE LEFT ILIAC FOSSA

Usually + guarding = localized peritionitis

Contraindications to conservative management
(intestinal obstruction; spread of symptoms or signs)

No contraindications to conservative management

Conservative management

Worse

Better

General laparotomy

Investigations
(sigmoidoscopy;
barium enema)

Rarely, some other lesion

Usually, mass in rectosigmoid

Positive

Negative

Treat as necessary

**Treat as
necessary**
(Chapter 12)

**See once
more, then
discharge**

Generalized peritonitis

No generalized peritonitis

Clean peritoneum

**Proximal colostomy
and resection**

**Paul-Mikulicz
resection**
(no possibility
of carcinoma)

Further reading

Cohen, M.M. (1971). Treatment and mortality of perforated peptic ulcer: a survey of 852 cases. *Canadian Medical Association Journal* **105**, 263–9.

Eusebio, E.B. and Eisenberg, M.M. (1973). Natural history of diverticular disease of the colon in young patients. *American Journal of Surgery* **125**, 308–11.

Howie, J.G.R. (1968). The place of appendicectomy in the treatment of young adult patients with possible appendicitis. *Lancet* **i**, 1365–7.

Pledger, H.G. and Buchan, R., (1969). Deaths in children with acute appendicitis. *British Medical Journal* **4**, 466–70.

Ross, F.P. and Dunphy, J.E. (1970). Studies in acute cholecystitis. II. Cholecystostomy: indications and technique. *New England Journal of Medicine* **242**, 359–64.

Thomas, D.R. (1970). Conservative management of the appendix mass. *Surgery* **73**, 677–80.

Thorpe, C.D. (1973). Emergency intravenous cholangiography in patients with acute abdominal pain. *American Journal of Surgery* **125**, 26–50.

Van der Linden, W. and Sunzel, H. (1970). Early versus delayed operation for acute cholecystitis: a controlled clinical trial. *American Journal of Surgery* **120**, 7–13.

Chapter 28

The Acute Abdomen and the Genitourinary Tract

There are four important situations: first, after trauma to the trunk that may have involved the urinary tract; secondly, renal colic and pain; thirdly, lower abdominal peritonitis with symptoms or signs suggestive of genitourinary tract disease; and fourthly, laparotomy at which gynaecological abnormalties are found.

The question of trauma and the urinary tract is discussed in Chapter 15 (page 176).

Renal Pain and Colic

The distinguishing characteristic of pain originating in the upper urinary tract (kidneys and ureters) is its distribution. In the typical case, the pain starts in the loin and spreads downwards and forwards along the flank and iliac fossa to reach the groin and thence the testis or labium. Other important features are that the patient writhes around his bed in an effort to find a comfortable position, his abdomen is distended by swallowed air and there may be nausea or vomiting. About half the patients in whom the pain is due to obstruction of the tract complain of colicky (intermittent) pain, with complete remission between the spasms of pain; in the other half the pain is continuous although there may be colicky exacerbations.

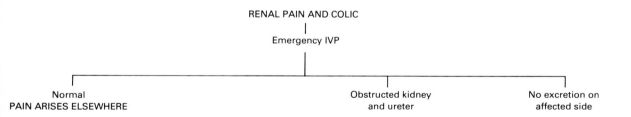

RENAL PAIN AND COLIC

Emergency IVP

Normal — PAIN ARISES ELSEWHERE   Obstructed kidney and ureter   No excretion on affected side

Value of intravenous pyelography

Although in most cases the clinical features are sufficiently typical to allow a confident clinical diagnosis to be made, in many they are not clear-cut: particularly when the pain is right-sided, one must remember the possibility of such diseases as acute appendicitis mimicking renal pain. The best confirmation is provided by immediate intravenous pyelography (IVP). There is no question of waiting for the 24 hours required by the preparation of the patient for the routine pyelography: the essence of the value of this examination lies in its being performed while the patient is in pain, and the pain may have disappeared within a few hours. The usual plain abdominal x-ray is taken first, since most calculi are radio-opaque and therefore likely to be seen in this film. Contrast medium is injected intravenously, and a film taken 20 minutes later. If the patient is still having pain and the 20-minute film shows normal excretion on both sides, then

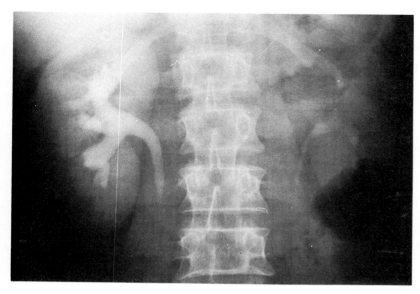

Fig. 28.1 Emergency intravenous pyelogram: 2-hour film. The normal, left, kidney showed well in earlier films but its pelvis and calyces are now scarcely visible. However, the right kidney, which had not been visible in earlier films, is now visualized. Note the nephrogram effect, the dilated pelvicalyceal system, and the apparent obstruction in the right ureter at the lower border of the third lumbar vertebra — presumably due to a stone.

it is almost inconceivable that the pain arises in the urinary tract. If there is normal excretion of contrast in the pelvis and ureter of the opposite side and no excretion visible on the affected side, it is almost certain that the upper renal tract is obstructed, although congenital absence of the kidney is a theoretical, but in these circumstances highly remote, possibility. Occasionally, a dilated pelvis and ureter are shown on the affected side, down to a point short of the entry of the ureter into the bladder, with no contrast in the ureter below this point so that this is clearly the point of the obstruction, and a radio-opaque calculus may be seen at this point. Finally, if no contrast shows on the affected side, it is wise to take further films at 1 and 2 hours after the injection,

and again the following morning: if one perseveres, in the end one does see contrast in the dilated tract, sufficiently well to form an impression of the site of the obstruction.

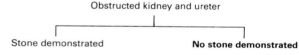

Even if the emergency pyelogram does not demonstrate a ureteric calculus, patients in whom the films confirm ureteric obstruction can be assumed to be suffering from this condition unless there are any pointers to the contrary.

No stone demonstrated

Nothing suggests alternative diagnosis   **Suggestion of alternative diagnosis**

One cause of radiolucent obstruction of the ureter is blood clot, which may form due to slow bleeding from a lesion higher up such as a carcinoma of the pelviureteric epithelium. Suggestive features such as a visible abnormality of the configuration of the pelvicalyceal system or proximal ureter, or frank haematuria (as distinct from the microscope haematuria which occurs in most patients with calculous disease) should lead to urgent further investigations such as cystoscopy and retrograde pyelography, or renal arterio-

graphy. Another possibility is a sloughed renal papilla following necrotic changes in the papilla due to such predisposing diseases as diabetes mellitus and sickle-cell disease, and poisoning with certain drugs such as phenacetin. An important diagnostic trap may also arise if the later films are not taken and the radiographic evidence is limited to absence of excretion on the affected side in the 20-minute film. The failure of renal excretory power may be due to a unilateral reduction in renal artery flow such as may occur in combination with loin pain during the asymmetric development of clot in an abdominal aortic aneurysm approaching rupture, or in renal vein thrombosis. Evidence of shock is incompatible with a diagnosis of simple obstruction due to a ureteric calculus.

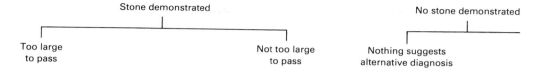

Subsequent management

In the absence of such pointers, the patient is treated conservatively: he is asked to maintain his normal daily intake of fluids (the traditional advice to increase fluid intake has not been shown to be beneficial and may be harmful if obstruction is complete), pethidine is given as necessary to relieve pain, the temperature is taken 4-hourly, and every sample of urine is collected and strained in search of the calculus. Should the stone be recovered, the fact that it is indeed the whole of the obstructing agent is checked by repeating the plain x-ray (if the stone was radio-opaque), or the 20-minute film while the stone itself is sent for chemical examination. If the stone does not pass but the pain subsides, then provided that the emergency pyelogram did not show marked obstruction of the kidney, the patient can be discharged to follow-up in the out-patient clinic. Indications to abandon conservative management are the persistence of severe pain, marked obstruction of the upper renal tract as shown by distensions of the renal pelvis and clubbing of the calyces, and infection, as demonstrated by pyrexia and possibly rigors, and by the results of culture of the urine. A relative indication is that a radio-opaque stone seems too large, or too irregular in shape, to be likely to pass. Judgement of this indication requires much experience, and when in doubt one should tend towards conservatism.

The nature of the intervention required depends upon the exact site at which the calculus has impacted. The pelviureteric junction and upper third of the ureter are approached via a loin incision, the middle third by an extraperitoneal approach via the iliac fossa, and the lower third similarly through a paramedian or transverse suprapubic (Pfannenstiel) incision. The stone is removed through a small longitudial incision in the overlying wall of the ureter. The incision does not need to be sutured, but the site is drained for 5–10 days. It is vital that the absence of any residual obstruction should be checked by passing a bougie distally into the bladder. The most difficult part of the ureter to reach is the intramural part, the terminal 2 cm lying obliquely in the wall of the bladder. A stone in the lower third of the ureter can sometimes be extracted via the cystoscope, by passing an instrument up the ureter to engage the stone so that it can be pulled downwards with the instrument. The Dormia basket, for example, consists of several steel strands that can be used to enmesh the stone. Such techniques are potentially dangerous (rupture of the ureter is a real possibility) and should be attempted only by experienced urologists. With a stone presenting almost at the ureteric orifice, it may suffice to enlarge the orifice by slitting it upwards for 0.5 – 1 cm with a fine-pointed diathermy electrode through the cystoscope: unfortunately, this operation is likely to produce ureteric reflux. Recently a number of exciting new techniques have become available for dealing with stones in the urinary tract. A flexible fibreoptic ureteroscope can be passed via a cystoscope in the bladder so that the stones can be seen and removed under direct vision. If the stone is causing obstruction, a similar technique can be used via a percutaneous nephrostomy (p. 181). Stones can also be broken up into small fragments by the oscillatory shock waves of an ultrasound emitter. This can be applied closely to the stone by either of the above routes, or even from the exterior — in a modern German invention, the patient sits in a water-bath and the ultrasound waves are focussed on the stone. Sometimes the residual fragments themselves impact and have to be removed, but with the increasing availablity and application of these methods it will not be long before an operation to remove a calculus from the urinary tract becomes a surgical museum-piece.

The chemical nature of the calculus occasionally influences management. Cystine stones draw attention to an inborn error of the metabolism of cystine. Urate stones, like cystine stones, are only relatively insoluble, and the patient can usually protect himself from a recurrence by increasing his fluid intake, especially in the middle of the night by waking himself with an alarm clock to drink extra fluid, and by keeping the urine alkaline with sodium bicarbonate. However, most calculi are essentially calcium oxolate. Oxolate stones may be associated with oxaluria, but one cannot influence this by removing from the diet substances rich in oxalates. In most patients with oxalate stones there is no demonstrable disorder of oxalate metabolism. Calcium phosphate stones are associated with urinary tract infections, particularly with Proteus.

Surgically the most important, though rare, cause of renal stone formation is hyperparathyroidism: the excess production of parathyroid hormone by the gland increases plasma calcium concentration and urinary calcium excretion, thus predisposing to stone formation. Since severe hypercalcaemia causes grave metabolic disturbances which can culminate in coma and death, and since the hyperparathyroidism is occasionally associated with the excess secretion of other hormones such as gastrin (Zollinger – Ellison syndrome, p. 104) which can themselves have dangerous consequences (the so-called pluriglandular or multiple endocrine adenoma syndrome), an early diagnosis is desirable. All patients who have renal calculi should therefore be fully investigated on the first occasion; three consecutive fasting blood samples should be taken for calcium and phosphate estimations. Calcium in the plasma is present not only in the ionized, but also in forms bound to the plasma proteins. Taking the samples without stasis and studying the patient in the fasting state are procedures intended to stabilize the plasma protein concentration. Corrections can be made for changes in the plasma protein concentration, which should therefore also be routinely measured. The total calcium concentration must then be considered carefully in relation to the normal range for the particular laboratory concerned — say, 2.20 – 2.25 mmol/1 (8.8 – 10.2 mg/100ml). A simultaneous plasma phosphate concentration lower than normal supports the diagnosis.

If the screening test is positive, more refined studies are undertaken. Nowadays, parathyroid hormone concentrations in the plasma can be measured at special centres, and these occasionally clinch the diagnosis. It is even possible under radiographic control to catheterize selectively various veins draining different parts of the parathyroid region, and measure hormone concentrations in these veins. In this way preoperative evidence can be obtained of an excess production of hormone coming uniformly from all four glands (hyperplasia), or of localization of the production to a single gland (parathyroid adenoma). Such foreknowledge can be useful to the surgeon when he explores the neck in an attempt to cure the hyperparathyroidism: for a single adenoma, removal of the affected gland should be curative, but for hyperplasia only a small portion of one or two of the parathyroids should be left *in situ*.

Lower abdominal peritonitis and the genitourary tract

Patients with localized pain, tenderness and guarding in one or other iliac fossa often have symptoms or signs that direct attention to the genitourinary tract. The importance of this situation is that the right-sided peritonitis in particular may require urgent laparotomy if it is not due to disease of the genitourinary system, but operation may be contraindicated if it is. For example, acute appendicitis should be operated on, acute salpingitis should not. Another important point is that even if the operation is indicated, it might be preferable that it were performed by a gynaecologist rather than by a general surgeon, or at least that a gynaecologist were available for consultation if necessary during the operation.

Urinary tract disturbances

The usual problem here is, does the patient have acute appendicitis or acute pyelonephritis? Features suggestive of the latter include pyrexia of 38°C or higher, rigors, frequency of micturition, alterations in the pain produced by the act of micturition, and an excess of leucocytes in the spun deposit of a sample of urine. However, all these features can be manifestations of acute appendicitis, the pyrexia and rigors due to a complicating septicaemia, and the urinary manifestations due to the inflamed appendix happening to lie in the pelvis and irritating a nearby ureter. One should therefore weight one's decision on the side of operating rather than not operating.

Genital tract disturbances

Features suggestive of disease of the genitourinary tract include a history of menstrual disturbances, especially recent amenorrhoea, findings on vaginal examination that there is a mass in the pouch of Douglas or a purulent or sanguinous discharge from the cervical os, or that moving the cervix with the examining finger is very painful for the patient. Severe shock with a lower abdominal peritonitis, especially if the patient also complains of the referred shoulder-tip pain of diaphragmatic irritation, also suggests a gynaecological disorder — a ruptured ectopic pregnancy with bleeding into the peritoneal cavity — but one should resuscitate and proceed to laparotomy as soon as possible, and without

Flow-chart 28.1

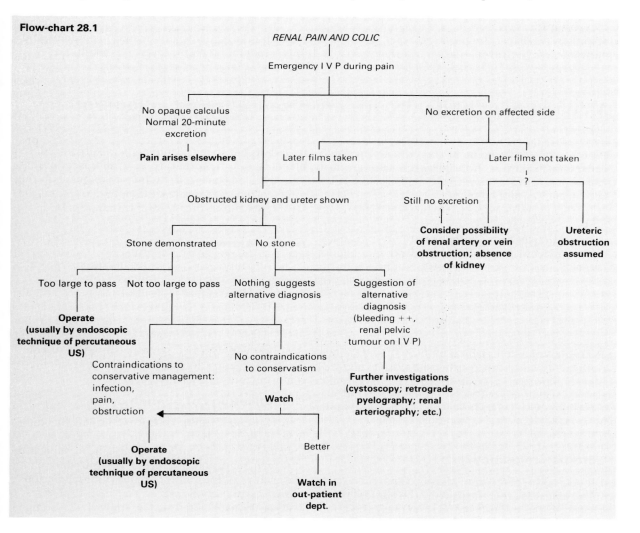

waiting for a gynaecological opinion if there is any delay in getting one.

Should any of the less urgent features be present, one should, if possible, make a joint decision with the gynaecologist about management: the remarks which follow are meant to indicate guidelines should a gynaecological opinion not be available.

A mass in the pouch of Douglas may be a tumour, probably of ovarian origin, that has become twisted on its vascular pedicle to the point of infarction (strangulation), thus producing the signs of peritonism; another possibility is that the mass is a localized collection of blood, collecting in the pouch as a result of slow bleeding from the tubal mole type of ectopic gestation (see below). In either case, laparotomy is indicated, although where the facilities exist this is the sort of case in which laparoscopy can be helpful. The laparoscope is inserted into the peritoneal cavity through a small incision in the anterior abdominal wall, and often gives a good view of many of the intra-abdominal organs, including those in the pelvis. Bleeding from the cervical os indicates an ectopic pregnancy, or occasionally trauma from an attempt to procure an abortion; except in the latter instance, such bleeding is therefore also a strong indication for operation. Pain on tilting the cervix occurs both in tubal pregnancy and in salpingitis, and is therefore a less helpful sign. A purulent discharge from the os usually indicates salpingitis, which should be treated conservatively with antibiotics after swabs have been taken for culture from urethra, vagina and rectum, bearing in mind that the common aetiology (except after birth or abortion) is gonococcal. However, occasionally there is some doubt about the diagnosis, and it is then wise to operate: operating on a patient with acute salpingitis does no harm, but failing to operate on a patient with acute appendicitis and lower abdominal peritonitis can be fatal.

Management of genitourinary disease found at laparotomy

Whether or not the general surgeon has operated expecting to find genitourinary disease, he must be prepared to deal with it. The following rules are very important.

In the premenopausal woman, ovarian tissue must be conserved if at all possible. In particular, if the sugeon who has operated for a diagnosis of acute appendicitis finds the appendix normal, he must resist the temptation to remove the right ovary simply because it contains one or a number of small cysts. These may well be bilateral, and in any case are probably not responsible for the patient's symptoms. An ovarian cyst can usually be easily enucleated, leaving the ovary intact. Finally, the anatomy of the uterus, both tubes and both ovaries should be fully displayed before any tissue is excised or vascular pedicle clamped. This statement should be extended to apply to the ureters if manipulations are necessary near their course.

Ectopic pregnancy

Blood is evacuated and the affected tube carefully assessed together with the other pelvic organs. If the opposite tube is healthy, the affected tube is removed, but the ovary is retained unless it has been completely disorganized by bleeding. If the other tube is diseased or has already been removed, an incision is made in the affected tube at the site of the pregnancy and the latter evacuated; the incision is then repaired.

Acute salpingitis

If the abdominal ostia are occluded, incisions are made to ensure free drainage into the peritoneum. Pus is squeezed out of the tubes and all exudate collected in the pouch of Douglas is cleared out. If a pyosalpinx has formed, the tube is irreparably damaged and should be removed. A tubo-ovarian abscess may also result in complete disorganization of the ovary, and salpingo-oöphorectomy is indicated.

Complications of ovarian cysts

The two complications are torsion and bleeding into the cyst. Both can produce very severe lower abdominal pain. Torsion can be subacute and recurrent, and produce a very puzzling clinical picture of intermittent pain with long periods of severe exacerbations.

A torsion, if present, is untwisted. Benign cysts should be enucleated if the ovary proper is viable, but this may not be the case after torsion so that oöphorectomy should then be performed. The neoplastic nature of a cyst may be obvious; for example, widespread metastatic deposits may be present in the peritoneum. The standard treatment for malignant cysts is bilateral salpingo-oöphorectomy and hysterectomy. Help in distinguishing between benign and malignant cysts can be obtained from frozen-section examination of a biopsy. In cases of doubt, the general surgeon operating for acute abdominal symptoms should clearly tend towards conservatism; the definitive treatment for cancer can, if necessary, be undertaken later by a specialist gynaecologist.

Further reading

Blandy, J.P. (1980) Urethral stricture. *Postgraduate medical Journal* **56,** 383–418

Burke, M. and Buck, P. (1976). Ectopic Pregnancy: a changing picture. *British Journal of Hospital Medicine* **15,** 552–65

Cameron, M.D. (1976). Gynaecological problems and the general surgeon. In: *Current Surgical Practice*, Vol 1, pp. 202–17, Ed. by G.J. Hadfield and M. Hobsley. London, Edward Arnold.

Gilmore, O.J.A., Brodribb, A.J.M., Browett, J.P., Cooke, T.J.C., Griffin, P.H., Higgs, M.J., Ross, I.K. and Williamson, C.N. (1975). Appendicitis and mimicking conditions. *Lancet* **ii** 421–4.

Mitchell, J.P. (1971). Trauma to the urinary tract. *British Medical Journal* **2,** 567–73.

Smiddy, F.G. (1976). Ancillary methods in the treatment of stones in the urinary tract. In: *The Medical Management of the Surgical Patient*, pp. 228–35. London, Edward Arnold.

Sunden, B. (1950). The results of conservative treatment of salpingitis diagnosed at laparotomy and laparoscopy. *Acta Obstetrica et Gynaecologica Scandinavica* **38,** 286–96.

Warwick, R.T.T. (1968). Diagnosis and management of calculi. *British Journal of Hospital Medicine* **2,** 1035–45.

Warwick, R.T.T. (1973). Observations on the treatment of traumatic urethral injuries and the value of the fenestrated urethral catheter. *British Journal of Surgery* **60,** 775–81.

Chapter 29

Acute ischaemia of the limbs

Acute massive ischaemia in the limbs presents with symptoms and signs which constitute what should be an unmistakable clinical picture. The picture is the same in both the arm and the leg, and may involve one or both limbs. However, for a number of reasons, ischaemia is so much commoner in the legs that this chapter contains scant reference to the problems of the upper limb.

Clinical picture

The patient complains of a sudden, severe pain, usually of a constricting or numbing quality, and of coldness and deadness of the limb. On examination there is pallor and coolness of the skin, the veins are collapsed, one can elicit hypoaesthesia or anaesthesia to pin-prick and paresis or paralysis of voluntary movement, and the distal pulses disappear. As time passes the skin becomes marbled: the waxy white appearance is mottled with areas of dusky cyanosis where capillaries have died as a result of anoxia and allowed their small contents of deoxygenated blood to extravasate into the tissue spaces. Once the tissues are stained, the changes are irreversible. With further progression, areas of gangrene appear, usually first at the tips of the digits which start with the least adequate blood supply, or at points where local damage has been allowed to occur by pressure.

Site of arterial obstruction

The point at which the arterial system is obstructed is usually higher than the upper limit of subjective and visible disturbance. The site of the obstruction can be determined by feeling the pulses. If neither groin pulse can be felt, this means that the aortic bifurcation is blocked. If one groin pulse cannot be felt, this indicates an obstruction somewhere between the aortic bifurcation and the beginning of the femoral artery. If both groin pulses can be felt, but the popliteal artery behind the knee, on one or both sides, does not pulsate, this locates the obstruction to the femoral artery in the thigh. In practice, this is much the commonest situation which is encountered. If the groin and knee pulses are absent, the foot pulses will also be absent. Occasionally it happens that all pulses to knee (popliteal) level are palpable, but the foot is pulseless. This indicates a block in the small vessels, which in practice suggests diabetes or collagen disease. The most extreme case of all is the patient whose symtoms are those of deficient blood supply to his muscles, but whose pulses can all be felt: this represents a real diagnostic challenge.

Refinements can be introduced with auscultation at the groin: the turbulence produced by a partial obstruction in an iliac artery is transmitted distally along the vessel to produce an audible murmur at the groin. Such refinements are less useful than they used to be because the modern operative approach is less dependent on precise knowledge of the site of the block (p. 351).

Acute arterial insufficiency may result in death of the limb unless the obstruction is relieved within a few hours. The diagnosis must be made clinically, without recourse to complicated methods of investigation such as arteriography that might delay treatment.

Focal acute ischaemia can also occur, e.g. a small embolus occluding a digital artery.

Care of the limb

Immediate positive action must be undertaken to minimize damage to the ischaemic limb. Ischaemic tissues are sensitive to pressure, and their oxygen requirements increase with temperature. The limb is therefore carefully protected from external pressure, and kept cool. Broad slings under the thigh and calf can be used to suspend the lower limb with an even distribution of weight, and take the weight off the usual pressure areas of the heel, etc., or nests of cotton wool or lamb's fleece can be employed. The affected limb should be kept cool by leaving it exposed without bedclothes and, if necessary, in the path of the draught from an electric fan. The place of vasodilator drugs, sympathectomy and sympathetic block is doubtful.

The correct handling of the limb is crucial to the success of the management policy. There is no point in relieving the arterial obstruction if the affected tissues have already suffered irreversible damage that necessitates a major amputation.

The limb is protected in this way, and a decision has next to be made on whether operative intervention should be taken.

Further management

The most important factor deciding further management is whether or not the arterial obstruction has arisen as a result of trauma.

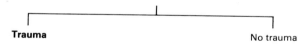

Trauma   No trauma

Traumatic ischaemia

If the ischaemic limb has been acutely injured, immediate operation to explore the region of the obstruction is mandatory. This statement applies whether the injury is open or closed, or whether it involves a fracture of bone or not. It is true that the commonest cause of traumatic arterial obstruction is pressure on the artery from displaced fragments of bone, but similar obstruction can develop from soft tissue injury such as an expanding haematoma in the surrounding tissues or even in the wall of the artery itself. It used to be taught that arterial spasm in response to direct trauma can produce ischaemia, and that various injections of anti-spasmodic drugs around the artery would relieve the spasm. This teaching has resulted in procrastination while such attempts were carried out, and an increased chance of death of the limb. The facts are that such a degree of persistent arterial spasm as to cause ischaemia peripherally is a most unusual event, and the safe rule is to explore all post-traumatic cases.

Associated nervous injury

Coincident damage to neighbouring nerves is notoriously difficult to diagnose in such patients, because the ischaemia produces a global (glove or stocking) type of interference with sensation and muscular function that obscures the characteristic patterns of such deficiencies associated with injury to a particular nerve. It is important, therefore, to be particularly thorough in the clinical testing of nervous functions, and even if clinical evidence is lacking the operator must remember to explore neighbouring nerves for possible damage.

Exploration for traumatic ischaemia

The important principle guiding the operator is that exploration must be adequate. This means long incisions, usually placed axially along the limb but modified at major flexures such as the groins or popliteal fossae to avoid a right-angled crossing of the flexure that might lead later to a contracture.

The usual debridement of all dead or foreign matieral is carried out, and in patients with fractures it is essential to immobilize the bones first. The artery is dissected carefully out of its surroundings until it is clear that there is no question of extrinsic pressure from deformed neighbouring structures such as fractured bones or haematomas expanding in tight fascial compartments. If at the end of this procedure the artery is visibly and palpably pulsating along the whole of its exposed length, and if the pulses distal to this region have reappeared, nothing further need be done from the viewpoint of the arterial injury. However, if the evidence points to continued arterial obstruction, the operator proceeds to explore the vessel itself. The site of obstruction may be obvious to external examination as a place where the normal proximal pulsation disappears, or as an area of swelling or bruising of the wall. In difficult cases with a long segment of the vessel damaged, help in pinpointing the obstruction may be gained from arteriography on the operating table. Control of haemorrhage is obtained by passing slings round the vessel above and below the site of damage, and similar measures should be taken with any major branch that takes origin from the vessel in the segment to be isolated. A small longitudinal incision is then made in the artery and the cause of the obstruction identified. Often the lesion is an intimal tear resulting in the elevation of a flap that obstructs the lumen. The obstructing agent is removed and the artery repaired. A Fogarty catheter can be useful (p. 351).

Sometimes the damage to the artery is more extensive, and it is necessary to excise the affected segment. Repair may be possible by end-to-end anastomosis of the proximal and distal ends, but failing this the artery must be repaired by some form of graft or prosthesis. A segment of long saphenous vein, reversed in direction so that its valves do not obstruct the flow of arterial blood distally, is a popular technique, and safer than an arterial prosthesis of man-made fibre such as Dacron, particularly if the wound has been open and there is a high risk of infection.

Whatever manoeuvre is necessary to relieve the obstruction, some surgeons inject 5000 units of heparin into the isolated segment and remove the distal sling first, then the proximal sling so that the heparin is carried distally into the regions of the limb which have temporarily been deprived of their blood supply. They hope that this measure will reduce any tendency to arterial thrombosis in the distal territory of the damaged vessel.

Whether or not arteriography was used before the arteriotomy was performed, it is certainly useful after exploration as it can provide objective evidence that the obstruction has indeed been relieved. Newer and potentially less damaging techniques are also available, such as Doppler ultrasound.

Occasionally, the extent of arterial damage, or of concomitant injuries to other structures, or the degree of contamination and associated risk of infection, are so great that the vessel must simply be tied. In the case of a major artery, and particularly where the damage is to the lower rather than the upper limb, gangrene of the distal part of the limb may be judged to be inevitable and an amputation may be performed to forestall this event.

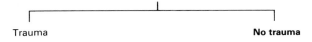

Trauma   **No trauma**

Non-traumatic ischaemia

Patients who suffer embolic or thrombotic occlusive disease are likely to have atheroma elsewhere in their cardiovascular system, and evidence of coronary or cerebral artery disease should be sought. Diabetes mellitus is also a common association.

If there is no history or physical evidence of trauma, the crucial decision to make is whether to explore or to treat the condition conservatively. In practice, non-traumatic acute arterial obstruction is due to thrombosis or embolism: patients with thrombosis tend to do badly if operated upon, but embolism is much more amenable to surgical intervention.

Three major factors help in making this decision.

1 Degree of acuteness

Within the framework of an acute onset there are degrees of suddenness. The embolus impacts and immediately transforms a limb with normal circulation into an ischaemic one. In the case of thrombosis, the final act of obstruction is usually the laying down of a soft thrombus on a pre-existing area of atherosclerosis which, by its narrowing of the lumen, may have produced chronic ischaemic symptoms (Chapter 16).

A confusing, though very rare, factor arises when an embolus impacts for a short time at a proximal site, and then breaks into one or more large fragments that may impact at more distal sites, leaving the proximal site clear. In the circumstances, an early episode of widespread ischaemia may be succeeded by some apparent recovery in the proximal parts of the limb (or limbs) and then by further and more intense ischaemia distally. Unless the history is taken very carefully, this course of events may be mistakenly interpreted as a less acute type of onset due to thrombosis.

2 Cause for embolism

If the patient presents an obvious possible cause for embolism, the chances are high that embolism is indeed the cause of the clinical picture of arterial obstruction. The embolus is often a detached thrombus, and thrombi are likely to form in stagnant backwaters of the circulation. Venous thrombi, if they become detached, travel back to the right side of the heart and thence, via the pulmonary trunk, to the lungs where they impact in the branchings of the pulmonary artery as pulmonary emboli. However, if there is present a congenital (or, very occasionally, post-cardiac infarction) septal defect between atria or ventricles, the very rare *paradoxical arterial embolus* may result from a venous thrombosis. Usually, the cause of the arterial embolus is a thrombus forming in the left atrium in a patient with atrial fibrillation, or in an aortic aneurysm. In atrial fibrillation, the uncoordinated and ineffective contractions of the left atrium leave the contents of the left atrial appendage largely undisturbed, and thrombus forms in this area. Similarly, the periphery of an expanding aortic aneurysm is remote from the mainstream of flow through the aorta, and thrombus becomes laid down which may at any stage become detached. Other causes of arterial embolism are rare, except that one must bear in mind that foreign material, such as a prosthetic heart valve, or the combination of a diseased heart valve plus infection, as in bacterial endocarditis, can result in local thrombus formation and subsequent minor embolism.

3 Evidence of collateral circulation

Sometimes nature is already dealing adequately with the situation by the time the patient presents. If, in terms of history and examination, there is evidence that the circulation in the limb is improving, it would clearly be meddlesome to operate unless it later became apparent that the improvement had ceased and the viability of the limb was still in doubt. The possible collateral circulation is anatomically and functionally much more effective in the upper than in the lower limb, and in the upper limb it is safe to await spontaneous improvement provided that there is no actual gangrene of the extremities and that observation for an hour reveals no deterioration. Even in the lower limb, after a definite decision to operate has been made, it is worth reassessing the patient at the end of the usual hour of pre-medication before actually proceeding with the operation.

Management of non-traumatic ischaemia

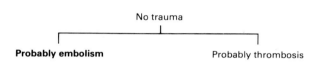

On the basis of the preceding considerations, a decision is made whether to operate or to manage conservatively. The decision is not necessarily inevitable, at least up to the moment that an operation is commenced: frequent review and a readiness to change the original plan are important features of management.

Conservative measures have already been described (p. 189).

Operation

The femoral artery is exposed in the groin and tapes passed around it at the upper and lower extremities of the exposure, about 8 cm apart. While haemorrhage is controlled by pulling on the tapes, a small (1 cm) incision is made longitudinally in the artery and a Fogarty catheter inserted downwards into the vessel. The Fogarty catheter has an inflatable balloon mounted symmetrically near its tip: inflation of the balloon can be achieved via a separate channel within the catheter. For obstruction below the groin, the catheter is passed distally down the

Flow-chart 29.1

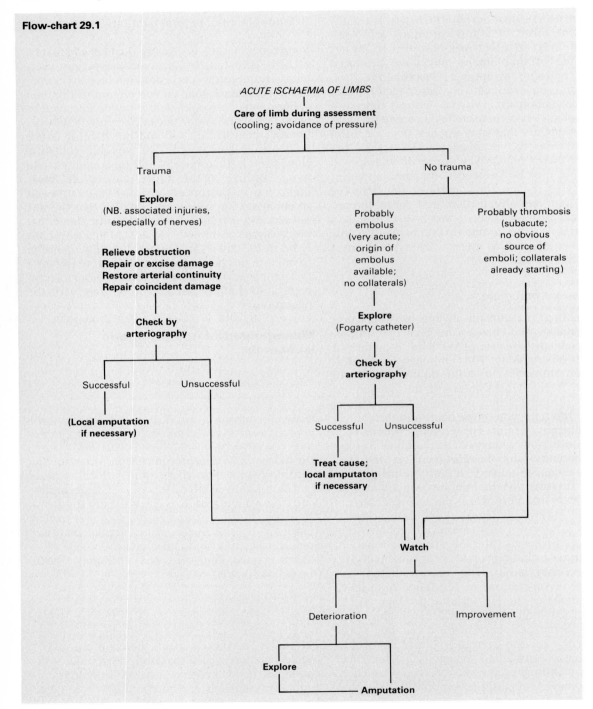

ACUTE ISCHAEMIA OF LIMBS

Care of limb during assessment
(cooling; avoidance of pressure)

Trauma

Explore
(NB. associated injuries,
especially of nerves)

Relieve obstruction
Repair or excise damage
Restore arterial continuity
Repair coincident damage

Check by
arteriography

Successful   Unsuccessful

(Local amputation
if necessary)

No trauma

Probably
embolus
(very acute;
origin of
embolus
available;
no collaterals)

Probably thrombosis
(subacute;
no obvious
source of
emboli; collaterals
already starting)

Explore
(Fogarty catheter)

Check by
arteriography

Successful   Unsuccessful

Treat cause;
local amputaton
if necessary

Watch

Deterioration   Improvement

Explore

Amputation

main (superficial) femoral artery as far as it will reach; the balloon is then gradually inflated with fluid from a syringe till it can be felt to be gently distending the walls of the surrounding artery. The catheter is then slowly withdrawn, bringing fragments of embolus with it. The procedure can be repeated till the surgeon has cleared the vessel as completely as possible. The arteriotomy is closed, and the tapes removed.

If there is any possibility of obstruction in the vessels proximal to the groin, it is a good practice to pass the catheter proximally first, while good control is maintained distally so that any fragments of embolus dislodged by the catheter cannot find their way into the distal arteries of the limbs. The distal exploration is performed later.

If the Fogarty manoeuvre is unsuccessful at the groin, it is worth trying again at the knee.

In those rare cases where emboli in the upper limb require exploration, the usual site for the arteriotomy is the brachial artery at the elbow. The principles involved are identical with those followed in operating on the lower limbs.

The after-care of a patient who has undergone exploration includes immediate confirmation of the restoration of peripheral patency, and careful observation to note any reobstruction, a phenomenon that is not too unusual and may require a further exploration.

Results of operation

If the operation has been carried out within 6 hours of the onset of the obstruction, and a full circulation to the affected limb has been achieved, complete recovery is usual, though the lateral popliteal nerve injury (foot drop) may continue for several weeks. Where gangrene of the extremity has already occurred, a further operation will be required to remove the dead tissue. It is usually wise not to perform this toilet amputation too soon; once the arterial supply has been restored, it is extraordinary how much tissue that looks irreparably damaged ultimately recovers, and the final amputation may turn out to be considerably less extensive than originally appeared inevitable. For further discussion of amputation, see p. 190.

Late management

Once the fate of the limb has been decided, and either conservative or operative treatment has been successful or an amputation has been necessary, consideration can be given to dealing with the cause of the embolus. In cases of atrial fibrillation, it is important that no attempt be made to restore normal rhythm until and unless the left atrial appendage has been amputated so as to remove the source of further emboli.

Further reading

Gardham, J.R.C. (1976). The ischaemic leg. *British Journal of Hospital Medicine* **16**, 43–52.

Martin P., King, R.B. and Stephenson, C.B.S. (1969). On arterial embolism of the limbs. *British Journal of Surgery* **56**, 882–4

Newcombe, J.F. (1978). Presentation and management of the ischaemic lower limb. In: *Current Surgical Practice* Vol 2. Hadfield, J. and Hobsley, M. (Ed). London, Edward Arnold.

Rob, C. and Kenyon, J.R. (1960). Dissecting aneurysms. *British Medical Journal* **1**, 1384–8.

Taylor, G.W. (1973). Chronic arterial occlusion. In: *Peripheral Vascular Surgery*, pp. 211–34. Ed. by M. Birnstingl. London, Heinemann Medical.

Thompson, J.E., Sigler, L., Raut, P.S., Austin, D.J. and Patman, R.D. (1970). Arterial embolectomy: a 20-year experience with 163 cases. *Surgery* **67**, 212–19.

Index

Index